BODY IMAGE

BODY IMAGE

A Handbook of Science, Practice, and Prevention

second edition

Edited by
THOMAS F. CASH
LINDA SMOLAK

THE GUILFORD PRESS
New York   London

Paperback edition 2012

Printed in the United States of America

This book is printed on acid-free paper.

Last digit is print number: 9 8 7 6 5

The authors have checked with sources believed to be reliable in their efforts to provide
information that is complete and generally in accord with the standards of practice that
are accepted at the time of publication. However, in view of the possibility of human
error or changes in behavioral, mental health, or medical sciences, neither the authors,
nor the editor and publisher, nor any other party who has been involved in the preparation or publication of this work warrants that the information contained herein is in every
respect accurate or complete, and they are not responsible for any errors or omissions or
the results obtained from the use of such information. Readers are encouraged to confirm
the information contained in this book with other sources.

Library of Congress Cataloging-in-Publication Data

Body image : a handbook of science, practice, and prevention / edited by Thomas F. Cash,
Linda Smolak. — 2nd ed.
    p. cm.
  Rev. ed. of: Body image : a handbook of theory, research, and clinical practice / edited by
Thomas F. Cash, Thomas Pruzinsky. c2002.
  Includes bibliographical references and index.
  ISBN 978-1-60918-182-6 (hbk. : alk. paper)
  ISBN 978-1-4625-0958-4 (pbk. : alk. paper)
  1. Body image. 2. Body image disturbance. I. Cash, Thomas F. II. Smolak, Linda, 1951–
BF697.5.B63B617 2011
306.4′613—dc22

2011009429

About the Editors

Thomas F. Cash, PhD, is Professor Emeritus of Psychology at Old Dominion University in Norfolk, Virginia. His research focuses on influences of physical appearance and body image on psychosocial functioning, including such topics as body image development, assessment, and treatment; obesity; eating disorders; cosmetic surgery; appearance-altering conditions; and appearance stereotyping and discrimination. He has authored or edited seven books and over 200 journal articles and book chapters. Dr. Cash has developed an empirically supported cognitive-behavioral program for body image improvement, as well as over a dozen validated assessments of dimensions of body image. He is the founder and Editor-in-Chief of *Body Image: An International Journal of Research* and an elected Fellow of the Association for Psychological Science. Dr. Cash resides in Naples, Florida. His website is *www.body-images.com*.

Linda Smolak, PhD, is Professor Emerita at Kenyon College in Gambier, Ohio. Her research focuses on the development of body image and disordered eating, including such topics as media and familial influences on children's body image; child sexual abuse and body image; muscle building among adolescent boys; eating disorder prevention programs; athletic participation and body image; and gender roles and body image. She has been involved in the development of several body image–related scales. Dr. Smolak is author or editor of seven books and dozens of journal articles and book chapters. She is an Associate Editor of *Body Image: An International Journal of Research* and serves on the editorial board for *Eating Disorders: A Journal of Treatment and Prevention*.

Contributors

Eileen P. Anderson-Fye, EdD, is Assistant Professor of Anthropology at Case Western Reserve University and Assistant Research Anthropologist at the University of California, Los Angeles. Her research focuses on adolescent well-being and mental health in contexts of cultural change, with a particular focus on eating and body image concerns and psychiatric medications.

Jakki Bailey, MA, is a research assistant in the Department of Psychiatry and Behavioral Sciences at Stanford University. She is interested in the intersection between psychological theory and the use of technology in education practices.

Rebecca L. Bassett, MSc, is a doctoral candidate studying health and exercise psychology in the Department of Kinesiology at McMaster University in Canada. Her research addresses body image concerns in relation to motivation for exercise behavior, particularly among men and women with spinal cord injury.

Marion Bilich, PhD, is a psychologist in private practice and has written books, articles, and papers, and conducted workshops on eating disorders, women's issues, dissociative identity disorder, and collaboration between therapists and clergy.

Thomas F. Cash, PhD. See "About the Editors."

Kelsey Chapman, BA, is a graduate student at Marshall University. She is interested in body image and eating disorders, as well as pro-eating disorder websites.

Canice E. Crerand, PhD, is a psychologist in the Division of Plastic Surgery at the Children's Hospital of Philadelphia. Her research interests include body image in youth with craniofacial conditions and the psychological aspects of plastic surgery.

Janis H. Crowther, PhD, is Professor of Psychology at Kent State University. She has authored numerous publications on body image and eating disorders.

Sherrie Selwyn Delinsky, PhD, is a clinical psychologist in private practice in Wellesley, Massachusetts, Assistant Psychologist at McLean Hospital, and Instructor at Harvard Medical School. Her clinical and research interests pertain to the development and implementation of effective treatments for eating and weight disorders and body image disturbance.

Rebecca J. Dilks, RD, is a Registered Dietitian and Research Coordinator at the Center for Weight and Eating Disorders in the Department of Psychiatry at the University of Pennsylvania School of Medicine. Her clinical and research interests are in the treatment of obesity.

James A. Fauerbach, PhD, is Associate Professor in the Department of Psychiatry and Behavioral Science at Johns Hopkins University School of Medicine. His research interests concern understanding the psychosocial recovery process from severe burns and heart attacks and optimizing psychosocial rehabilitation from these medical problems.

Debra L. Franko, PhD, is Professor in the Department of Counseling and Applied Educational Psychology at Northeastern University and Associate Director of the Harris Center for Education and Advocacy in Eating Disorders at Massachusetts General Hospital. Her research interests include ethnic and cultural differences and the prevention of eating disorders in children, adolescents, and young adults.

Rick M. Gardner, PhD, is Professor Emeritus in the Department of Psychology at the University of Colorado, Denver. His research interests are in the development and application of methodological techniques to measure the perceptual and attitudinal aspects of body image in a variety of populations.

Kathleen A. Martin Ginis, PhD, is Professor of Health and Exercise Psychology in the Department of Kinesiology at McMaster University in Canada. Her research focuses on body image concerns and other psychological factors related to exercise adoption and adherence. She has a particular interest in exercise and psychological well-being among people with chronic disease and disability.

Christy Greenleaf, PhD, is Associate Professor in the Department of Kinesiology, Health Promotion, and Recreation at the University of North Texas. Her research examines the psychosocial aspects of body image, eating, and physical activity.

Sarah Grogan, PhD, is Professor of Health Psychology in the Centre for Health Psychology at Staffordshire University, Stoke on Trent, United Kingdom. Her research focuses on understanding the impact of body image on health-related behaviors such as smoking and anabolic steroid use, and the impact of aging on body image.

Diana Harcourt, PhD, is Reader in Health Psychology and Co-Director of the Centre for Appearance Research at the University of the West of England, Bristol, United Kingdom. Her research focuses on psychosocial issues around disfigurement, with a particular interest in the impact of an altered appearance due to treatment for cancer.

Tom Hildebrandt, PsyD, is Director of the Eating and Weight Disorders Program and the Program for Appearance and Performance Enhancing Drug Use Research at the Mount Sinai School of Medicine. His research spans the eating disorders and addiction fields, with a specialty in gender differences, male body image disturbance, and hormonal contributions to these forms of psychopathology.

Andrew J. Hill, PhD, is Professor of Medical Psychology at Leeds University School of Medicine in the United Kingdom. His main research interests include children's self-perception relating to shape and weight, psychological issues in obesity and eating disorders, and appetite control.

Caroline Hood, MN, is a Head and Neck Cancer Clinical Nurse Specialist in Ayrshire and Arran, Scotland. Her interests include the psychological aspects of oncology and more specifically the experience of body image change(s) in people with head and neck cancer. She has recently led a project with Macmillan Cancer Support on body image and cancer.

Joshua I. Hrabosky, PsyD, is a clinical psychologist at the Weight Loss and Diabetes Center at Greenwich Hospital in Connecticut. His research and clinical interests include the evaluation and treatment of body image and disordered eating in obesity and bariatric surgery.

Josée L. Jarry, PhD, is Associate Professor in the Department of Psychology at the University of Windsor in Canada, where she heads the Studies of the Psychology of Appearance laboratory. Her main areas of research concern factors affecting body image and psychotherapy outcome research.

Meenakshi Jolly, MD, is Assistant Professor in Rheumatology, Department of Medicine and Department of Behavioral Medicine at Rush University. Her clinical and research interests are the psychosocial and health outcomes of lupus, especially body image and patient-reported health outcomes.

Diane Carlson Jones, PhD, is Professor Emerita of Human Development and Cognition in Educational Psychology at the University of Washington, Seattle. Her research interests include gender and body image issues during adolescence. She specializes in the contributions of friends and peers to body image development.

Kathleen Y. Kawamura, PhD, is a clinical psychologist in private practice in Mission Viejo, California. She has published articles and chapters on perfectionism, parenting styles, and body image in the general and Asian American populations. Her clinical specialties are in anxiety disorders, perfectionism, body image, and multicultural issues.

Leeana Kent, PhD, is a research supervisor with Central Queensland University and a practicing psychologist in Cairns, Australia. Her research interests center on the social psychological correlates of body art and the practice of body modification.

Kelly L. Klump, PhD, is Associate Professor in the Department of Psychology at Michigan State University. Her research interests include developmental differences in genetic, neurobiological, and environmental influences on eating pathology across adolescence and adulthood.

Ross Krawczyk, MA, is a graduate student at the University of South Florida. Her research interests include influences of media on body image, male body image, and obesity.

Justine Lai, BA, is a senior research coordinator of both the Eating and Weight Disorders Program and the Program for Appearance and Performance Enhancing Drug Use Research at the Mount Sinai School of Medicine. Her interests include the relationship between body image and appearance- and performance-enhancing drug use and the provision of mental health services to underserved populations.

Janet D. Latner, PhD, is Associate Professor in the Department of Psychology at the University of Hawaii at Manoa. Her areas of research interest include the assessment and amelioration of obesity, eating disorders, and weight bias.

John W. Lawrence, PhD, is Associate Professor at the College of Staten Island, The City University of New York. His research focuses on the assessment and treatment of body image and social integration difficulties following a severe burn.

Michael P. Levine, PhD, FAED, is Samuel B. Cummings Jr. Professor of Psychology at Kenyon College. His special interest is body image and eating problems and their links with preventive education, mass media, and social justice in the context of community psychology and public health.

Danielle M. Lindner, MS, is a graduate student in the Clinical Psychology Doctoral Program at the University of Central Florida. Her primary research interests include body image theoretical perspectives (e.g., social comparison theory, objectification theory), men's body image, and the impact of body image on social functioning.

Lynda S. Lowry, MA, is a graduate student in the Department of Psychology at the University of the Pacific. Her research interests pertain to women's issues including body image and sexuality and the role of sociocultural factors in developmental psychopathology.

Nina Mafrici, MA, is a doctoral candidate in Counselling Psychology at the Ontario Institute for Studies in Education, University of Toronto, in Canada. Her research focuses on the development of body image in adolescent girls, and how social discourses relating to gender influence girls' and women's experiences in their bodies.

Leanne Magee, PhD, is a Postdoctoral Fellow in Psychology in the Division of Plastic Surgery at the Children's Hospital of Philadelphia. Her research interests include body image and social anxiety in cosmetic and reconstructive surgery patients.

Marita P. McCabe, PhD, is Professor in the School of Psychology, Deakin University, Melbourne, Australia. Her research interests pertain to the development of body image and body change strategies across the lifespan, and obesity, culture, and sexuality.

Donald R. McCreary, PhD, is Adjunct Professor of Psychology at both Brock University (St. Catharines, Ontario, Canada) and York University (Toronto, Ontario, Canada). His research interests are focused in the area of men's health and men's body image, as well as gender roles and the social psychology of health.

Jessica M. McCutcheon, BSc, is a master's student in applied social psychology at the University of Saskatchewan in Canada. Her research interests include attitudes toward sexual minorities, heterosexism, gender role nonconformity, and women's studies.

Nita Mary McKinley, PhD, is Associate Professor in the Interdisciplinary Arts and Sciences program at the University of Washington, Tacoma. She teaches psychology of women, lifespan development, and women's study courses. Her current research examines age differences in objectified body consciousness in adults.

Jessie E. Menzel, MA, is a graduate student at the University of South Florida. Her research interests include the study of positive body image, the relationship between body image and exercise, and protective factors against the development of disordered eating and body image disturbances.

Todd G. Morrison, PhD, is Associate Professor of Applied Social Psychology at the University of Saskatchewan in Canada. His research interests include male body image (in particular, the drive for muscularity), sociocultural theory and the body, psychometrics, and gay and lesbian psychology.

Sarah K. Murnen, PhD, is Professor of Psychology at Kenyon College. She has published empirical articles and theoretical chapters examining how gendered experiences help shape the occurrence of body dissatisfaction and eating-disordered attitudes. This body of work is informed by a feminist, sociocultural theoretical perspective.

Dianne Neumark-Sztainer, PhD, MPH, RD, is Professor in the Division of Epidemiology and Community Health, School of Public Health, University of Minnesota. She conducts epidemiological and qualitative research aimed at understanding factors associated with eating and weight-related outcomes in adolescents and intervention research aimed at preventing weight-related problems in youth.

Jennifer A. O'Dea, MPH, PhD, is Associate Professor in the Faculty of Education and Social Work at the University of Sydney, Australia. Her research interests pertain to understanding body image perceptions among male and female schoolchildren, adolescents, and college students, and the implementation of programs to reduce body image difficulties and eating disorders.

Susan J. Paxton, PhD, is Professor and Head of School in the School of Psychological Science, La Trobe University, Melbourne, Australia. Her research interests include risk factors, prevention, early intervention, and treatment for body image and eating concerns in adolescent girls, adults, and women in midlife. She has been a member of Victorian and National Ministerial Advisory Committees advising on public policy measures to prevent body dissatisfaction.

Trent A. Petrie, PhD, is Professor in the Department of Psychology and Director of the Center for Sport Psychology at the University of North Texas. His research examines physical and psychosocial antecedents of eating disorders and body image, particularly within the sport environment.

Katharine A. Phillips, MD, is Director of the Body Dysmorphic Disorder Program and Director of Research for Adult Psychiatry at Rhode Island Hospital, and Professor of Psychiatry and Human Behavior at the Alpert Medical School of Brown University. Her research focuses on body dysmorphic disorder, particularly its psychopathology and treatment.

Niva Piran, PhD, is Professor in the Department of Adult Education and Counselling Psychology of the Ontario Institute for Studies in Education, University of Toronto, Canada, and a Fellow of the Academy for Eating Disorders. She has worked as a consultant on body image to the National Ballet School of Canada and other schools. Her publications include three coedited books on the prevention and treatment of eating disorders.

Judith Ruskay Rabinor, PhD, is Founder and Director of the American Eating Disorder Center of Long Island. She has authored numerous books, articles, and chapters on eating and body image disorders. She also lectures and trains therapists nationwide and has a private practice in New York City and on Long Island.

Lina A. Ricciardelli, PhD, is Associate Professor in the School of Psychology, Deakin University, Melbourne, Australia. Her research interests pertain to the understanding of body image and body change strategies among children and adolescents, with a particular focus on boys, and the role of both culture and sociocultural factors.

James P. Roehrig, MA, is a doctoral candidate in the Department of Counseling and Applied Educational Psychology at Northeastern University. His research interests include prevention, stigma, and treatment outcome in eating disorders.

Nichola Rumsey, PhD, is VTCT Professor of Appearance Psychology and Co-Director of the Centre for Appearance Research at the University of the West of England, Bristol, United Kingdom. Her research interests relate to the psychological impact of disfigurement, and interventions to meet the needs of those adversely affected.

David B. Sarwer, PhD, is Associate Professor of Psychology in the Departments of Psychiatry and Surgery at the University of Pennsylvania School of Medicine. His research interests include the psychological aspects of plastic surgery and bariatric surgery.

Deborah Schooler, PhD, is Assistant Professor in the Department of Psychology at the University of the Pacific. Her research focuses on cultural influences on adolescent body image, including gender, ethnicity, and media.

Helen Skouteris, PhD, is a Senior Research Fellow in the School of Psychology at Deakin University, Melbourne, Australia. Her research interests pertain to understanding factors that influence maternal and child health and well-being, including body image concerns, ante- and postnatal depression, excessive gestational weight gain, and postpartum weight retention.

Linda Smolak, PhD. See "About the Editors."

Jacqueline C. Spitzer, MS, is a Research Coordinator at the Center for Weight and Eating Disorders in the Department of Psychiatry at the University of Pennsylvania School of Medicine. Her research interests include the treatment of obesity and health-related quality of life.

Jessica L. Suisman, MA, is a clinical psychology graduate student at Michigan State University. Her research interests focus on understanding the interplay between genes and the environment in the etiology of eating disorders.

Viren Swami, PhD, is Reader in the Department of Psychology at the University of Westminster in London, United Kingdom. His research interests are focused on the psychology of interpersonal attraction, with a specific interest in cross-cultural differences in beauty ideals.

Stacey Tantleff-Dunn, PhD, is Associate Professor in the Department of Psychology at the University of Central Florida. Her research focuses on eating behavior and body image, with particular emphasis on media effects, interpersonal influences, and men's body image. She is also in private practice specializing in couples and family coaching.

C. Barr Taylor, MD, is Professor of Psychiatry at Stanford University School of Medicine, where he serves as Director of the Laboratory for the Study of Behavioral Medicine. His research has focused on developing strategies for and evaluating innovative techniques for prevention of various disorders.

Andrew R. Thompson, DClinPsych, is Senior Clinical Lecturer and Chartered Clinical and Health Psychologist in the University of Sheffield/NHS Clinical Psychology Training Unit, United Kingdom, and he provides a clinical service in Rotherham NHS Foundation Trust. His research and clinical work focus on understanding and facilitating adjustment to disfigurement, particularly in relation to long-term health conditions and traumatically acquired injuries.

J. Kevin Thompson, PhD, is Professor of Psychology in the Department of Psychology at the University of South Florida. His research interests include eating disorders, obesity, and body image. Current body image research includes the study of etiological models, assessment development, and tanning and cosmetic surgery attitudes.

Marika Tiggemann, PhD, is Professor of Psychology at Flinders University in South Australia. Her research interests cover body image broadly, and include the sociocultural antecedents (particularly media) of weight, dieting, and body image issues among both adults and children.

Tracy L. Tylka, PhD, is Associate Professor of Counseling Psychology at the Columbus and Marion campuses of The Ohio State University. Her research and clinical interests include understanding, assessing, and modeling body image and eating behavior among women and men of various ages, sexual orientations, and cultural backgrounds. In these endeavors, she focuses on positive and negative body image as well as adaptive and maladaptive eating.

Hannah Weisman, BA, is a research assistant in the Department of Psychiatry and Behavioral Sciences at Stanford University. Her interests include the psychology of gender roles and marginalized groups and the use of technology in prevention and treatment programs.

Eleanor H. Wertheim, PhD, is Professor (Personal Chair) in the School of Psychological Science, La Trobe University, Melbourne, Australia. Her research interests cover the etiology, treatment, and prevention of body image disturbances and disordered eating throughout the lifespan.

Craig A. White, PhD, is Professor of Psychological Therapies at the University of the West of Scotland and Assistant Director of Healthcare Quality with NHS Ayrshire and Arran. He was the first Consultant in Psychosocial Oncology in the National Health Service in Scotland and has clinical and research interests in specialist psychological care.

Michael W. Wiederman, PhD, is Professor of Psychology at Columbia College, an all-women's college in Columbia, South Carolina. His teaching and research interests include human sexuality, gender, body image, and disordered eating.

Nicole M. Williams, MA, is a doctoral candidate in the graduate program in clinical psychology at Kent State University. Her research interests are in body image and eating disorders.

Rebecca E. Wilson, BA, is a doctoral student in the Department of Psychology at the University of Hawaii at Manoa. Her areas of research interest include understanding the correlates of body image, and the nature and consequences of dietary restraint.

Andrew Winzelberg, PhD, is a researcher in the Department of Psychiatry and Behavioral Sciences at Stanford University School of Medicine. His research focuses on the development and evaluation of technology-enhanced programs for the prevention and treatment of health problems.

Zali Yager, PhD, is a lecturer in the Faculty of Education at La Trobe University, Australia. Her research interests focus on body image, eating disorders, and exercise disorders among physical education teachers. Her work demonstrates how best to implement educational programs for teachers' ability to be effective change agents in school-based body image programs.

Preface

Nearly a decade has passed since the publication of the first edition of this comprehensive volume. During this time, the field has continued to grow in the dissemination of scientific research on the multidimensional concept of body image and its implications and applications. Body image, the psychological experience of embodiment, profoundly influences the quality of human life. Historically, much research has focused on body image in relation to eating disorders and disturbances among adolescent girls and young women in Western cultures. However, as conveyed in this volume and its previous edition, increasing topical diversity and sophistication are evident in body image scholarship. Research has expanded to consider body image development and difficulties among boys and men and body image functioning in various cultures. The validation of new body image assessments has proliferated. Appearance-altering conditions within medical contexts are increasingly studied in terms of body image. Our knowledge has grown further regarding the prevention and treatment of body image problems. Simply stated, we know much more about body image than we knew a decade ago.

In this handbook, internationally recognized experts skillfully distilled their scientific wisdom into concise, insightful reviews of specific topics that address the richness and complexity of body image experiences. As in the earlier edition, chapters are meaningfully organized into nine sections. Some topics are novel to this second edition. In Part I, "Conceptual Foundations," there are new chapters to provide contemporary sociocultural, evolutionary, genetic/neuroscientific, and positive psychology perspectives on human appearance and body image. In Part II, "Developmental Perspectives and Influences," there are now separate chapters concerning body image development in adolescent boys and girls. Part III, "Body Image Assessment," includes a new chapter on crucial issues in body image assessment. In Part IV, "Individual and Cultural Differences," and Part V, "Body Image Dysfunctions and Disorders," chapters have been added covering body image in non-Western cultures, body image and binge-eating disorder, body image and appearance- and performance-enhancing drug use, and separate chapters on obesity in youth and in adulthood. In Part VI, "Body Image Issues in Medical Contexts," there are new chapters that focus on body image issues in rheumatology and those associated with burn injuries. Part VII, "Changing the Body: Medical, Surgical, and Other Approaches," includes a new chapter on body art. And in Part VIII, "Changing Body Images: Psychosocial Interventions for Treatment and Prevention," the coverage of prevention has been expanded to four chapters.

For both seasoned and aspiring professionals, this second edition of *Body Image* is a distinctively comprehensive, scientifically up-to-date, and clinically valuable resource, particularly for scientists and practitioners in psychology and mental health, as well as those in medical and allied health fields. As editors, we made certain that chapters informatively cross-reference one another. As catalysts for further discovery, each chapter offers an annotated bibliography of "Informative Readings."

Readers familiar with the first edition of this handbook will notice a change in the editorship of the work. Tom Pruzinsky was a coeditor of the first edition. Since that time, he has gradually transitioned to other personally important pursuits. Nevertheless, the present version of the handbook continues to reflect his long-standing devotion to the field, especially his clinical health psychology interests in appearance-altering medical conditions.

In addition to our esteemed contributing authors, many people were vital in the production of this work. As always, The Guilford Press was a superlative publisher. We appreciate their support, and particularly thank Jim Nageotte, Jane Keislar, Carolyn Graham, Anna Nelson, Katherine Lieber, and Paul Gordon. Each editor also personally wishes to recognize certain persons who were instrumental to this work:

Tom Cash: First and foremost, I am grateful to Tom Pruzinsky, my valued friend and colleague for over 20 years. The opportunity to know and collaborate with him has always been inspiring and fulfilling. Tom is one of the most caring and genuine people I have ever known. I sincerely thank my new coeditor, Linda Smolak, for the wisdom, diligence, upbeat attitude, and friendship she brought to this work. From 1973 to 2008, I had the exceptional good fortune to spend my academic career in the Department of Psychology at Old Dominion University. I treasure my experiences there, with the faculty and many undergraduate and graduate students who were integral to my satisfying career. Of course, I am especially grateful to my family—my deceased parents, who always believed in me; my adult sons, who make me proud; my grandchildren, who keep me hopeful; and my wonderful wife, Natalie, who makes me smile every day.

Linda Smolak: I want to first thank Tom Cash for his continued passionate dedication to the field of body image and for the vision that became this book. It is an honor to have been invited to work on it. Tom brought intelligence, thoroughness, and, importantly, good humor to this endeavor. Second, the contributors to this book, many of whom are long-time friends, were timely and professional in sharing their expertise in these chapters. They made it possible to produce such a rich volume. Kenyon College has been my professional home since 1980. I continue to value my colleagues there despite my recent retirement. In particular, I want to thank my Kenyon friends Michael Levine, Sarah Murnen, and Dana Krieg. Finally, I want to thank my husband, Jim Keeler, for his patience and support throughout this project. He makes my work possible and every day a pleasure. My children—Marlyce, Jesse, and Meghan—and grandchildren—Sabrina, Nathan, Iz, and Lydie—continue to remind me why this work is important and to provide laughter in my life.

Reflecting the rapid expansion of the field, this handbook is testimony to the central importance of body image in the full range of human experience. Our hope is that this volume contributes, in science and clinical practice and prevention, to the alleviation of body image suffering and the promotion of body image acceptance.

Thomas F. Cash, PhD
Linda Smolak, PhD

Contents

PART II. DEVELOPMENTAL PERSPECTIVES AND INFLUENCES

PART III. BODY IMAGE ASSESSMENT

PART IV. INDIVIDUAL AND CULTURAL DIFFERENCES

PART V. BODY IMAGE DYSFUNCTIONS AND DISORDERS

PART VIII. CHANGING BODY IMAGES: PSYCHOSOCIAL INTERVENTIONS FOR TREATMENT AND PREVENTION

PART IX. CONCLUSIONS AND DIRECTIONS

PART I

CONCEPTUAL FOUNDATIONS

CHAPTER 1

Understanding Body Images
Historical and
Contemporary Perspectives

THOMAS F. CASH
LINDA SMOLAK

Introduction

Looking back over a century of scholarly efforts to understand the profoundly human experience of embodiment that defines "body image," we find a very rich and inspiring history. From diverse perspectives, behavioral scientists, physicians, and philosophers have theorized about the nature and significance of body image. Researchers have made systematic observations to test their ideas and discover the meanings of body image. Clinical practitioners have pursued remedies, both body changing and mind changing, to help people whose quality of life is diminished by their body image experiences. Other applied researchers have developed interventions for the prevention of body image problems among youth.

This introductory chapter offers a historical and conceptual context for the volume. We highlight important milestones in body image scholarship during the 20th century and first decade of this century. We identify specific published books that reflect the growth of knowledge in the field. Finally, we articulate contemporary perspectives on body image by summarizing the organization and contents of this handbook, which speak to its rationale and uniqueness.

3

Milestones in Body Image Scholarship

20th-Century Legacies

Understanding modern perspectives on body image requires insight into the lineage of the body image construct. Early in the 1900s, neurologists studying and treating brain injuries sought to make sense of a variety of unusual forms of body perception and experience reported by their patients. There was also considerable effort to understand "phantom limb," in which amputees report sensory experiences associated with the missing limb. Early "body image" research was dominated by investigation of what Henry Head termed *the body schema*, a hypothetical neural mechanism whereby changes in body posture and movement were proposed to be centrally coordinated. Little consideration was given to psychological variables in theorizing about body image.

Paul Schilder, who was trained as a neurologist, was "single-handedly" responsible for moving the study of body image beyond the exclusive domain of neuropathology and was "the first to devote entire volumes to the topic of body image" (Fisher, 1990, p. 12). In his 1935 *The Image and Appearance of the Human Body*, Schilder presciently argued for a biopsychosocial approach to body image, emphasizing the need to examine its neurological, psychological, and sociocultural elements. Historically, one of the most important body image scholars was Seymour Fisher who, with his colleague Sidney Cleveland, published two editions of the text *Body Image and Personality* in 1958 and 1968. Their work reflected the then pervasive psychodynamic views of body image, especially Fisher's theorizing about the construct of *body image boundaries*. Their empirical research focused on the "barrier" and "penetration" boundary dimensions posited to reflect the strength or permeability of body boundaries. These investigations, with "normal" subjects as well as psychiatric and medical patients, almost invariably used projective methodologies, including the Holtzman or Rorschach Inkblot Tests. Fisher's 1986 two-volume opus, *Development and Structure of the Body Image*, is the apex of the portion of his career devoted to body image scholarship. Volume 1 consists of a comprehensive review of research from 1969 through 1985. Volume 2 analyzes and synthesizes data pertinent to Fisher's own concepts, including "body image boundary, assignment of meaning to specific body areas, general body awareness, and distortions in body perception" (p. xi). Seymour Fisher died in 1996, yet these works remain testimony to his insightful and prolific contributions to the field.

Franklin Shontz, in his 1969 *Perceptual and Cognitive Aspects of Body Experience* and in later writings, was a pioneer in directing body image research away from the domination of a psychodynamic paradigm. Shontz argued that the shift from neurological to psychodynamic conceptions had removed "body" from body image. He also critically noted that Fisher's psychodynamic view of body image as "a projection screen for emotional learning and experience" served to eradicate the "image" from body image by operationally defining it as a manifestation of perceiving inkblots or other ambiguous stimuli (see Shontz, 1990, p. 156). Shontz redressed these limitations in several ways as he argued for the study of multifaceted "body experience." He postulated seven functions of body image experience and four or more levels of these functions. He emphasized the use of diverse scientific methods and encouraged expansion and integration of theoretical developments, especially from field theory, Gestalt psychology, and cognitive theory. Furthermore, Shontz sought to put the body back into body image, partly by applying body image concepts to the study of physical disability and health psychology. He endeavored to return the image to body image by articulating cognitive and perceptual dimensions of body experience.

The Productive 1990s

The 1990s was a pivotal decade in the evolution of body image scholarship. This was a productive period of conceptual, psychometric, and psychotherapeutic developments. In 1990 Cash and Pruzinsky published *Body Images: Development, Deviance, and Change*, an edited volume that stressed the multidimensionality of body image and expanded its application into areas of investigation previously inadequately explored—for example, disfigurement, disability and rehabilitation, and cosmetic and reconstructive surgery. In the same year, J. Kevin Thompson authored *Body Image Disturbance: Assessment and Treatment*, followed by his 1996 edited book, *Body Image, Eating Disorders, and Obesity: An Integrative Guide for Assessment and Treatment*. Reflecting the burgeoning scientific and clinical interest in eating disorders and obesity, these works enhanced our knowledge of the assessment and treatment of body image disorders. Reflecting a growing clinical interest in body dysmorphic disorder, in 1996, Katharine Phillips published an informative volume, *The Broken Mirror: Understanding and Treating Body Dysmorphic Disorder* (revised in 2005).

In 1999, *Exacting Beauty: Theory, Assessment, and Treatment of Body Image Disturbance*, written by Thompson, Heinberg, Altabe, and Tantleff-Dunn, provided a needed compilation and synthesis of the extensive progress in body image research. Sarah Grogan's 1999 book, *Body Image: Understanding Body Dissatisfaction in Men, Women, and Children*, similarly offered a detailed and scholarly review of the literature.

Emergent in this decade was the development and scientific evaluation of a cognitive-behavioral treatment approach to body image problems. In 1991, Cash published his *Body Image Therapy* program as an audiotape series with client and clinician manuals. Subsequent versions of the program appeared in 1995 as *What Do You See When You Look in the Mirror?* and in 1997 as *The Body Image Workbook*.

The New Millennium

During this century's initial decade, body image scholarship continued to flourish. Perhaps the most significant milestone has been the publication of a peer-reviewed scientific journal, *Body Image: An International Journal of Research*. Launched in 2004, this quarterly journal has provided a dedicated home for high-quality body image research from the behavioral sciences as well as the medical/health sciences. Evident in the pages of the journal is the growth in the investigation of body image among boys and men, among diverse cultures, and among persons with a range of psychological disorders and appearance-altering medical disorders. Also apparent is the expansion of work to develop better assessments of body image as a multidimensional construct and to evaluate interventions to treat and prevent body image problems.

In 2001, Thompson and Smolak edited a long-overdue volume about body image in childhood and adolescence and the prevention of body image problems, *Body Image, Eating Disorders, and Obesity in Youth: Assessment, Prevention, and Treatment*. They published their second edition of this work in 2009. Grogan also published the second edition of her comprehensive book in 2008. Thompson's edited 2004 *Handbook of Eating Disorders and Obesity* thoroughly incorporated a consideration of body image. The decade brought new attention to male body image issues with *The Adonis Complex: The Secret Crisis of Male Body Obsession* published by Pope, Phillips, and Olivardia in 2000. Advances in this area are also evident in *The Muscular Ideal* that Thompson and Cafri edited in 2007. Castle and Phillips edited their informative *Disorders of Body Image* in 2002. Another overdue volume was Rumsey and Harcourt's 2005 *The Psychology of Appearance*, which provides a valuable understanding of the body image and social experiences of persons with disfiguring conditions. Furthermore, reflecting the editorial collaboration of three psychologists and three plastic surgeons, in 2006 David Sarwer and his colleagues assembled a unique book entitled *Psychological Aspects of Reconstructive and Cosmetic Plastic Surgery*.

During the past few years, the clinical treatment of body image disorders and difficulties continues to receive attention. For example, in 2008 Cash published the second edition of his *Body Image Workbook* that details a cognitive-behavioral program for body image change. Several workbooks and manuals to assist persons with body dysmorphic disorder have been published, including Veale and Neziroglu's detailed *Body Dysmorphic Disorder* treatment manual in 2010.

Contemporary Perspectives on Body Image: Organization and Contents of the Handbook

In the first edition of this handbook in 2002, Cash and Pruzinsky presented evidence that confirmed the continuous growth in body image research over the previous 50 years, from 1951 to 2000. This growth has clearly persisted in the first decade of the 21st century. A search of two prominent research databases, PsycINFO and Medline, indicates that the number of body image publications in each database more than doubled from 2000 through 2010 relative to the 1990s. Not long ago, most body image research focused on eating pathology and weight/shape concerns among White female college students. The variety of contexts and populations in which body image is explored has broadened considerably. These impressive developments are expounded and elucidated by the contributors to this handbook. We have organized their chapters into eight substantive sections:

Conceptual Foundations

This first section of the book presents an array of conceptual approaches for understanding human appearance and body image. Our contributors present important, wide-ranging perspectives, including sociocultural, evolutionary, genetic and neuroscientic, cognitive-behavioral, and feminist (objectification theory) viewpoints, as well as a chapter discussing positive psychology perspectives on body image. In this section, authors thoughtfully articulate concepts, principles, and propositions applicable to the empirical data and clinical observations presented throughout the book.

Developmental Perspectives and Influences

In the second section, seven chapters describe the development of body image across the lifespan, with special emphasis on understanding the unique body experiences of childhood, adolescence, and adulthood in both males and females. These body image trajectories are further elucidated in chapters that carefully examine the influences of cultural media, family systems, and other interpersonal relationships as well as the impact of sexual abuse. The developmental context is essential for understanding virtually all body image experiences, whether adaptive or dysfunctional.

Body Image Assessment

The scientific study of body image requires thoughtful and precise measurement of its components and dimensions. This section begins with a chapter on crucial considerations in the assessment of body image. It is followed by a chapter on assessing body image among children and two chapters on assessments for adolescents and adults. One targets perceptual body image measures and discusses both the pitfalls and the progress associated with these types of assessments. The other provides a practical compendium of both new and commonly used validated assessments of various facets of the attitudinal body image construct. Collectively, these chapters offer comprehensive yet concise guidelines for scientists and practitioners to understand methodological, psychometric, and practical issues in measuring body image.

Individual and Cultural Differences

A genuine understanding of body image requires a deep appreciation for the diversity of cultural and personal contexts of embodiment. Building upon the foundations of the handbook's reviews of conceptual and developmental perspectives, this extensive section offers 11 chapters that examine a range of cultural and individual differences in body image experiences. These chapters summarize literatures on body image diversity related to gender, sexual orientation, and ethnicity. They include consideration of the expanding research on non-Western societies. To elucidate individual differences in body image functioning, they examine the influences of adiposity, muscularity, athleticism, and disfiguring congenital conditions on body image functioning.

Body Image Dysfunctions and Disorders

Many students of body image are interested in the myriad difficulties and disorders of body experience. In this section of the handbook, contributors review the explosive growth of observations and evidence in the study of body image dysfunctions and disorders. This section's seven chapters highlight difficulties that range from "common" body image discontent to more severe disturbances, including body dysmorphic disorder and eating disorders (i.e., anorexia nervosa, bulimia nervosa, and binge-eating disorder). Chapters consider the importance of body image to both social functioning and sexual functioning as well as in relation to appearance- and performance-enhancing drug use.

Body Image Issues in Medical Contexts

One of the new frontiers of scholarship is the elucidation of the body image challenges associated with physical diseases and disorders. An obvious but oft-neglected fact is that body image issues accompany changes in the appearance and functioning of the human body, and that these changes can dramatically affect quality of life. Such issues are routinely encountered in many medical specialties. This section of the handbook samples five of these areas: dermatology, oncology, obstetrics and gynecology, rheumatology, and medical specialties associated with the treatment of burn injuries. Contributors summarize the state of our scientific knowledge of body image in these specialties and offer constructive guidance for future research, as well as clinical practice.

Changing the Body: Medical, Surgical, and Other Approaches

This first of two sections on body image change focuses on one central question: Does changing the body lead to a changed body image? The chapters in this section review the scientific evidence regarding body image changes as a result of physical interventions, such as weight loss (including bariatric surgery), systematic exercise regimens, cosmetic surgery for "elective" appearance changes, and reconstructive surgeries for congenital and acquired disfiguring conditions. Included in this section is a chapter that uniquely considers another form of body modification— body art (e.g., tattooing and piercing).

Changing Body Images: Psychosocial Interventions for Treatment and Prevention

This second section on body image change offers an array of psychotherapeutic and psychoeducational interventions. The empirically validated cognitive-behavioral approaches to body image change are reviewed, as well as less well-researched but clinically common experiential approaches. Four chapters tackle the imperative topic of prevention—how to effectively prevent body image problems that themselves threaten quality of life and also are risk factors for other difficulties such as eating disorders and depression. One chapter delineates school-based psychoeducational interventions. The second considers computer-based interventions. The third articulates ecological and activism approaches to prevention and the fourth discusses changes in public policy to prevent body image problems and their consequences.

Conclusions and Directions

The handbook's final section contains the editors' chapter "Future Challenges for Body Image Science, Practice, and Prevention." Drawing upon the contents of the volume, this chapter offers an organized series of epigrammatic statements regarding the most important future directions for body image research and its application to treatment and prevention.

Conclusions

The scientific study of body image has a fascinating history and continues to be a rapidly growing field. Human experiences of embodiment affect many aspects of psychosocial functioning and quality of life. This volume provides the state of the science vis-à-vis our knowledge of body image development and functioning, as well as our knowledge of the prevention and change of body image difficulties and disorders. The contents of this handbook make it clear that body image transcends a singular experience. It is complex and multidimensional. It is gendered. It is ethnic and cultural. It is age dependent. It depends on the state of the body and the state of the mind. Much has been learned since the first edition of this handbook was published in 2002. Much remains to be learned.

Informative Readings

This chapter identifies numerous scholarly works on body image over the past century. The references below include some of the most recent reference sources:

Cash, T. F. (2004). Body image: Past, present, and future (editorial). *Body Image: An International Journal of Research, 1*, 1–5.—Provides the editor's perspective on the field for the journal's inaugural issue, which includes nine review articles on core topics about body image.

Fisher, S. (1990). The evolution of psychological concepts about the body. In T. F. Cash & T. Pruzinsky (Eds.), *Body images: Development, deviance and change* (pp. 3–20). New York: Guilford Press.—An excellent historical view of the body image construct from an influential scholar in the field.

Grogan, S. (2008). *Body image: Understanding body dissatisfaction in men, women, and children* (2nd ed.). East Sussex, UK: Routledge.—Offers an extensive and detailed overview of the field.

Rumsey, N., & Harcourt, D. (2005). *The psychology of appearance*. Maidenhead, UK: Open University Press.—A review of human appearance and body image with a particular focus on visible differences.

Sarwer, D. B., Pruzinsky, T., Cash, T. F., Goldwyn, R. M., Persing, J. A., & Whitaker, L. A. (Eds.). (2006). *Psychological aspects of reconstructive and cosmetic plastic surgery: Clinical, empirical, and ethical perspectives*. Philadelphia: Lippincott, Williams and Wilkins.—Provides an integrated consideration of body image in relation to reconstructive and cosmetic surgery.

Shontz, F. C. (1990). Body image and physical disability. In T. F. Cash & T. Pruzinsky (Eds.), *Body images: Development, deviance, and change* (pp. 149–169). New York: Guilford Press.—Summarizes the history of body image concepts and their application to physical disabilities.

Smolak, L., & Thompson, J. K. (Eds.). (2009). *Body image, eating disorders, and obesity in youth: Assessment, prevention, and treatment* (2nd ed.). Washington, DC: American Psychological Association.—Details research literatures on body image in relation to eating disorders and obesity among children and adolescents.

Thompson, J. K. (Ed.). (2004). *Handbook of eating disorders and obesity*. Hoboken, NJ: Wiley.—An extensive volume on eating disorders and obesity with an integral consideration of body image.

Thompson, J. K., & Cafri, G. (Eds.). (2007). *The muscular ideal: Psychological, social, and*

medical perspectives. Washington, DC: American Psychological Association.—
Considers how cultural and personal ideals and pursuits of a muscular physique affect men (and some women).

Veale, D., & Neziroglu, F. (2010). *Body dysmorphic disorder: A treatment manual.* West
Sussex, UK: Wiley-Blackwell.—A volume that integrates theory and science
on body dysmorphic disorder and delineates the elements of treatment.

CHAPTER 2

Sociocultural Perspectives on Human Appearance and Body Image

MARIKA TIGGEMANN

Introduction

Appearance in general and body image in particular have become very important constructs in contemporary Western societies. The strong emphasis on appearance is abundantly displayed—on billboards, in any shop window, in any magazine, in the ordinary conversations of individuals, in the amount of money, time, and effort invested in the pursuit of beauty through clothes, hair, dieting, and other everyday grooming practices, and in the increasing popularity of cosmetic surgical procedures (see Chapter 45). Further, there is a great deal of evidence that body image is experienced negatively by the majority of women and girls. Many are dissatisfied with their body, particularly with their body size and weight and wish to be thinner, so much so that weight has been aptly described as "a normative discontent" for women. There is also increasing evidence that men and boys too are beginning to experience body dissatisfaction—in the direction of wishing to be more muscular—albeit at lower rates (for the moment) than their female counterparts. Finally, appearance esteem and body satisfaction represent probably the major contributors to overall levels of global self-esteem; that is, they are very important components of how individuals feel about themselves as a whole.

This chapter sets out to introduce and describe what has become in the literature one of the dominant theoretical frameworks for viewing body image, namely, the sociocultural perspective. This perspective holds sociocultural ideals and pressures as paramount to the genesis of body image disturbance, and so is in accord with many lay or everyday explanations. In reviewing evidence supporting the sociocultural model, the chapter seeks not only to present what is known, but also to identify gaps in the existing research on sociocultural influences.

The Sociocultural Model

Although there exist several more specific forms of the sociocultural model, the perspective is perhaps best thought of as a heuristic or conceptual model providing a general framework for viewing and investigating body image and disordered eating. At its simplest, the sociocultural model holds that (1) there exist societal ideals of beauty (within a particular culture) that are (2) transmitted via a variety of sociocultural channels. These ideals are then (3) internalized by individuals, so that (4) satisfaction (or dissatisfaction) with appearance will be a function of the extent to which individuals do (or do not) meet the ideal prescription.

How does this operate in current Western society? A casual flick through any women's fashion magazine will reveal a plethora of young, tall, long-legged, large-eyed, moderately large-breasted, tanned but not too tanned, and clear-skinned women with usually White features. But perhaps the most obvious and consistent physical characteristic shared by these models is that they are also very thin. Not only are they naturally thin, but digital modification techniques are often used to further slice off pounds and inches from waists, hips, and thighs. Thus current societal standards for female beauty inordinately emphasize the desirability of thinness. These ideals are then transmitted by powerful and pervasive sociocultural influences, most notably the media, family, and peers, and hence the sociocultural model is sometimes referred to as the tripartite model. Despite the thin ideal being impossible for most women to achieve by healthy means, it is nevertheless accepted and internalized by many; that is, it is adopted and incorporated by the woman as the reference point against which to judge herself. As it is virtually impossible for women to match up to this thin ideal, they are invariably disappointed, resulting in body dissatisfaction. This, in turn, may lead to dieting and other usually futile (and most often unhealthy) attempts to pursue thinness, ultimately resulting in disordered eating symptoms.

A parallel process operates for men, but in this case the ideal that is socioculturally transmitted is a mesomorphic and muscular V-shaped body, with broad shoulders, well-developed upper body, flat but muscular stomach ("six-pack abs"), and narrow waist and hips. Again, this hypermuscular ideal is impossible for most men to achieve by healthy means. Nevertheless, it is internalized by many, resulting in body dissatisfaction and a potentially unhealthy pursuit of muscularity (via compulsive exercise, supplements, or steroids).

A Couple of Caveats

The sociocultural model has been applied primarily in the realm of body weight and shape. In principle, it can be applied equally well to other features such as skin color, breast size, or size of eyes, or indeed to any attribute about which people can feel themselves deficient.

Second, in its simplest form, the sociocultural model would have *everyone* suffering from extreme body dissatisfaction and eating disorders, which is clearly not the case. There are a number of genetic and other biological (see Chapter 4) and psychological influences that potentially moderate the links of the model, and ultimately determine an individual's degree of vulnerability to sociocultural pressures. For example, the extent to which an individual internalizes or absorbs the societal thin ideal might be moderated by levels of self-esteem (or autonomy), such that women with high self-esteem will be less influenced by societal ideals and pressures.

Evidence in Support of the Model

The sociocultural model offers a relatively simple, easily understood, and face-valid framework for understanding contemporary body image. What is the research evidence for the steps of the model?

Evidence for the Existence of Sociocultural Ideals

A number of converging lines of evidence point to the importance of sociocultural ideals of appearance. First, there is a great deal of research indicating that the societal beauty ideal for women has become increasingly thin over recent decades. For example, one analysis of Miss America pageant winners and *Playboy* centerfolds documented a significant decrease in body size from the 1950s to 1990s, by which time the majority had weights that were more than 15% below their expected weight for height. Other formal content analyses of visual media including fashion magazines, film, television, and video games confirm this trend. Further, there is no doubt that these levels of thinness have not abated but continued as the ideal into the 2000s, but with a greater focus on having at least a medium bust size and being toned, in addition to being thin. One estimate is that the average fashion model has a body mass index (BMI) of 16.3, well below the normal healthy range of 18.5–24.9.

In men, there is similar evidence that the cultural norm for the ideal body has become increasingly muscular. For example, one study found that *Playgirl* centerfold (male) models increased in both BMI and muscularity (fat-free mass index) across the 1970s–1990s, with some male ideals exceeding the upper limit of muscularity attainable without the use of anabolic steroids. More generally there has been a documented increase in the use of young, lean, bare-chested, and muscled male bodies in fashion magazines and advertising.

Second, the same sociocultural ideals are reflected in media specifically marketed at children, and in children's toys. For example, the Barbie doll represents a cultural icon of female beauty that is owned by over 90% of 3- to 10-year-old girls. Yet Barbie's weight and body proportions are completely unrealistic. In a unique experimental study with children, Dittmar and colleagues showed that 5- to 8-year-old girls reported lower body esteem and greater desire for a thinner shape after brief exposure to images of the Barbie doll. Many boys, on the other hand, play with male action toys—small plastic figures of various adventure heroes (e.g., GI Joe, Luke Skywalker)—that can likewise be taken as representations of the sociocultural ideal for male body image. Studies have documented that these figures have become increasingly muscular during the last two decades, with many contemporary figures exceeding the levels of muscularity of any human.

Third, the prevalence of different sociocultural ideals has been examined in different cultures. Although earlier cross-cultural comparisons suggested adherence to the thin ideal was lower in developing or non-Western societies, there is now increasing consensus that it has become a transnational phenomenon, usually attributed to proliferation of Western media. In the largest cross-cultural survey of body ideals to date (International Body Project, with a convenience sample of more than 4,000 women and 3,000 men from 26 countries), there was little difference in ratings of attractive or ideal female figures or body dissatisfaction across 10 world geographic regions. Importantly, in non-Western societies, more self-reported exposure to Western media was associated with preference for a thinner female figure (by both men and women), in a way that exposure to local media was not.

Fourth, within Western cultures, differences in occupation or interest have been related to body image. In particular, research has documented that members of subcultures where ideal body pressures are amplified (e.g., ballet dancers, fashion models, athletes in "lean" or "aesthetic" sports, gymnasts, members of fitness centers, gay men) do indeed have higher rates of body dissatisfaction and eating disorders.

Evidence Concerning Sociocultural Transmission of Ideals and Its Effects

The three sociocultural influences that have been identified as important transmitters of sociocultural ideals are parents, peers, and the media (see

Chapters 12 and 13). The role of each of these has now been supported by a large body of correlational research. For example, there is evidence that parents can influence the body image of their children in both direct (parental commentary about the child's weight or appearance, or the imposition of particular food rules) and indirect ways (through unintended parental modeling of their own weight concerns and dieting behaviors).

The role of peers has been mostly studied among adolescents, but is also relevant to younger children and to adult women, for example, through "fat talk," a script in which women or girls seek reassurance for their anxieties about being or becoming fat. Among adolescent girls, there is evidence that girls who are part of a particular friendship group have similar levels of body image concern and dietary restraint. Specific peer influences that have been demonstrated include comments from peers about weight and shape (teasing is an extreme form of this), the modeling of weight concerns and weight control techniques, perceived peer norms, conversations among peers about weight or appearance, and the belief that popularity is dependent on conforming to the thin (or muscular) ideal.

However, the most powerful and pervasive transmitter of the sociocultural ideals of beauty are the mass media (see Chapter 12). Extensive correlational, experimental, and meta-analytic evidence supports the link between exposure to fashion magazines and particular forms of television (notably soap operas and music videos) and the outcomes of internalization of the thin ideal, body dissatisfaction, and eating disorder symptomatology for adult and adolescent women. A smaller meta-analysis has confirmed that media exposure (or perceived pressure from media) is also associated with negative body image for men. As yet, however, little research has addressed newer media (e.g., the Internet), even though there exist many sites with an appearance focus, including health, beauty, clothing, and celebrity sites as well as pro-ana (anorexia) or pornography sites.

While the media, family, and peers have been identified as major conveyors of sociocultural ideals, there are many other potential sources of influence, including teachers, sports coaches, ministers, and medical practitioners. Furthermore, these multiple agents can exert influence concurrently, and can also interact. For example, Jones and colleagues showed that adolescent girls exist in "an appearance culture" where media ideals and peer conversations about appearance-related topics reinforce each other.

Evidence on Mediating Mechanisms

The existence of particular societal ideals does not by definition mean that there will be negative psychological consequences for people who do not meet these ideals. Several mediating mechanisms have been proposed by which societal messages from parents, peers, and the media lead to body dissatisfaction. The earlier versions of the sociocultural model postulated internalization of ideals (i.e., acceptance and adoption of societal ideals as goals for oneself) as the major mediating mechanism. More recently, this has been supplemented by the process of social comparison, whereby women compare their appearance with the idealized media images and almost invariably find themselves lacking. Other mediating variables, such as perceived pressure from the media, have also been proposed.

There is a large amount of evidence, including data from longitudinal studies, that the above variables correlate with body dissatisfaction. There is also a smaller body of evidence that they actually mediate (i.e., can account for or explain) the relationships between peer and media influences and body dissatisfaction.

Evaluation of the Complete Model

Thompson and colleagues have attempted to test the whole sociocultural model as it applies to women by structural equation modeling in a series of adolescent and young adult samples. In general, their modeling shows that perceived influence from parents, peers, and the media leads to internalization and appearance comparison that, in turn, lead to body dissatisfaction and finally to disturbed eating patterns. Usually, a direct effect from media influence to restrictive eating has also been found. These results indicate overall support for the sociocultural model. Less systematic tests of aspects of the model in male samples indicate that the model appears also to apply to men's body image.

Limitations

In the main, the claims of the sociocultural model have been investigated among White adolescent and young adult (college-age) women. Although there is growing interest in the body image of men, the experience of other groups (preadolescent children, adult men and women, more ethnically diverse samples) warrants more research attention. The influence of other sociocultural agents, such as sports coaches and medical practitioners, as well as newer forms of the media (e.g., the Internet), should also be addressed. An important remaining task is the identification of moderating variables, those individual differences (biological, psychological, or social) that make some people vulnerable to sociocultural pressures to conform to the ideal, but others more resilient to the same pressures.

But perhaps the largest limitation in the existing research is that it is primarily correlational and hence cannot determine causal directions. For the effects of media, for example, while it is tempting to conclude that exposure to a large dose of thin idealized images leads to body dissatisfaction in accord with the causal sequence proposed in the sociocultural model, the converse causal assumption is equally plausible: Body dissatisfaction may lead to heightened use of the media. Yet there is surprisingly little longitudinal evidence indicating that sociocultural influences actually *precede* body concerns in time, a necessary condition for causality. In particular, there is virtually no evidence that media exposure is temporally antecedent to body dissatisfaction in adolescent or adult women, although two recent studies show television to be predictive across a 1-year time period in quite young children. Most likely the relationship between sociocultural influences and body image will be complex, multiply determined, and bidirectional.

For effects of family and peers, a program of research by Dianne Neumark-Sztainer and colleagues (Project EAT—Eating Among Teens) in a large cohort of ethnically diverse adolescents over a 5-year time span) furnishes valuable information, although measures were necessarily simple and single-itemed. The variables identified that actually predicted body dissatisfaction or eating disturbance 5 years later included BMI, weight-related teasing by family or peers, parental weight-related concerns and behaviors, and friend dieting. On the other hand, frequent family meals, positive atmosphere at family meals, and frequent lunch intake emerged as protective factors. These findings need to be qualified, however, as typically they applied to some but not all age and gender subsamples, indicating that different predictors may emerge at different stages of development (e.g., early vs. middle adolescence).

Conclusions

The primary purpose of any theoretical model is to increase understanding and to generate testable hypotheses. In this, the sociocultural model has performed well. Although more longitudinal evidence is required, many aspects of the model have received considerable support. Accordingly, the sociocultural perspective has proved a very useful general framework for viewing contemporary body image.

Informative Readings

Clark, L., & Tiggemann, M. (2007). Sociocultural influences and body image in 9- to 12-year-old girls: The role of appearance schemas. *Journal of Clinical Child and Adolescent Psychology, 36,* 76–86.—A test of interrelated peer and media influences on the body image of children.
Dohnt, H., & Tiggemann, M. (2006). The contribution of peer and media influences to the development of body satisfaction and self-esteem in young girls: A prospective study. *Developmental Psychology, 42,* 929–936.—A prospective study demonstrating the predictive role of both media and peer influences in the body image of 5- to 8-year-old girls.

Jones, D. C., Vigfusdottir, T. H., & Lee, Y. (2004). Body image and the appearance culture among adolescent girls and boys. *Journal of Adolescent Research, 19,* 323–339.—Introduction to the concept of "appearance culture," whereby media, peer, and other sociocultural influences reinforce each other.

Levine, M. P., & Murnen, S. K. (2009). "Everybody knows that mass media are/are not [pick one] a cause of eating disorders": A critical review of evidence for a causal link between media, negative body image, and disordered eating in females. *Journal of Social and Clinical Psychology, 28,* 9–42.—A comprehensive analysis of the evidence for media effects; clearly sets out different forms of evidence and the criteria for a causal risk factor.

Neumark-Sztainer, D. R., Wall, M. M., Haines, J. I., Story, M. T., Sherwood, N. E., & van den Berg, P. A. (2007). Shared risk and protective factors for overweight and disordered eating in adolescents. *American Journal of Preventative Medicine, 33,* 359–369.—One in a series of reports of a large-scale longitudinal investigation of adolescents over a 5-year time span.

Shroff, H., & Thompson, J. K. (2006). The tripartite influence model of body dissatisfaction and eating disturbance: A replication with adolescent girls. *Body Image: An International Journal of Research, 3,* 17–23.—A structural equation modeling confirmation of the general sociocultural model.

Smolak, L., & Levine, M. (2001). Body image in children. In J. K. Thompson & L. Smolak (Eds.), *Body image, eating disorders, and obesity in youth: Assessment, prevention, and treatment* (pp. 41–66). Washington, DC: American Psychological Association.—A specific and elaborated sociocultural model of the development of body image in children.

Stice, E. (1994). Review of the evidence for a sociocultural model of bulimia nervosa and an exploration of the mechanisms of action. *Clinical Psychology Review, 14,* 633–661.—Perhaps the earliest articulation of a specific sociocultural model for body dissatisfaction and disordered eating.

Swami, V., Frederick, D. A., Aavik, T., Alcalay, L., Allik, J., Anderson, D., et al. (2010). The attractive female body weight and female body dissatisfaction in 26 countries across 10 world regions: Results of the International Body Project I. *Personality and Social Psychology Bulletin, 36,* 309–325.—The largest existing cross-national comparison of body image ideals.

Sypeck, M. F., Gray, J. J., & Ahrens, A. H. (2004). No longer just a pretty face: Fashion magazines' depictions of ideal female beauty from 1959 to 1999. *International Journal of Eating Disorders, 36,* 342–347.—A content analysis of 1920 magazine covers.

Thompson, J. K., & Stice, E. (2001). Thin-ideal internalization: Mounting evidence for a new risk factor for body-image disturbance and eating pathology. *Current Directions in Psychological Science, 10,* 181–183.—A review presenting correlational, experimental, and prospective evidence for the role of internalization in body image and eating disturbance.

Wertheim, E. H., Paxton, S. J., & Blaney, S. (2004). Risk factors for the development of body image disturbances. In J. K. Thompson (Ed.), *Handbook of eating disorders and obesity* (pp. 463–494). Hoboken, NJ: Wiley.—Includes a summary of longitudinal research on sociocultural factors and multifactorial models.

CHAPTER 3

Evolutionary Perspectives on Human Appearance and Body Image

VIREN SWAMI

Introduction

An evolutionary approach provides a useful theoretical basis for understanding a wide array of human behaviors that are related to appearance, attractiveness, and body image. Specifically, under the rubric of sexual selection, evolutionary psychologists have suggested that some traits in humans evolved, not because they confer any survival advantage but rather because they are related to fitness-enhancing benefits or because they are used in competition for access to potential mates. In other words, some traits are perceived and used by individuals to assess the quality and desirability of potential mates in order to enhance their own chances of reproductive success.

Since the theory of sexual selection was first introduced by Charles Darwin in *The Origin of Species*, it has been used to explain some of the most remarkable physical and behavioral displays in animals, such as the peacock's tail, the courtship displays of some bird species, and deer antlers. By contrast, humans do not possess any obviously sexually selected physical traits, although there is evidence that some phenotypic traits in humans act as fitness indicators and are used when forming judgments of attractiveness. In practice, the focus has been on various components of the human face and body, as shown in this chapter, but some scholars have suggested that many human behaviors, including humor, musical ability, and verbal creativity, are courtship adaptations that have evolved through sexual selection.

Facial Attractiveness

Fluctuating Asymmetry

Fluctuating asymmetries (FAs) refer to random deviations from perfect symmetry in bilateral traits that are, on average, symmetric at the population level. Within populations, there is a high degree of variability in FA, which arises as a result of stressors, such as reduced nutrition and disease, during the developmental process. On this basis, some evolutionary psychologists have suggested that FA reflects the degree to which individuals are able to maintain developmental stability in the face of environmental and genetic stressors. Furthermore, it is suggested that selection of potential mates on the basis of low FA may be adaptive, insofar as it increases reproductive success.

Indeed, preferences for symmetrical ornaments have been documented in a variety of species, including barn swallows and cerambycid beetles. Moreover, there is evidence to suggest that symmetry is preferred in human mate choice decisions. Thus, recent studies have reported that symmetric male and female faces are rated as more physically attractive than slightly asymmetric faces, and that this effect remains stable even after controlling for the effects of facial averageness and skin texture. There is also evidence to show that lower FA is associated with a higher number of lifetime and extra-pair sexual partners (i.e., a partner outside one's primary relationship) among men, and that women paired with men of low facial FA report a higher frequency of copulatory orgasms than women partnered with men of high facial FA.

However, in her review of the literature, Rhodes pointed out that the effect sizes of facial symmetry are small to medium at best and that symmetry may matter very little in relation to other facial characteristics, such as sexually dimorphic traits (see below). It has also been suggested that the appeal of symmetric faces may not be driven by perceptions of symmetry. For instance, some studies report that facial symmetry predicts ratings of men's attractiveness just as well as the attractiveness of half-faces, where cues of symmetry are minimal. In explanation, some scholars have suggested that it is the covariation of symmetry with factors such as jaw size and skin texture that explains the association of the former with attractiveness.

Facial Sexual Dimorphism

Sexually dimorphic facial traits are secondary sexual characteristics that differ between women and men and that generally emerge during puberty. Among men, testosterone stimulates the development of typically masculine facial traits (such as a pronounced jaw, chin, cheekbones, and brow ridges), whereas in women, estrogen stimulates the development of typically feminine traits (such as large eyes and lips, and a small nose and chin). Some evolutionary psychologists have proposed that sexually dimorphic traits may be a useful indicator of mate quality, insofar as only high-quality individuals are able to support the costs associated with the growth and maintenance of these secondary sexual traits.

Consistent with this hypothesis, numerous studies have reported that feminine facial traits are perceived as attractive on female faces, that average composite faces with feminine features are rated as more attractive than average composites, and that exaggerating femininity increases ratings of women's attractiveness. Early theorizing suggested that these effects may be driven by a preference for neoteny or "babyness" but more recent work has pointed out that some attractive feminine features are not neotenous (such as the high cheekbone in attractive female faces in contrast to the puffy cheeks of babies). On the other hand, studies of male facial masculinity and attractiveness are more equivocal, with some studies showing that exaggerated masculine traits are attractive in male faces (although the associations are weaker than for femininity) and other work reporting a female preference for feminized male faces.

A number of suggestions have been put forward to explain these equivocal results in relation to masculine faces. Thus, some authors have pointed out that high levels of testosterone are associated with a higher number of sexual partners, an increase in the likelihood of having extra-pair sex, and lower spousal investment and poorer father–child relationships. Based on these associations, it is suggested that a female mate-selection strategy that emphasizes male facial masculinity may sacrifice the potential benefits of spousal and paternal investment. In other words, women appear to seek a "trade-off" between good mates and good fathers, and this is consistent with studies showing that facial masculinity is associated with lower ratings of honesty, parental quality, and suitability as a partner.

In a similar vein, there are a slew of studies showing that women's preferences for facial masculinity vary across the menstrual cycle. Specifically, women show a stronger preference for masculine faces during the follicular, or fertile, phase of the menstrual cycle compared with the luteal, or infertile, phase. Corroborating evidence comes from studies showing that, when women are close to ovulation, they also provide higher ratings of the scent of symmetrical men, deep (masculine) voices, masculine walking gaits, and more intersexually competitive male behaviors. It has been proposed that these shifts in preferences arise because cues of masculinity are more valued when women are fertile and able to maximize the benefits of "good genes."

Bodily Attractiveness

The Waist-to-Hip Ratio

The literature on facial attractiveness demonstrates some of the more developed applications of evolutionary psychology to the topic of human appearance. In contrast, the available research on bodily attractiveness, until recently at least, lacked the same degree of rigor. One example of evolutionary psychology applied to bodily attractiveness is the waist-to-hip ratio (WHR) hypothesis of women's attractiveness, which asserts that low female WHRs (i.e., a more curvaceous figure) are universally attractive because they are associated with better health and fertility outcomes. The key pillar of this hypothesis is studies reporting a negative correlation between the WHRs of line-drawn figures and men's ratings of women's attractiveness (i.e., line drawings with low WHRs, typically 0.70, are judged the most attractive, and ratings decrease with increasing WHR).

Although some scholars continue to defend this hypothesis, the majority of researchers in the field are somewhat more skeptical. For one thing, a growing body of work has raised methodological concerns about the line-drawn stimuli that have been used to derive conclusions. For example, stimulus sets used in studies of the WHR hypothesis suffer from poor ecological validity (i.e., they do not fully capture the range of bodily variation that can be perceived in real-life figures and may overly simplify the way in which judgments of attractiveness are made) and further confound WHR with other phenotypic traits, primarily body weight. The latter problem is notable, as almost all early studies of the WHR hypothesis inadvertently made this error, making it difficult to say conclusively whether the importance attributed to WHR in these studies was an artifact of the covariation between WHR and body weight.

To investigate the relative importance of body weight and WHR in the perception of women's attractiveness, Tovée and Cornelissen designed a new set of stimuli consisting of real images of women, for whom body mass index (BMI; a measure of weight scaled for height) and WHR were known precisely. Their analyses showed that, although both BMI and WHR were significant predictors of women's attractiveness, BMI accounted for about 35 times more variance in attractiveness ratings than WHR. These results remain stable when women are presented in profile (rather than in frontal view) and when different methodological designs are used, including three-dimensional images and video clips. Nor are these results an artifact of the stimulus set, as comparable studies show that body shape (specifically the waist-to-chest-ratio) emerges as a more important predictor of men's attractiveness than BMI.

Moreover, there is now a large and continually growing body of evidence documenting cross-cultural, cross-ethnic, and cross-national differences in what is considered an attractive WHR. While low WHRs are typically judged to be attractive, healthy, and fertile in contexts of high socioeconomic status (SES), high WHRs are judged more positively in contexts of low SES (after controlling for the effect of body weight). To put it simply, a heavier female body is considered the height of beauty in contexts of low SES, and this is even the case when participants in otherwise affluent environments are made to feel "poor." For example, some recent work has shown that participants in contexts of high SES who are made to feel hungry or financially dissatisfied (both proxies for resource availability) idealize a higher female BMI and WHR.

A Combined Perspective

It may be possible to explain these combined findings from an evolutionary psychological perspective. Thus, one argument suggests that humans are capable of calibrating their attractiveness preferences to local conditions. For example, in recent cross-cultural studies, Swami and colleagues have shown that there is an inverse relationship between SES and ideal body size, such that heavier body sizes are perceived as more physically attractive in contexts of low SES. Moreover, when migrants move from contexts of low to high SES, there appears to be a shift in their body size ideals, such that thinner bodies come to be perceived as more physically attractive. This relationship has been explained as a function of observers "tailoring" their body size ideals in response to changing socioeconomic conditions, resource availability, and so on.

This explanation relies on a general evolutionary perspective, that is, that cross-cultural differences in body size ideals emerge because of variations in optimal body size in terms of health and fertility. However, it also accepts that cultural norms, such as gender role stereotypes, educational and political systems, and dietary factors, play a role in influencing what is considered a locally attractive body shape. Thus, Tovée and colleagues reported that a heavier body size may have been perceived as more attractive in rural South Africa because of the combined effects of a heavier body weight being healthier in that context, as well as the social connotations associated with a thin figure (e.g., HIV/AIDS infection being associated with thinness). In short, it appears to be the case that mate-selection criteria are calibrated according to local conditions, leading to cross-cultural variance in ideal body size.

Recent work has further overturned the once-prevalent notion that there are few, if any, within-culture differences in what is perceived as the ideal body size. Thus, several studies have reported differences in the strength of preferences for low WHRs as a function of a "power motive" (a predisposition to strive for status and power), ethnic identity, and sociosexuality. Related work has shown that individual difference traits including personality factors, sexist attitudes, and social conformity may influence what is perceived as the ideal body size. Also of note, some recent research has shown that men involved in particular subcultures, such as "fat admirers," may idealize significantly heavier body sizes, suggesting that there may be marked within-culture differences in body size preferences even within a single culture.

Body Image and Eating Disorders

A handful of recent studies have attempted to apply an evolutionary perspective to body image and eating disorders specifically, although it should be noted at the outset that these theories are still in their infancy. Thus, one theory postulates that anorexia nervosa is an adaptive attempt at reproductive suppression by the affected individual, particularly when environmental conditions are unfavorable. A related theory suggests that anorexia is a manifestation of reproductive suppression of subordinates by dominant women within a process of female intrasexual competition. These theories are distinctive in that they limit themselves to explaining the distal cause of anorexia, suggesting that the disorder serves an adaptive purpose.

On the other hand, the "sexual competition hypothesis" suggests that eating disorders, as well as the pursuit of thinness by women more generally, stems from intrasexual female competition. This hypothesis postulates that, as a result of declining fertility rates in contexts of high SES, the proliferation of idealized beauty, greater female autonomy, and other factors, women have to compete with other women primarily through the display of signs of health and fertility. It is further hypothesized that, in well-nourished populations, slimness is emblematic of maximal health and youthfulness (an association that is intensified by the increasing thinness of media images). A drive for thinness, therefore, develops among women as an adaptive strategy to maximize fitness by focusing on their appearance and attempting to display signs of health and youthfulness. Body dissatisfaction and eating disorders may develop among some women as an extreme variant of this tendency, as the adaptive process becomes maladaptive.

The same phenomena may also be applicable to explanations of drive for muscularity among men. Thus, studies have shown that muscular men are rated as physically attractive by women and that upper-body strength is (or was) likely beneficial in intrasexual male competition. Combined with the increasing prevalence of media images of muscular men (i.e., images of high-quality competitors rather than just role models to be emulated), men may compete with each other through displays of muscularity. In some cases, such competition may manifest itself as a maladaptive drive for muscularity, leading to body dissatisfaction and body dysmorphic disorder.

As I have indicated above, however, there are only a handful of studies that have evaluated this hypothesis and those that have, typically suggest that the association between intrasexual competition and body image may be more complicated. For example, recent work has suggested that female competition for status may only have an indirect causal effect on eating disorders, mediated through the influence of perfectionism. In other words, women who are high on intrasexual competition may be achievement oriented and perfectionistic, which results in their attempting to reduce their body weight as a means of securing mates. Even so, the available evidence does appear to support intrasexual competition among women as a distal factor influencing body dissatisfaction and ultimately eating disorders.

Conclusions and Future Directions

It is undeniable that evolutionary perspectives have helped to stimulate and advance our understanding of phenomena related to appearance, attractiveness, and body image. However, future work utilizing evolutionary frameworks must be guided by more consistent conceptual frameworks and rely less on a posteriori hypothesizing. A prerequisite for the development of an evolutionary psychological framework on attractiveness, in my view, will be its ability to generate hypotheses that are testable and that are embedded in a solid theoretical framework. Furthermore, as more sophisticated technologies become available to researchers, these should be used to explicate the evolutionary underpinnings of attractiveness, as is slowly happening in relation to work on bodily attractiveness.

Most importantly, however, it is essential that scholars begin to put together the distal focus of evolutionary psychological explanations with more proximate sociocultural and individual difference factors. As an example, the male-taller norm in height preferences (where both Western women and men report preferring to be in relationships where the male is taller than the woman) has almost exclusively been explained in terms of an evolutionary adaptation, where height in men is assumed to signal preferred traits. However, recent work has also shown that proximate factors, such as sexist beliefs and attitudes, reliably predict the male-taller norm, which is consistent with the feminist argument that patriarchal beliefs shape beauty ideals in contemporary societies.

In short, the available research does not deny a role for distal-evolved psychologies in explaining phenomena such as physical attractiveness. However, such perspectives must now attempt to incorporate and account for an array of proximate factors that similarly shape beauty ideals and practices. It is the combination of evolutionary, sociocultural, and individual difference perspectives that will likely result in a more comprehensive account of human appearance and body image.

Informative Readings

Cunningham, M. R., Barbee, A. P., & Philhower, C. L. (2002). Dimensions of facial physical attractiveness: The intersection of biology and culture. In G. Rhodes

& L. A. Zebrowitz (Eds.), *Advances in visual cognition: Vol. 1. Facial attractiveness: Evolutionary, cognitive, and social perspectives* (pp. 193–238). Westport, CT: Ablex.—An overview of facial attractiveness from evolutionary and sociocultural perspectives.

Faer, L. M., Hendriks, A., Abed, R. T., & Figueredo, A. J. (2005). The evolutionary psychology of eating disorders: Female competition for mates or for status? *Psychology and Psychotherapy: Theory, Research, and Practice, 78,* 397–417.—An empirical study examining the hypothesis that female intrasexual competition influences eating disorders and body image.

Frederick, D. A., & Haselton, M. G. (2007). Why is muscularity sexy? Tests of the fitness indicator hypothesis. *Personality and Social Psychology Bulletin, 33,* 1167–1183.—A comprehensive overview and test of evolutionary hypotheses concerning the importance of muscularity in men's physical attractiveness.

Rhodes, G. (2006). The evolutionary psychology of facial beauty. *Annual Review of Psychology, 57,* 199–226.—A comprehensive review of the biological factors influencing facial attractiveness.

Singh, D. (1993). Adaptive significance of female physical attractiveness: Role of waist-to-hip ratio. *Journal of Personality and Social Psychology, 65,* 292–307.—Seminal paper on the influence of the female waist-to-hip ratio on judgments of physical attractiveness.

Swami, V. (2011). Love at first sight? Individual differences and the psychology of initial romantic attraction. In T. Chamorro-Premuzic, A. Furnham, & S. von Stumm (Eds.), *Handbook of individual differences.* Oxford, UK: Wiley-Blackwell.—A review of the literature on individual difference and personality traits that affect the attraction process.

Swami, V., & Furnham, A. (2008). *The psychology of physical attraction.* London: Routledge.—A book-length review of the evolutionary psychology of physical attraction, with specific chapters on the waist-to-hip ratio hypothesis and cross-cultural ideals.

Swami, V., & Salem, N. (2011). The evolutionary psychology of human beauty. In V. Swami (Ed.), *Evolutionary psychology: A critical introduction* (pp. 131–182). Oxford, UK: Wiley-Blackwell.—A comprehensive critique of the waist-to-hip ratio hypothesis of female attractiveness.

Swami, V., & Tovée, M. J. (2005). Female physical attractiveness in Britain and Malaysia: A cross-cultural study. *Body Image: An International Journal of Research, 2,* 115–128.—An empirical study showing that body size ideals vary according to socioeconomic and cultural contexts.

Swami, V., & Tovée, M. J. (2006). Does hunger influence judgements of female physical attractiveness? *British Journal of Psychology, 97,* 353–363.—A study examining the effect of proprioceptive hunger on body size ideals within an affluent context.

Tovée, M. J., & Cornelissen, P. L. (2001). Female and male perceptions of female physical attractiveness in front view and profile. *British Journal of Psychology, 92,* 391–402.—A critique of the waist-to-hip ratio hypothesis and empirical work showing the greater importance of body mass index in relation to female physical attractiveness.

Tovée, M. J., Swami, V., Furnham, A., & Mangalparsad, R. (2006). Changing perceptions of attractiveness as observers are exposed to a different culture. *Evolution and Human Behavior*, *27*, 443–456.—An empirical paper documenting cross-cultural differences in body size ideals as well as the malleability of those ideals with changing socioeconomic context.

CHAPTER 4

Genetic and Neuroscientific Perspectives on Body Image

JESSICA L. SUISMAN
KELLY L. KLUMP

Introduction

Psychosocial factors have been the focus of theory and research on the development of body image. Although such factors are critical, researchers have argued that psychosocial influences are unlikely to explain *all* of the individual differences in body image and body image problems. They reason that, despite pressure from media, social relationships, and other sources for men and women to adhere to body ideals in Western society, only *some* individuals develop body image problems. It therefore has been hypothesized that genetic and/or biological factors may increase susceptibility to poor body image, in some, but not all, individuals.

To address this hypothesis, researchers have begun examining the role of genetic and biological factors in the development of body image problems. Behavioral genetic researchers have made use of twin and adoption study designs to demonstrate robust effects of genetic factors on body image problems. Molecular geneticists have begun to study particular genes that may influence body image disturbances. Finally, advances in neuroimaging techniques have allowed for the exploration of specific areas of the brain that may be implicated in body image problems.

Twin and Adoption Studies of Body Image

Twin and adoption studies are powerful tools for investigating genetic influences on a trait or disorder. These studies disentangle genetic from environmental effects by examining the degree of similarity on a psychological trait or characteristic between siblings who share differing amounts of genetic material. In the twin study design, the extent of similarity on a characteristic is compared between monozygotic (i.e., MZ or identical) twins, who share approximately 100% of their genes, and dizygotic (i.e., DZ or fraternal) twins, who share approximately 50% of their genes. Genetic influences are inferred when MZ twins are twice as similar to one another as DZ twins. By contrast, adoption studies compare adoptive siblings, who share none of their genes, to biological siblings, who share roughly 50% of their genes. Similar to twin studies, when biological siblings are twice as similar on a characteristic as adoptive siblings, genetic influences on the characteristic are inferred.

Body image problems including body dissatisfaction (i.e., dissatisfaction with one's weight and/or shape), weight preoccupation/drive for thinness (i.e., preoccupation with weight, dieting, and the pursuit of thinness), weight concerns (i.e., dissatisfaction and preoccupation with one's weight), and shape concerns (i.e., dissatisfaction and preoccupation with the shape of one's body) have been the focus of several twin studies and one adoption study to date. Unfortunately, body image problems that may be particularly common in men, such as drive for muscularity (i.e., preoccupation with achieving a muscular body), have not been examined in twin or adoption studies.

Table 4.1 includes estimates of genetic effects from twin and adoption studies of several types of body image problems. All studies used community-based samples of twins, and examined body image problems on a continuum, ranging from few body problems to clinically significant body image problems. Notably, studies are organized by sex and developmental stage, as research suggests that these variables may significantly impact estimates of genetic effects (see below).

Female Adolescents and Adults

As shown in Table 4.1, twin studies in adolescent and young adult females suggest moderate-to-large genetic influences on a range of body image problems. Heritability estimates were generally 50% or higher, suggesting that at least 50% of individual differences in body image problems within a population are due to genetic factors. Most studies controlled for body mass index (BMI) in analyses to ensure that the heritability of body image problems is not due to the well-known heritability of body weight. Indeed, body image problems were moderately heritable even after controlling for the effects of body weight. Twin study findings were recently replicated in the first adoption study of disordered eating attitudes and behaviors where the heritability of body dissatisfaction and weight preoccupation was found to be approximately 60%. Replications of genetic effects across samples and methodologies provide strong evidence for the presence of moderate-to-strong genetic effects on a range of body image problems.

TABLE 4.1. Estimates of Genetic and Environmental Influences on Body Image in Females and Males

Study	Measure	Heritability
	Female adolescents/adults	
Baker et al. (2009)	EDI Body Dissatisfaction	.57 (.30–.70)
	EDI Drive for Thinness	.61 (.33–.68)
Keski-Rahkonen et al. (2005)	EDI Body Dissatisfaction	.59 (.53–.65)
	EDI Drive for Thinness	.51 (.44–.58)
Klump et al. (2000)	MEBS Body Dissatisfaction	.60
	MEBS Weight Preoccupation	.52
Klump et al. (2009)[a]	MEBS Body Dissatisfaction	.59 (.06-1.0)
	MEBS Weight Preoccupation	.61 (.05-1.0)
Klump, Burt, et al. (2010)	EDEQ Weight/Shape Concerns (Combined Scale)	.54 (.40–.59)
Rutherford et al. (1993)	EDI Body Dissatisfaction	.52
	EDI Drive for Thinness	.44
Spanos et al. (2010)	EDEQ Shape Concerns	.64 (.50–.74)
	EDEQ Weight Concerns	.66 (.51–.76)
Wade et al. (1998)	EDE Shape Concerns	.62 (.50–.71)
	EDE Weight Concerns	.00
Wade et al. (2001)[b]	Figure Rating Scale—Current Body Size	.54–.65
	Figure Rating Scale—Desired Body Size	.20–.44
Wade et al. (2003)	Body Attitudes Questionnaire (BAQ) subscales	.37–.53
	Female preadolescents	
Klump, Burt, et al. (2010)	EDEQ Weight/Shape Concerns (Combined Scale)	.00 (.00–.44)
Klump et al. (2000)	MEBS Body Dissatisfaction	.49
	MEBS Weight Preoccupation	.47
	Males	
Baker et al. (2009)	EDI Body Dissatisfaction	.40 (.06–.57)
	EDI Drive for Thinness	.20 (.00–.43)
Keski-Rahkonen et al. (2005)	EDI Body Dissatisfaction	.00
	EDI Drive for Thinness	.00
Wade et al. (2001)[b]	Figure Rating Scale—Current Body Size	.00–.54
	Figure Rating Scale—Desired Body Size	.00–.25

Note. EDI, Eating Disorder Inventory; MEBS, Minnesota Eating Behavior Survey; EDEQ, Eating Disorder Examination Questionnaire; EDE, Eating Disorder Examination. When available, confidence intervals are printed in parentheses following the heritability estimates.

[a]This study is the only adoption study of body image problems conducted to date.

[b]This study examined heritability estimates in adults, with heritability estimates reported separately by decade (ages 18–30, 30–40, 40–50, etc.). The heritability estimates in the table represent the full range of heritability estimates obtained for ages 18–60 years.

Female Preadolescents

Only two studies have examined body image problems in preadolescent females, and results differ from findings in adolescence/adulthood. These studies found negligible genetic influences on weight/shape concerns (0%), and moderate genetic influences on body dissatisfaction (49%) and weight preoccupation (47%) during preadolescence. However, models demonstrated that there were significantly *smaller* genetic influences in preadolescence versus adolescence for weight/shape concerns (0% vs. 54%, respectively) and body dissatisfaction (47% vs. 60%, respectively). Results for weight preoccupation were less clear, as models indicated moderate heritability (47%) in both groups, although power to detect group differences was limited.

More research is needed to confirm the presence of developmental effects, where heritability of body image problems in preadolescence may be lower than that in adolescence/adulthood. If replicated, these results would fit into a larger literature on disordered eating in general. Several studies now indicate that there are minimal genetic influences on overall levels of disordered eating (including binge eating, compensatory behaviors, and weight/shape concerns) in preadolescence and prepuberty, but substantial genetic effects during puberty and adulthood. These findings suggest that puberty may be a critical period for the emergence of genetic influences on disordered eating and body image problems, and that biological/genetic factors associated with puberty may contribute to the genetic diathesis of disordered eating. Consistent with this hypothesis, Klump, Keel, Sisk, and Burt compared the heritability of disordered eating and body image problems in a group of female twins with *low* versus *high* circulating levels of estradiol during puberty. The "low-estradiol" group demonstrated little-to-no genetic effects on body dissatisfaction and weight preoccupation scores, whereas the "high-estradiol" group demonstrated significant genetic effects. Critically, results remained unchanged even after controlling for the effects of age, BMI, and the physical changes of puberty (e.g., growth spurts, breast development). Taken together, results are highly suggestive of a role for puberty and ovarian hormones in the genetic predisposition for body image problems, but much more research is needed to confirm these impressions and determine the types of body image problems (e.g., body dissatisfaction vs. weight concerns) that exhibit pubertal/hormone effects.

Males

To date, only three studies have examined genetic influences on body image problems in males. Findings across studies differ (see Table 4.1), with two studies suggesting significant genetic effects, whereas the remaining study found no evidence for these effects. Differences in methodology across studies may explain these discrepant findings. Specifically, Wade and colleagues used figural images to assess current and ideal body size in adults (ages 18–60 years old). They found evidence for genetic influences in males (0–54%), although not to the extent as found in females (20–65%). Two other studies examined body dissatisfaction and drive for thinness using the Eating Disorder Inventory (EDI). However, the EDI was used differently in each of these studies. Baker and colleagues found significant genetic influences (20–40%) using the EDI body dissatisfaction and drive for thinness scores as continuous measures of body image problems in adolescent males (ages 15–17). Keski-Rahkonen and colleagues found negligible genetic influences (0%) in young adult twins (ages 22–27) using the EDI body dissatisfaction scale and drive for thinness scales dichotomously (i.e., symptoms present or absent; see Table 4.1). Reasons for differences in genetic influences across these studies are unclear, although measurement issues may play a role. More specifically, the dichotomization of the EDI scales in the Keski-Rahkonen et al. study makes it difficult to directly compare these results to the continuous measures used in other studies of both males and females. Clearly, additional research is needed to confirm these impressions and determine the significance of genetic influences on body image problems in males.

Molecular Genetic Studies of Body Image

Given behavior genetic studies suggesting robust genetic influences on body image problems in females, and perhaps males, efforts are being made to identify specific genes that may be related to body image problems. Although limited to only two studies thus far, findings are promising in suggesting that higher levels of body dissatisfaction and drive for thinness may be associated with the S allele of the serotonin transporter gene (5-HTTLPR) in women with anorexia nervosa (AN) and bulimia nervosa (BN). These findings are interesting given that the S allele has been linked to higher levels of serotonin neurotransmission, and serotonin is implicated in the regulation of food intake and mood.

Likewise, another study found links between particular chromosomes (i.e., chromosomes 1 and 13) and AN and BN when stratifying subjects based on high levels of drive for thinness. These findings suggest that dividing patients with AN and BN into homogeneous groups (i.e., those high vs. low in drive for thinness) may lead to more robust links with particular chromosomes than when examining the full sample without subtyping. The importance of stratifying patients by drive for thinness in this study suggests that these body image problems may be linked with particular chromosomes even in nonclinical samples, although it is unclear whether the associations would be as strong as those found in these clinical samples. Continuing to identify risk genes for body image problems in the general population (in addition to patient populations) would significantly enhance etiological models across the spectrum of eating pathology.

Neuroimaging Studies of Body Image

Researchers have begun to directly investigate the brain to increase understanding of the specific neurobiological processes that may influence body image perception and body image problems. These studies used functional magnetic resonance imaging (fMRI) to examine brain regions that become activated when the subject is presented with stimuli relevant to body image. Stimuli used have varied across studies, but have been designed to evoke the negative cognitions/feelings that would be associated with poor body image. For example, studies asked participants to study their own digitally distorted body, where either overall body size or particular body parts such as thighs or stomach were enlarged. Participants have also been asked to examine negative words related to body image (e.g., *overweight*, *stumpy*), figural rating scales of bodies ranging from thin to overweight, and images of faces. Studies have examined women with AN and women without eating disorders, and one study examined men without eating disorders (i.e., no studies of men with eating disorders have been conducted). One study also examined men and women with body dysmorphic disorder (BDD), which is a disorder characterized by excessive preoccupation with a perceived defect in physical feature(s). Investigations of BDD could contribute to the understanding of body image problems given the severe difficulties individuals with this disorder have with body image concerns and perception.

Findings to date have suggested some specific patterns of activation in response to body image stimuli. In females (with and without AN) and males, activation of the fusiform gyrus has been observed when participants view the body image-related stimuli described above. The fusiform gyrus has been implicated in neural processes related to face and body recognition, and therefore it is reassuring and perhaps not surprising that this area would be reactive to body image-related stimuli. Studies of BDD suggested that patients showed increased left hemisphere activation in the prefrontal cortex and temporal lobe when examining faces. These brain regions are important in processing detail, and suggest that patients with BDD may be more detail oriented in face processing than controls.

There may also be increased activation in brain areas related to emotion and fear responses. For example, in women with AN, men and women with BDD, and in nonclinical populations, the amygdala and anterior cingulate cortex appear to become activated in response to negative body image-related or face stimuli. It is unclear whether differences between patients and controls exist in these patterns of activation, as two studies found the association in women with AN but not control women, while another study including only a nonclinical population also found the association. Interestingly, increased amygdala and anterior cingulate activation is associated with subjects' self-rated anxiety in response to viewing the body image stimuli and thus, may be due to the fear or anxiety evoked by negative body image stimuli. However, these activation patterns were not found in a nonclinical sample of males (without an eating disorder or BDD). This sex difference in activation indicates that women may process body image stimuli with an emotional, fear response that is not present in men. These findings suggest the intriguing possibility that an increased sensitivity to the thin ideal in women relative to men may be due to a neurologically based, emotional reactivity that contributes to gender differences in prevalence of body image problems and eating disorders (rates of 10:1–4:1 in women vs. men, respectively). Alternatively, it is possible that the increased sensitivity in women develops over the lifespan due to increased exposure to, and internalization of, the thin ideal in women. Future studies should continue to confirm these findings and also aim to delineate whether differences in men and women are inherent or develop over time.

Conclusions and Future Directions

It is clear from the research reviewed in this chapter that there are prominent genetic and neurobiological influences on body image in females. It is critical that this knowledge be used to enhance existing etiological models that tend to focus exclusively on psychosocial risk factors associated with body image (e.g., cultural, familial, or peer influences). In combination, genetic/biological and psychosocial models will ultimately form more nuanced models of risk and resilience for body image problems than any one influence could likely provide on its own.

Although genetic and biological findings to date are promising, more research is needed to further understand the etiology of body image problems. Behavior genetic studies that simultaneously examine preadolescent and adolescent/adult males and females would allow for the direct examination of similarities and differences across gender and developmental stage. Likewise, molecular genetic studies in clinical and nonclinical populations would increase understanding of the specific genes and chromosomal regions contributing to individual differences in body image problems across the spectrum of pathology. Finally, neuroimaging studies that examine women and men with and without eating disorders will extend neurobiological models developed thus far to understand sex differences in neural bases of risk. Incorporation of prospective designs would be particularly powerful, as they would allow researchers to delineate whether differences in neural processing precede the development of body image problems (suggesting a causal role of neural processing) or instead develop during or after body image problems begin (suggesting that an increase in body image problems leads to changes in neural processing).

Despite the significance of the biological influences discussed above, these factors do not negate the importance of psychosocial risk factors. Indeed, genetic and biological influences likely place certain individuals at increased risk for body image disturbances in the face of psychosocial risk. For example, two individuals may be exposed to the same risk factor (e.g., peer teasing), but only one individual may develop body dissatisfaction in response to this risk. The individual who develops body dissatisfaction may have higher genetic or biological risk that becomes activated in the face of the psychosocial stressor. These types of gene–environment interactions have yet to be investigated in the area of body image problems but are a critical avenue for future work.

Informative Readings

Articles identified with an asterisk (*) are included in Table 4.1.

Baker, J. H., Maes, H. H., Lissner, L., Aggen, S. H., Lichtenstein, P., & Kendler, K. S. (2009). Genetic risk factors for disordered eating in adolescent males and females. *Journal of Abnormal Psychology, 118*, 576–586.—One of the only existing twin studies of body image in males. (*)

Devlin, B., Bacanu, S., Klump, K., Bulik, C., Fichter, M., Halmi, K., et al. (2002). Linkage analysis of anorexia nervosa incorporating behavioral covariates. *Human Molecular Genetics, 11*, 689.—A study showing the association between certain chromosomes and AN, particularly when individuals were stratified based on degree of body image problems.

Feusner, J. D., Yaryura-Tobias, J., & Saxena, S. (2008). The pathophysiology of body dysmorphic disorder. *Body Image: An International Journal of Research, 5*, 3–12.—A review of genetic, neuroimaging, and cognitive research on BDD.

Friederich, H. C., Uher, R., Brooks, S., Giampietro, V., Brammer, M., Williams, S. C. R., et al. (2007). I'm not as slim as that girl: Neural bases of body shape self-comparison to media images. *NeuroImage, 37*, 674–681.—A brain imaging study examining neural responses to body image stimuli that includes a thoughtful review of other fMRI studies to date.

Frieling, H., Römer, K. D., Wilhelm, J., Hillemacher, T., Kornhuber, J., de Zwaan, M., et al. (2006). Association of catecholamine-O-methyltransferase and 5-HTTLPR genotype with eating disorder-related behavior and attitudes in females with eating disorders. *Psychiatric Genetics, 16*, 205.—A molecular genetics study demonstrating an association between serotonin genes and body image problems.

Keski-Rahkonen, A., Bulik, C. M., Neale, B. M., Rose, R. J., Rissanen, A., & Kaprio, J. (2005). Body dissatisfaction and drive for thinness in young adult twins.

International Journal of Eating Disorders, 37, 188–199.—A very large twin study of body image in adult males and females. (*)

Klump, K. L., Burt, S. A., Spanos, A., McGue, M., Iacono, W. G., & Wade, T. D. (2010). Age differences in genetic and environmental influences on weight and shape concerns. *International Journal of Eating Disorders, 43,* 679–688.— The first twin study to examine cross-sectional differences in the heritability of weight and shape concerns before and after puberty. (*)

Klump, K. L., Keel, P. K., Sisk, C. L., & Burt, S. A. (2010). Preliminary evidence that estradiol moderates genetic influences on disordered eating attitudes and behaviors during puberty. *Psychological Medicine, 40,* 1745–1753.—A pilot twin study directly investigating the influence of estradiol on changes in the heritability of body dissatisfaction in prepubertal and pubertal female twins.

Klump, K. L., McGue, M., & Iacono, W. G. (2000). Age differences in genetic and environmental influences on eating attitudes and behaviors in preadolescent and adolescent female twins. *Journal of Abnormal Psychology, 109,* 239–251.— The first twin study to demonstrate lower heritability of body image problems in preadolescence as compared to adolescence. (*)

Klump, K. L., Suisman, J. L., Burt, S. A., McGue, M., & Iacono, W. G. (2009). Genetic and environmental influences on disordered eating: An adoption study. *Journal of Abnormal Psychology, 118,* 797–805.—The only existing adoption study of body image problems. (*)

Rutherford, J., McGuffin, P., Katz, R. J., & Murray, R. M. (1993). Genetic influences on eating attitudes in a normal female twin population. *Psychological Medicine, 23,* 425–436.—One of the earliest twin studies of body image problems. (*)

Shirao, N., Okamoto, Y., Mantani, T., & Yamawaki, S. (2005). Gender differences in brain activity generated by unpleasant word stimuli concerning body image: An fMRI study. *British Journal of Psychiatry, 186,* 48.—The only existing fMRI study investigating sex differences in the neuronal networks related to body image.

Spanos, A., Burt, S. A., & Klump, K. L. (2010). Do weight and shape concerns exhibit genetic effects? Investigating discrepant findings. *International Journal of Eating Disorders, 43,* 29–34.—A review of previous literature on the heritability of weight and shape concerns and a significant contribution toward clarifying previous findings. (*)

Uher, R., Murphy, T., Friederich, H. C., Dalgleish, T., Brammer, M. J., Giampietro, V., et al. (2005). Functional neuroanatomy of body shape perception in healthy and eating-disordered women. *Biological Psychiatry, 58,* 990–997.—An fMRI study examining neuronal responses to figural rating scales in women with eating disorders and healthy controls.

Wade, T. D., Bulik, C. M., Heath, A. C., Martin, N. G., & Eaves, L. J. (2001). The influence of genetic and environmental factors in estimations of current body size, desired body size, and body dissatisfaction. *Twin Research and Human Genetics, 4,* 260–265.—The only twin study to investigate the heritability of ratings on figural rating scales in males and females. (*)

Wade, T., Martin, N. G., & Tiggemann, M. (1998). Genetic and environmental risk factors for the weight and shape concerns characteristic of bulimia nervosa. *Psychological Medicine, 28,* 761–771.—The only twin study to investigate heritability of body image using an interview-based rather than self-report measure of body image. (*)

Wade, T. D., Wilkinson, J., & Ben-Tovim, D. (2003). The genetic epidemiology of body attitudes, the attitudinal component of body image in women. *Psychological Medicine, 33,* 1395–1405.—A twin study using the Body Attitudes Questionnaire (BAQ) to examine genetic and environmental influences on body image problems in women. (*)

CHAPTER 5

Cognitive-Behavioral Perspectives on Body Image

THOMAS F. CASH

Introduction

Most contemporary research on body image derives directly or implicitly from cognitive and/or behavioral paradigms in psychology. An integrative cognitive-behavioral (CB) viewpoint reflects no single theory but rather draws upon an enduring tradition of ideas and empirical evidence that emphasize social learning and conditioning processes and the cognitive mediation of behaviors and emotions. This chapter conveys key concepts and processes inherent in cognitive and behavioral conceptions of body image.

To articulate basic elements of a CB model, I first distinguish historical factors from proximal or concurrent factors that shape body image development and functioning. Historical factors refer to past events, attributes, and experiences that predispose or influence how people come to think, feel, and act in relation to their body. Salient among these factors are cultural socialization, interpersonal experiences, physical characteristics and changes, and personality variables. Through various types of cognitive and social learning, historical factors instill fundamental body image attitudes, including dispositional body image evaluations and degrees of body image investment, including core self-schemas vis-à-vis one's physical appearance. *Body image evaluation* refers to individuals' satisfaction or dissatisfaction with their body and their evaluative beliefs about it. *Body image investment* refers to the cognitive, behavioral, and emotional importance of the body for self-evaluation. In the CB model, proximal body image factors pertain to current life events and consist of precipitating and maintaining influences on body image experiences, including information processing and internal dialogues, body image emotions, and self-regulatory actions.

Figure 5.1, which delineates the concepts and processes discussed in this chapter, must be viewed with three important caveats in mind. First, it is a heuristic model to help organize our thinking about body image and its multidimensionality. Secondly, the distinction between historical and proximal events is intended to differentiate prior cognitive social learning from more immediate events, experiences, and reactions. However, just as today inevitably becomes yesterday, proximal body image events may be stored and contribute to one's cumulative body image history. Finally, although Figure 5.1 is depicted with proposed, directional causal arrows, causality is believed to be complex and reflect what Albert Bandura, in his social cognitive theory, termed *triadic reciprocal causation*. Within individuals, there exists a reciprocally interactive causal loop among external environmental events, intrapersonal factors (cognitive and affective events), and the individual's own behaviors.

Historical and Developmental Influences

Historical factors largely pertain to socialization about the meaning of physical appearance and one's body-focused experiences during childhood and adolescence. However, people are not simply passive recipients of socialization. Formative body image experiences unfold as person–environment–behavior transactions. These experiences occur in the contexts of individuals' cognitive, social, emotional, and physical development. This book's detailed chapters in Part II on body image development and in Part IV on the influences of gender and culture elucidate some of the core forces that are foundations in the construction of body image.

Cultural Socialization

Throughout the world, cultures and subcultures possess and transmit information about the meanings of human appearance. Cultural messages convey "standards" or expectations about appearance—what physical characteristics are and are not socially valued and what it means to possess or lack these characteristics. Of course, developed cultures with extensive communication media powerfully create and disseminate these values. Cultural messages not only articulate and reinforce normative notions about physical attractiveness and unattractiveness, but they also express gender-based expectations, tying "femininity" and "masculinity"

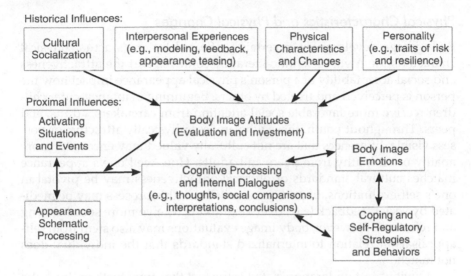

FIGURE 5.1. Body image: Dimensions, determinants, and processes.

to certain physical attributes. Culture may further prescribe body-altering means to attain societal expectations (e.g., by dieting, exercising, body-building, using beauty and fashion products, obtaining surgical and medical procedures). When understandably internalized by individuals, these strong, gender-related cultural messages and norms foster the acquisition of basic body image attitudes (e.g., body image evaluation and investment), which predispose how individuals construe and react to their own appearance and appearance-related life events.

Interpersonal Experiences

Socialization about the meaning of one's body involves more than exposure to media messages. Expectations, opinions, and verbal and nonverbal communications are conveyed in interactions with family members, friends and other peers, and even strangers. Parental role modeling, comments, and criticisms express the degree to which physical appearance is valued within the family, potentially establishing standards against which a child compares him- or herself. Moreover, siblings sometimes provide a social-comparison standard for the self-evaluative appraisal of a child's looks. Siblings, especially brothers, are also frequent perpetrators of appearance-related teasing or denigration. By their words and actions, peers are especially powerful purveyors of appearance norms and expectations. Appearance teasing by peers is a common childhood and adolescent experience, one that can predispose body image dissatisfaction.

Physical Characteristics and Physical Changes

Body image development is certainly affected by one's actual physical characteristics. A vast scientific literature confirms that the attractiveness and social acceptability of a person's physical appearance impact how the person is perceived and treated by others. Beginning in infancy, cuter children receive more favorable social attention from caretakers, adults, and peers. Throughout youth, those who are less physically attractive or possess visible differences that are not culturally valued may encounter more apathy or antipathy from peers and adults. How well one's appearance matches cultural standards of physical attractiveness may be pivotal in one's self-evaluations. In part, as noted above, this process may be mediated by social feedback (e.g., overweight kids receive more social teasing and rejection). However, body image evaluations may also stem from self-appraisals in relation to internalized standards that the individual does not match.

Obvious but underappreciated is the fact that from birth to death the human body changes. Changes in physical competence and appearance are especially dramatic during youth. For example, pubertal maturation in adolescence, a period marked by rapid physical change, can affect body image development. Weight is not the sole physical factor affecting body image formation. As other contributors to this handbook attest, countless characteristics can alter one's goodness of fit with personal and social expectations—deviations of stature and muscularity, conditions such as adolescent acne, and acquired disfigurements, to name a few. Aging in adulthood may bring physical changes such as weight gain, hair loss, and less elasticity in the skin. Simply stated, the body is a "moving target," which entails an ongoing process of adaptation to physical changes, for better or for worse.

Personality Factors

Individual personality attributes can also influence acquisition of body image attitudes. Some personality traits may represent risk factors for the development of body image problems. Some may foster resilience and promote positive body image attitudes. For example, a positive self-concept and strong social support may facilitate the development of a favorable evaluation of one's body and serve as a buffer against events threatening one's body image. Conversely, poor self-esteem and lack of social support may heighten one's body image vulnerability. Perfectionism, especially as related to one's standards for social self-presentation, is another potentially influential trait that may lead persons to invest self-worth in lofty or exacting physical ideals and risk feeling discontent. Public self-consciousness, a disposition of attentional self-focus on one's own observable appearance and behaviors (i.e., self as object), may increase one's monitoring and processing of appearance-related information. Public body consciousness is similar to "body surveillance" as articulated by objectification theory (see Chapter 6). Furthermore, as discussed in Chapter 30, an insecure interpersonal attachment system, whereby individuals seek love and acceptance yet feel unworthy, may foster dysfunctional body image attitudes. On the other hand, secure attachment may promote more favorable body image development. A final example of predisposing personality factors pertains to certain gender-role attitudes and values. Research suggests that women who endorse traditional gender attitudes in their relationships with men are more invested in their appearance, internalize cultural standards of beauty more fully, and hold more maladaptive beliefs about their looks.

Body Image Attitudes

Having examined the historical developmental variables that predispose the acquisition of body image attitudes, let's consider how these attitudes operate in everyday life. As Figure 5.1 shows, body image attitudes are central organizing constructs in the interplay of cognitive, emotional, and behavioral processes that occur within the context of environmental events. As mentioned previously, two basic attitudinal elements are body image investment and evaluation. Investment refers to the CB importance individuals place in their appearance. Evaluation refers to their positive-to-negative beliefs about and appraisals of their appearance (e.g., body satisfaction–dissatisfaction). As Cash and Szymanski showed in 1995 and subsequent researchers have verified, body image evaluations derive substantially from the degree of discrepancy or congruence between one's self-perceived physical characteristics and personally internalized and valued appearance ideals. Chapter 18 provides informative details about the most common validated assessments of body image attitudes.

An attitudinal body image construct that reflects one's body image investment involves self-schemas that are related to one's appearance. In 1977, Markus defined self-schemas as "cognitive generalizations about the self, derived from past experience, that organize and guide the processing of self-related information contained in an individual's social experience" (p. 64). A person who is schematic for a self-dimension (here, one's body and appearance) will process information pertinent to that dimension differently than someone who is not schematic. Furthermore, as cognitive theorist Aaron Beck explained, implicit attitudes, assumptions, beliefs, and rules comprise schematic content and dictate the substance of thought, emotion, and behavior.

Body image schemas reflect one's core affect-laden assumptions or beliefs about the importance and influence of one's appearance in life, including the centrality of appearance to one's sense of self. The Appearance Schemas Inventory—Revised (ASI-R), developed in 2004 by Cash,

Melnyk, and Hrabosky, assesses this construct. The ASI-R taps two related but different forms of self-schematic investment: (1) *self-evaluative salience* of appearance reflects the importance of appearance to one's sense of self-worth: Exemplary items are "In my everyday life, lots of things happen that make me think about what I look like," "When I meet people for the first time, I wonder what they think about how I look," and "By controlling my appearance, I can control many of the social and emotional events in my life"; and (2) *motivational salience* of appearance reflects the importance of having or maintaining an attractive appearance, with items such as "I try to be as physically attractive as I can be" and "I have never paid much attention to what I look like" (reverse scored). Research with the ASI-R indicates that the former type of investment is more dysfunctional than the latter, which is relatively benign or may actually be adaptive (i.e., taking "pride" in one's looks and grooming).

Proximal Events and Processes

Activating Events and Cognitive Processing

According to CB perspectives, specific situational cues or contextual events (including internal events) activate schema-driven processing of information about and self-evaluations of one's physical appearance. Thus, appearance-schematic individuals place more importance on, pay more attention to, and preferentially process information relevant to their appearance. Precipitating events may entail, for example, body exposure, mirror exposure, social scrutiny, social feedback, wearing certain clothing, weighing, exercising, mood states, or changes in appearance.

The resultant internal dialogues (sometimes termed *private body talk*) involve emotion-laden automatic thoughts, inferences, interpretations, and conclusions about one's looks. Among individuals with problematic body image attitudes and self-schemas, these inner dialogues are habitual, faulty, and dysphoric. Thought processes may reflect various errors or distortions, such as dichotomous thinking, emotional reasoning, biased social comparisons, arbitrary inferences, overgeneralization, overpersonalization, magnification of perceived defects, and minimization of assets. In 2006, Jakatdar and her colleagues developed and published the Assessment of Body-Image Cognitive Distortions, a validated measure of these distorted thought processes.

Adjustive and Self-Regulatory Processes

To manage or cope with distressing body image thoughts and emotions, whether anticipated or actual, individuals engage in a range of actions and reactions. These may involve well-learned cognitive strategies or behaviors to accommodate or adjust to perceived environmental events.

Adjustive reactions include avoidant and body-concealment behaviors, appearance-checking or appearance-correcting rituals, social reassurance seeking, and compensatory strategies. In 2009, Engle and her colleagues validated new measures of such body image behaviors. These reactive maneuvers serve to maintain body image attitudes via negative reinforcement, as they enable the individual temporarily to escape, reduce, or regulate body image discomfort.

Despite a vast literature on human coping processes, surprisingly little research has examined coping specifically in relation to body image. Until recently, no method for assessing body image coping has existed. To remedy this problem, in 2005 Cash and his colleagues constructed and published the Body Image Coping Strategies Inventory (BICSI). Three CB strategies for dealing with perceived body image threats or challenges were identified: (1) *experiential avoidance* involves attempts to avoid situations, thoughts, or feelings that are deemed threatening; (2) *appearance fixing* consists of efforts to alter or correct the aspects of one's appearance perceived as flawed; and (3) *positive rational acceptance* includes mental and behavioral activities that emphasize the use of positive self-care or rational self-talk and the acceptance of one's experiences. Research using the BICSI confirms that, in contrast to coping by body rational acceptance, coping by avoidance and appearance fixing are associated with less adaptive body image attitudes (e.g., negative evaluations and excessive investment), more body image dysphoria, and poorer psychosocial functioning (e.g., more eating pathology and lower self-esteem).

People also engage in proactive, purposeful self-regulatory behaviors to control evaluative body image and other self-reinforcing consequences. One class of self-regulating body image behaviors that has been seldom studied is appearance self-management. Appearance self-management is not always negatively motivated—only for concealment or correction of "offending" physical characteristics and avoidance of self-conscious thoughts and emotions. For many individuals, everyday grooming behaviors provide favorable and reinforcing affective, cognitive, and interpersonal consequences. Appearance self-management (with clothing, cosmetics, hairstyling, jewelry, etc.) is ubiquitous across cultures. People can experience pleasure and pride in their physical appearance. Human appearance is not entirely biogenetically assigned; it is also continually created by the individual.

Conclusions

CB perspectives have demonstrated considerable utility in our scientifically productive understanding of body image. Most chapters in this book delineate ideas and evidence that directly or indirectly emanate from this paradigm. CB viewpoints have further enhanced our understanding of eating disorders (see Chapters 32–34) and body dysmorphic disorder (Chapter 35), as well as human reactions to appearance-altering conditions (Chapters 29, 37, 38, 40, and 41). This fact attests not only to the validity of its principles and concepts but also to the scientific value system inherent in a CB viewpoint. The framework has served to guide the hypotheses of numerous investigations of body image. Moreover, it has been a catalyst for the development of many useful tools in the measurement of body image variables.

Chapters 49, 50, 51, and 52 of this handbook discuss the prevention of body image-related difficulties and disorders. Such interventions often tackle the "historical influences" described in Figure 5.1, seeking to alter those societal and social factors known to increase general population risks and vulnerable individual risks for the development of body image problems. Moreover, as discussed in Chapter 47, CB body image therapy is clearly the most extensively researched and empirically supported treatment for body image disturbances.

The study of body image has always been a pathology-focused endeavor—from historical attempts to understand the aberrant experiences of patients with brain injury or phantom limbs to the more recent boom in the investigation of eating disorders. One must realize, however, that a CB framework can be applied just as readily to understand the development and experience of a positive relationship between individuals and their body (see Chapter 7).

Informative Readings

Bandura, A. (1977). *Social learning theory.* Englewood Cliffs, NJ: Prentice Hall.—Discusses the foundations of Bandura's cognitive social learning perspective.

Bandura, A. (1986). *Social foundations of thought and action: A social cognitive theory.* Englewood Cliffs, NJ: Prentice Hall.—Explicates principles and processes in Bandura's theory.

Cash, T. F. (2002). The Situational Inventory of Body-Image Dysphoria: Psychometric evidence and development of a short form. *International Journal of Eating Disorders, 32,* 362–366.—Assesses the frequency of negative body image emotions as a function of situational context and tests hypotheses derived from a CB perspective.

Cash, T. F. (2008). *The body image workbook: An 8-step program for learning to like your looks* (2nd ed.). Oakland, CA: New Harbinger.—Cash's most recent version of his body image improvement program, which delineates and applies elements of a CB model.

Cash, T. F., Melnyk, S. E., & Hrabosky, J. I. (2004). The assessment of body-image investment: An extensive revision of the Appearance Schemas Inventory. *International Journal of Eating Disorders, 35,* 305–316.—Presents reliability, validity, and factor structure of a questionnaire to measure self-schematic investment in appearance.

Cash, T. F., Santos, M. T., & Williams, E. F. (2005). Coping with body-image threats and challenges: Validation of the Body Image Coping Strategies Inventory. *Journal of Psychosomatic Research, 58,* 191–199.—Provides reliability, validity, and factor structure of a novel assessment of how individuals cope with body image threats and challenges.

Cash, T. F., & Szymanski, M. L. (1995). The development and validation of the Body-Image Ideals Questionnaire. *Journal of Personality Assessment, 64,* 466–477.—Discusses and assesses evaluative body image in relation to self-ideal discrepancies.

Engle, E. K., Cash, T. F., & Jarry, J. L. (2009, November). *The Body-Image Behaviors Inventory-3: Development and validation of the Body-Image Compulsive Actions and Body-Image Avoidance Scales.* Poster presented at the convention of the Association for Behavioral and Cognitive Therapies, NY.—A summary (available from Cash) of reliability, validity, and structural information regarding these new body image assessments.

Fawkner, H. J. (2006). Body image attitudes in men: An examination of the antecedents and consequent adjustive strategies and behaviors. Dissertation Abstract and Summary in *Body Image: An International Journal of Research* (*www1.elsevier. com/homepage/sal/bodyimage/Vol3Iss1/BI-3-1-0005/index.html*).—Uses structural equation modeling to test certain elements of Cash's CB model of body image development and functioning.

Jakatdar, T. A., Cash, T. F., & Engle, E. K. (2006). Body-image thought processes: The development and initial validation of the Assessment of Body-Image Cognitive Distortions. *Body Image: An International Journal of Research, 3,* 325–333.—Provides reliability, validity, and factor structure of a novel assessment of cognitive distortions in the processing of appearance-relevant information.

Jarry, J. L., & Ip, K. (2005). The effectiveness of stand-alone cognitive-behavioural therapy for body image: A meta-analysis. *Body Image: An International Journal of Research, 2,* 317–331.—A quantitative review of evidence regarding outcomes (including their moderators) of CB therapy for body image dissatisfaction.

Smolak, L. (2009). Risk factors in the development of body image, eating problems, and obesity. In L. Smolak & J. K. Thompson (Eds.), *Body image, eating disorders, and obesity in youth* (2nd ed; pp. 135–155). Washington, DC: American Psychological Association.—Summarizes research evidence on risk factors associated with negative body image development in boys and girls.

Veale, D. (2004). Advances in a cognitive behavioural model of body dysmorphic disorder. *Body Image: An International Journal of Research, 1,* 113–125.—Discusses a model similar to the one presented in the present chapter.

Wertheim, E. H., Paxton, S. J., & Blaney, S. (2004). Risk factors for the development of body image disturbances. In J. K. Thompson (Ed.), *Handbook of eating disorders and obesity* (pp. 463–514). Hoboken, NJ: Wiley.—Reviews research on the biological, developmental, sociocultural, and individual psychological factors associated with a negative body image.

CHAPTER 6

Feminist Perspectives on Body Image

NITA MARY McKINLEY

Introduction

Feminist social critique has historically pointed out how the body has served as a locus of control in women's lives. Current feminist theory contends that women's normative body dissatisfaction is not a function of individual pathology, but a systemic social phenomenon. In this chapter, I review this feminist theory, outline the use of this theory to understand women's body experience, report empirical evidence supporting this theory, and make suggestions for future research and prevention of negative body experience.

Feminist Theory: Social Objectification of Women's Bodies

Feminist theorists have found the social construction perspective useful in understanding women's body experience and its relationship to gendered power relations. This perspective particularly fits a feminist understanding of women's lives because it stresses the social context of women's discontent, rather than individual pathology, and because it stresses the power inherent in social constructions that normalize gender inequities.

Western societies construct a duality between body and mind, and women are associated with the body and men with the mind, with the mind and men being more valued than the body and women. This allocation presumably occurs because of women's reproductive function, a "truth" that ignores the fact that many men are also reproductive and not all women are. Western societies also define men's bodies as the standard against which women's bodies are judged, and women's bodies are constructed as deviant in comparison. This creates a context that encourages the construction of women and girls as objects to be watched and evaluated in terms of how their body fits cultural standards. From infancy, girls are encouraged to focus on what they wear, how their hair is styled, and other factors related to appearance. They are praised for their appearance and learn that they are judged by how they appear to others. Girls learn to watch their own body from this outside perspective to avoid negative judgment. This construction of women as objects to be watched and evaluated both shapes women's consciousness and makes them dependent on others for approval.

Objectified Body Consciousness Theory and Early Empirical Work

A rich body of psychological research has developed from this feminist understanding of how women and girls come to view their body, particularly in terms of self-objectification (viewing the self in terms of appearance) and the consequent body surveillance (monitoring the appearance). My own work has emphasized what I call *objectified body consciousness* (OBC). OBC consists of body surveillance, internalization of cultural body standards, and appearance control beliefs.

Body surveillance is paying attention to one's self in terms of how one appears to others. Watching one's appearance is presumably associated with self-love and individual achievement for women. However, research shows that when people pay attention to how others perceive them, they try to meet relevant standards, feel bad if standards are not met, and are susceptible to influence by others. Fredrickson and Roberts argue that habitual self-monitoring of the body shapes women's psychological experience, increasing shame and anxiety while reducing flow, that is, peak motivational states and awareness of internal bodily states.

Internalization of cultural body standards makes it appear as though cultural standards come from individual women's own desires. This makes the standards difficult to challenge and conceals the external pressure to conform, such as the discrimination against women who do not achieve these standards. Further, this internalization predisposes women to connect achievement of these standards with their sense of self-worth. Because the standards are narrow and difficult to achieve, women experience a sense of empowerment as they approximate them, but more often shame when they do not. In OBC studies, internalization is measured using body shame. Women who are high on body shame do not simply feel dissatisfied with their body, but rather feel that not achieving appearance standards means they are a bad person.

Appearance control beliefs assure one that, given enough effort, cultural body standards can be achieved. To establish the legitimacy of judging women in terms of their body, body standards must be believed to be attainable. Regardless of the extent to which women actually control their appearance, control beliefs may benefit women by relieving the stress of working to attain sometimes impossible standards and giving them a sense of competence in controlling their body.

Early work validated the ability of OBC theory to predict women's body experience through survey data with predominantly European American undergraduate women. In this population, higher body surveillance was associated with lower body satisfaction, more eating problems, and lower levels of some measures of psychological well-being. Higher body shame was associated with greater endorsement of cultural body standards and is more strongly related to body satisfaction than endorsement of standards. Body shame is also related to higher body surveillance, lower body satisfaction, lower psychological well-being, and more eating problems. Control beliefs have less consistent relationships with predicted variables, with higher levels being associated with more eating problems, but usually they are unrelated to body surveillance or body shame and are associated with *increased* body satisfaction and psychological well-being in some samples. This is consistent with the claim that control beliefs serve to help women feel good about themselves in a context of cultural demand for body control. Survey data have also established that the relationships among body surveillance, body shame, and body satisfaction are stronger for undergraduate women than for undergraduate men and that women have higher levels of body surveillance and body shame than do men.

Experimental data have also confirmed the importance of body objectification in women's body experience and demonstrated that this experience may be influenced by immediate situational factors interacting with the sociocultural context that encourages objectification in women. The earliest version of these experimental data was the swimsuit study conducted by Fredrickson and her colleagues in which undergraduate women and men tried on either a swimming suit or a sweater in the context of a "consumer study." Trying on the swimsuit was presumed to evoke self-consciousness in terms of appearance, similar to body surveillance. Compared to the women in the sweater group, the swimsuit group had increased body shame, ate less, and also had decreased performance on a math test. These relationships were not found for men. These findings are especially important because the relationship of body practices to cognitive function is an understudied, but consequential, component of women's body experience.

Recent Empirical Work

More recent empirical work has extended our knowledge of self-objectification and OBC, including studying more diverse groups of women, age differences in OBC, and theorized correlates of body surveillance. Studied correlates include body satisfaction, psychological well-being, flow, health-related behaviors, and experiences of sexual objectification.

OBC in Diverse Women

A limited amount of research has compared women of different ethnicities and sexual orientations. These studies have generally shown similarities across groups, but a few studies find differences. Individual studies have found higher body surveillance among low-income women who were European American compared to those who were African American or Latino, higher body surveillance among lesbian women compared to heterosexual women, and skin tone surveillance uniquely related to body shame in African American women. Clearly, much more research is needed to clarify differences and similarities across groups of women including differences in social class. Differences in how gender-based objectification plays out among diverse women may reflect the interactions of objectification with other factors. For example, lesbians may monitor their body more because of heterosexism, yet intentionally challenge gender roles, providing protection from increased body dissatisfaction.

Age Differences in OBC

I have argued elsewhere that we need to take a lifespan approach to understanding women's body experience. Objectifying experiences and expectations are likely to vary as a function of the interactions between biology, psychology, and social context. We know very little about the developmental precursors to OBC. However, limited cross-sectional research has found lower levels of body surveillance and body shame in preteen girls compared to adolescents or undergraduate women, but among preteens, girls already had higher levels of body surveillance, but not body shame, compared to boys. More research has examined age-related differences from young adulthood to middle age. In my own research examining the experiences of young women and their middle-aged mothers, I have found undergraduate women to have higher levels of body surveillance and body shame than the middle-aged women. In the middle-aged women, body surveillance was not related to body satisfaction as it was in the young women. In a 10-year longitudinal follow-up study, I found body surveillance and body shame had decreased for the young women and there were no longer age differences in these variables. However, body surveillance continued to predict body esteem for the younger women.

Only one study has examined OBC in older women and has found their levels of body surveillance lower than younger women.

Theorized Correlates of OBC

Moradi and Huang have reviewed research on the relationship of body surveillance and its proposed consequences, including body satisfaction, eating problems, psychological well-being, and flow. Multiple correlational studies have shown associations among body surveillance, body shame, and body satisfaction. Correlational studies have confirmed the relationship of body surveillance and body shame to eating problems including desire to change weight and eating disorder symptomology. Findings are mixed in regard to the relationship of body surveillance and body shame to self-esteem, with some studies finding this relationship and others not. Reduction in flow experiences is one of the consequences proposed by Fredrickson and Roberts of the self-surveillance associated with OBC. Moradi and Huang point out some limitations of this line of research as it stands, but there is limited evidence that flow may be correlated with body surveillance.

In addition to eating problems, body surveillance and body shame have been shown to be correlated with other health behaviors, such as smoking and risky sexual behavior. For example, Impett and her colleagues have found body objectification to be related to less condom use (and also less sexual experience) in adolescent girls.

Moradi and Huang review studies showing that body surveillance and self-objectification mediate the relationship between being exposed to sexually objectifying experiences and negative outcomes. Outcomes such as eating problems and psychological well-being are no longer related to sexually objectifying experiences when body surveillance and/or self-objectification are controlled. Additionally, women who are high on body surveillance and/or self-objectification have a greater increase in body dissatisfaction when exposed to sexually objectifying media compared to women low on these variables.

Preventing Body Image Disturbance

Fredrickson and Roberts make a convincing case that an objectified view of the self can account for many of the mental health risks associated with being female, including depression, sexual dysfunction, and eating problems. An understanding of how OBC shapes women's experience allows us to account for the tenacity of women's body discontent.

We need to think of women's body problems as a social justice issue for women. Working to achieve cultural body standards deprives women of time, energy, and economic resources. We also know that standards for women's bodies reflect biases of race and ethnicity, class, age, sexual orientation, and ability. Given these biases, the definition of women in terms of the body helps maintain status differences among women.

An excellent example of the use of feminist theory to design intervention programs is Piran's study with adolescent girls (see Chapter 51). This study utilized participatory action research to help adolescent girls explore their body experiences to develop critical theory and activist approaches to generate change. For example, focus groups identified the lack of tampons in girls' bathrooms and the need to get permission to get tampons from the pharmacy as demonstrating a lack of respect for girls' bodies and the lack of personal ownership of their body. The girls successfully petitioned the school staff to place tampons in the girls' bathroom.

Feminism focuses on changing social systems rather than the individual (see Chapter 19). The social construction perspective underlines the belief that the source of women's negative body experience lies in the social context, rather than in individual pathology. Individual women may feel better about themselves by learning a cultural analysis of women's body issues and strategies for resistance. However, changing the context itself through political activism and the creation of body-positive communities may also be important for changing women's body experience.

Conclusions and Future Directions

Theories of OBC and objectification have generated a rich literature on women and their body experience within a feminist framework. In the last 15 years, our understanding and knowledge has expanded significantly. Still, there are many areas that need replication, expansion, and further theorizing.

We need more data on diverse women, including women of color, lesbians, bisexual women, women of nonprivileged social classes, women with disabilities, girls, and older women. Data showing similarities and differences between different groups of women are needed, as is additional theorizing to account for these findings. For example, I have argued elsewhere that lifespan developmental theory can inform our understanding of age-related differences in women's body experience.

Social constructions are not monolithic; at any given time, multiple meanings may coexist. We need more research to understand how diverse women think about their body and how women resist narrow definitions of themselves as bodies. For example, there is some evidence of that women who identify as feminist have lower body shame. Studying resistance helps to clarify how dominant constructions work as well as how they can be effectively counteracted. However, we also need to remember the power differentials that exist between institutionally supported social constructions and individual resistance. Changing how she thinks or acts will not change the very real patterns of discrimination a woman faces based on her appearance.

Although it is important to document women's objectification of their own body and the psychological consequences of this body consciousness, we also need to acknowledge that this focus creates a context in which body dissatisfaction and OBC continue to be understood as *psychological problems of individual women*. This frame leads to an assumption that the solution is one of simply helping women change how they think about their body. Thinking about themselves differently may sometimes be useful to certain women, but this strategy ignores the very real social pressures women experience not only to display a certain type of body but even to think about their body in certain ways. We need to expand our theorizing and research to include the social context itself: how particular types of social situations might encourage women and men to objectify other women, and how this objectification of women is learned (see Chapters 19 and 51). Without this broad research agenda, we risk simply changing labels—from "women like their bodies less than men" to "women objectify their bodies more than men"—without addressing greater social issues.

Informative Readings

Bartky, S. L. (1988). Foucault, femininity, and the modernization of patriarchal power. In I. Diamond & L. Quinby (Eds.), *Feminism and Foucault: Reflections on resistance* (pp. 61–86). Boston: Northeastern University Press.—A Foucaultian analysis of women's body experience and how surveillance is translated into social control.

Fredrickson, B. L., & Roberts, T. (1997). Objectification theory: Toward understanding women's lived experiences and mental health risks. *Psychology of Women Quarterly, 21,* 173–206.—A theoretical analysis of the pervasive relationship of objectification to women's psychological well-being.

Fredrickson, B. L., Roberts, T., Noll, S. M., Quinn, D. M., & Twenge, J. M. (1998). That swimsuit becomes you: Sex differences in self-objectification, restrained eating, and math performance. *Journal of Personality and Social Psychology, 75,* 269–284.—An experimental study showing a causal relationship between surveillance, eating behavior, and cognitive performance.

Impett, E. A., Schooler, D., & Tolman, D. L. (2006). To be seen and not heard: Femininity ideology and adolescent girls' sexual health. *Archives of Sexual Behavior, 35,* 131–144.—A correlational study showing the association of body objectification to sexual health.

Kozee, H., & Tylka, T. (2006). A test of objectification theory with lesbian women. *Psychology of Women Quarterly, 30,* 348–357.—Demonstrates that objectification theory appears to apply differently to lesbian and heterosexual women.

McKinley, N. M. (2006). The developmental and cultural contexts of objectified body consciousness: A longitudinal analysis of two cohorts of women. *Devel-*

opmental Psychology, 54, 159–173.—Longitudinal follow-up to the original survey data comparing undergraduate women and their middle-aged mothers.

McKinley, N. M. (2006). Longitudinal gender differences in objectified body consciousness and weight control: Cultural and developmental contexts in the transition from college. *Sex Roles: A Journal of Research, 54,* 159–173.—Longitudinal follow-up of original survey data comparing undergraduate women and men.

McKinley, N. M. (2010). Continuity and change in self-objectification: Taking a lifespan approach to women's experiences of objectified body consciousness. In R. Calogero, S. Tantleff-Dunn, & J. K. Thompson (Eds.), *Self-objectification of women: Causes, consequences, and counteractions* (pp. 101–115). Washington, DC: American Psychological Association.—A theoretical argument for the use of lifespan theory to inform studies of objectification and OBC and a review of relevant research.

McKinley, N. M., & Hyde, J. S. (1996). The Objectified Body Consciousness Scale: Development and validation. *Psychology of Women Quarterly, 20,* 181–215.—Theoretical introduction of OBC and psychometric analyses of the OBC scales in young and middle-aged women.

Moradi, B., & Huang, Y. (2008). Objectification theory and psychology of women: A decade of advances and future directions. *Psychology of Women Quarterly, 32,* 377–398.—A complete review of research on objectification and OBC to date.

Piran, N. (2001). Re-inhabiting the body from the inside out: Girls transform their school environment. In D. L. Tolman & M. Brydon-Miller (Eds.), *From subjects to subjectivities: A handbook of interpretive and participatory methods* (pp. 218–238). New York: New York University Press.—A description of a participatory action research project with adolescent girls where the girls develop critical body-based theory and engage in activism to create change.

Wolf, N. (1991). *The beauty myth: How images of beauty are used against women.* New York: Anchor Press.—A popular account of the political context of women's body experience.

CHAPTER 7

Positive Psychology Perspectives on Body Image

TRACY L. TYLKA

Introduction

Body image is a multidimensional construct with positive and negative features. Yet, theory, research, and practice have focused on understanding, preventing, and treating its negative features. In the first edition of this handbook, Cash and Pruzinsky recognized this lopsided approach, labeling it "pathology-driven." They called for a paradigm shift—to examine the experience of positive body image and identify factors that promote and emerge from it.

Ten years later, there are a handful of published studies on positive body image. This chapter synthesizes these findings and discusses how positive body image can be assessed and promoted—all in hope of encouraging additional research in this area. This research is imperative, as understanding positive body image is crucial for prevention and treatment efforts. Without this knowledge, current interventions designed to reduce negative body image may result in neutral body image. Practitioners need to take treatment even further—to help people appreciate, respect, celebrate, and honor their body.

Positive Psychology Perspective

Positive psychology, a perspective rooted in hygiology (the promotion of health), offers a framework to guide the study of positive body image.

Proponents of this perspective, including Martin Seligman, Shane Lopez, Sonya Lyubomirsky, and Barbara Fredrickson, argue that removing negative/maladaptive characteristics but not teaching positive/adaptive characteristics will likely create intermediate mental health characterized by a lack of pathology but the absence of vitality.

Deconstructing negative body image, then, will not automatically construct positive body image. Accordingly, positive body image should not be characterized simply as the opposite pole of a "single body image dimension" anchored at the other end by negative body image. Many other constructs do not share a single structural dimension. For instance, positive affect (e.g., joy, contentment) includes more features than low levels of negative affect (e.g., depression, anger). Positive affect also produces flexible thinking, enhances interpersonal relationships, promotes altruistic behavior, wards against illness, and builds hardiness.

Low Negative Body Image ≠ Positive Body Image

Striegel-Moore and Cachelin theorized that some characteristics of positive body image may be unique and not simply opposite of those associated with negative body image. Yet, scholars sometimes erroneously conclude that low body dissatisfaction, low body preoccupation, and low actual–ideal body size discrepancy automatically reflect positive body image. Research shows that positive body image is more complex.

Using cluster analysis, Williams and colleagues found three distinct body image groups of women: positive (44%), negative (30%), and neutral (26%). The positive body image group reported optimism, self-esteem, social support, adaptive coping, and weight stability. Hence, women with positive body image flourished and were empirically distinct from both women with neutral and negative body image.

Avalos and colleagues examined the body image literature and extracted four themes suggestive of positive body image: favorable opinions of the body regardless of actual appearance; acceptance of the body despite weight, body shape, and imperfections; respect of the body by attending to its needs and engaging in healthy behaviors; and protection of the body by rejecting unrealistic media images. The Body Appreciation Scale (BAS) was constructed to reflect these themes. In women, body appreciation predicted several indices of well-being (self-esteem, optimism, proactive coping) above and beyond commonly used measures of negative body image.

Therefore, consonant with the positive psychology perspective, positive body image is not equivalent to low negative body image. We cannot take all findings on negative body image and conclude that the opposite applies for positive body image. Two additional studies, both qualitative, reveal its connection with flourishing.

Characteristics of Positive Body Image

Wood-Barcalow and colleagues analyzed interviews from 15 young adult U.S. college women classified as having positive body image and five experts in the field of body image. Frisén and Holmqvist analyzed interviews from 30 adolescent girls and boys from Sweden with positive body image. Although the age, gender, and geographic region of the samples differed, similar characteristics emerged. These characteristics are included in Table 7.1. Quantitative studies have begun to support the connection of positive body image to many of these characteristics (e.g., spirituality, inner positivity, and broadly conceptualizing beauty).

These characteristics can be divided into core features of positive body image as well as factors that promote, maintain, and emerge from it. A synthesis of its core features suggests that positive body image reflects love and respect for the body. It permits individuals to appreciate how their body is unique and the functions that it performs for them. It provides a cognitive schema to help individuals interpret incoming information in a body-protective manner, whereby most positive information is internalized and most negative information is rejected or reframed. It reflects acceptance of the body, including aspects that are inconsistent with idealized images. Body assets are emphasized, whereas body imperfections are minimized. Individuals who hold a positive body image feel beautiful, comfortable, confident, and happy with their body, which is often expressed as an outer radiance, or "glow." They have a mindful connection with their body, which allows them to detect and fulfill their body's needs.

Characteristics that seem to promote positive body image include unconditional acceptance from important others, media literacy, environments/cultures that broadly conceptualize beauty, and the belief that a higher power thoughtfully designs each person to be unique. Characteristics that emerge from positive body image include inner positivity, engaging in adaptive self-care behaviors, and mentoring others to love their body. These precursors and consequences may be associated with positive body image in a cyclical manner, in that they help maintain favorable body image once it has developed. Reframing body-related information as neutral or positive and continued contact with others who have a positive body image may also preserve positive body image.

Processes of Positive Body Image

Although environmental factors shape body image, people with a positive body image also shape their environments in a growth-enhancing way, in a *reciprocal* process. They seek partners and friends who accept

TABLE 7.1. Characteristics of Positive Body Image Noted in Qualitative and Quantitative Research

Body appreciation

- Appreciating the functionality, health, and features of the body
- Praising the body for what it is able to do more so than its appearance

Body acceptance and love

- Expressing comfort with and love for the body, despite not being completely satisfied with all aspects of the body
- Choosing to focus on body assets rather than perceived body flaws
- Avoiding potentially hazardous means to alter appearance (e.g., cosmetic surgery)

Inner positivity influencing outer demeanor

- Feeling that positive inner qualities "shine through" to outer appearance and behavior
- Experiencing inner positivity (e.g., feeling good about oneself, being optimistic and happy), which manifests as helping others, smiling, asserting oneself, holding the "head up high," and emanating a "special glow" or "outer radiance" (e.g., "sparkle in the eye")

Broadly conceptualizing beauty

- Perceiving a diversity of weights, shapes, and appearances as beautiful
- Believing that what makes people beautiful is having the "special glow" or carrying the self well (e.g., being well-groomed, confident), not any one particular appearance
- Believing that individuals' appearances should not be compared; beauty is not a relative term—many people can be beautiful in various ways

Media literate

- Being aware of the unrealistic and fabricated nature of media images
- Rejecting and/or challenging images (e.g., pictures of thin models) and messages (e.g., appearance-related comments) that could endanger body image on a regular basis

Unconditional acceptance from others

- Perceiving body acceptance from important others (e.g., partners, family, friends)
- Feeling loved, special, and valued for authentic qualities not contingent on appearance (when appearance is mentioned by others, it is usually complimentary and related to interchangeable aspects, like clothes and hairstyle)

Finding others with a positive body image

- Choosing to surround the self with others who also hold a positive body image

Spirituality/religion

- Believing that a higher power designed them to be "special" and wants them to accept their body with its idiosyncrasies—this helps them cherish their unique qualities
- Showing respect by maintaining their health and their body as it was designed
- Feeling loved and accepted by a higher power buffers against body dissatisfaction

(continued)

TABLE 7.1. (continued)

Listening to and taking care of the body

- Engaging in pleasurable exercise and adaptive stress relief (e.g., yoga) on a regular basis
- Seeking medical care for preventative and remedial purposes
- Pampering the body (e.g., massages) on occasion
- Taking a flexible approach to eating—trusting the body to determine when and how much to eat; eating foods that are enjoyable, healthy, and help the body perform well
- Maintaining a stable weight (based on their body type) that is often in the normal range

their body. They encourage others to love their bodies, which in turn, helps them feel even more appreciative and respectful of their body. They avoid or minimize their exposure to media that promote the thin ideal.

Confronted with images and messages daily, people must choose whether to accept or reject this body-related information. Individuals with positive body image engage in *protective filtering*, whereby they hold a schema that helps them accept most positive information and reject most negative information.

Protective filtering is not foolproof. Negative information may be internalized at times, which temporarily increases body investment and shifts body evaluation from positive to negative. When individuals work to reframe this information as neutral or positive, their body investment returns to a healthy focus on the body's needs, and body evaluation returns to positive. *Fluidity* reflects this temporary flux in body image.

Measuring Positive Body Image

The BAS holds promise as a measure of positive body image. Its reliability and validity has been supported with women and men of various ethnicities from different geographical regions. However, it does not capture every feature in Table 7.1. Items could be developed to assess these remaining characteristics and used in conjunction with BAS items for a more comprehensive assessment of positive body image.

Other body image measures (e.g., appearance evaluation scales, body part satisfaction scales) limit their focus to one facet of the positive body image construct. Because positive body image is more complex than the opposite of negative body image, low scores on body dissatisfaction scales should not be used to infer positive body image.

Cultural and Gender Considerations

African and Hispanic cultural identification may promote positive body image. Proportionally more African American women than Caucasian women were classified in Williams et al.'s positive body image group. Half of the participants classified as having positive body image in Wood-Barcalow et al.'s study were African American; they indicated wanting to be "thick" and viewed this body ideal as realistic and the thin ideal as impossible. Parker and colleagues revealed that African American girls, when compared to Caucasian girls, were more flexible when defining beauty. They were more likely to emphasize their best qualities—being well groomed, adopting a personal style, and exuding inner positivity/confidence that establishes their presence—rather than try to achieve someone else's standard. In studies using the BAS in the United Kingdom, Hispanic women had the highest body appreciation, followed by Black, White, and South Asian women, respectively. Interestingly, Swedish adolescents described themselves as "average looking" (perhaps due to *Jante-law*, the cultural norm to not consider oneself better than others), whereas U.S. women described themselves as beautiful.

Men typically report slightly higher body appreciation than women. Swedish adolescents share similar characteristics of positive body image as emerging adult U.S. women, although it seems to be more difficult for boys to articulate what they like and dislike about their body.

Promoting Positive Body Image

Eighty percent of the women in Wood-Barcalow et al.'s study reported overcoming a negative body image; this provides hope that individuals can transition from a negative to a positive body image. It would benefit therapists and clients to know women can adopt a positive body image via protective filtering, interpersonal support, associating with and modeling others who are proud of their body, and embracing an inclusive definition of beauty. Furthermore, clients would benefit from knowing characteristics and processes of positive body image. For instance, recognizing when they are having a "bad body image day" could be a signal to redirect their thoughts to protect their positive body image.

Interventions promoting embodiment (body awareness and responsiveness), body functionality, and body acceptance (e.g., Hatha yoga) could be integrated into treatment. Clients could practice accepting positive information and framing information in a self-preserving rather than a self-destructive manner. Media literacy could help clients reject media messages (see Chapters 12 and 49). Pointing out that media definitions of beauty change over generations and with fashion trends will help clients understand that media body ideals are transient. Clients could be encouraged to develop a broad personal definition of beauty rather than allow societal ideals to determine what is beautiful for them.

Emphasizing the connection between positive body image and health (e.g., weight stability, normal-range body mass index), well-being (e.g., inner positivity), and intuitive eating (i.e., an adaptive eating style based on connection with internal hunger and satiety cues) may motivate clients to commit to adaptive self-care. Body appreciation is strongly related to intuitive eating; thus, healthy eating is connected to respecting the body rather than disliking it. Adaptive changes in eating, then, could be enhanced via positive body image.

Professionals could help form positive peer networks that focus on inner strengths, body functionality, and social support rather than appearance and body disparagement (e.g., "fat talk"). Having clients mentor others by discussing the characteristics and benefits of positive body image could help them and their protégés. Community programs could be developed to discuss the importance and appropriate expression of unconditional acceptance.

Conclusions and Future Directions

Research on positive body image has only just begun. This area has many implications for repositioning clients from a negative or neutral body image to a positive body orientation. Because positive body image is intimately connected to well-being, research in this area could enrich individuals' life satisfaction. Some questions for future research include:

1. If qualitative studies on positive body image were conducted on other age groups, cultures, or men, would additional and/or different characteristics emerge?
2. Would gender, age, ethnic identification, and sexual orientation, as well as individual difference variables (e.g., current eating and exercise behavior, personality, and stage of identity development) impact the expression of positive body image?
3. How does "filtering" become protective? How do we transition from a negative body image to a positive body image?
4. What are the strongest predictors and consequences of positive body image? Longitudinal studies examining models of positive body image are needed.
5. Is positive body image related to being more attentive to the body and the detection of disease (e.g., doing more breast and skin cancer self-screenings and awareness that something is wrong with the body)?

6. How can positive body image be nurtured in overweight individuals who are teased and who face weight discrimination?
7. Can positive body image prevent eating in the absence of hunger and binge eating?

Informative Readings

Avalos, L., & Tylka, T. L. (2006). Exploring a model of intuitive eating with college women. *Journal of Counseling Psychology, 53*, 486–497.—Examines positive body image within a model: Functional body orientation and unconditional body acceptance predict body appreciation, which then predicts intuitive eating.

Avalos, L., Tylka, T. L., & Wood-Barcalow, N. (2005). The Body Appreciation Scale: Development and psychometric evaluation. *Body Image: An International Journal of Research, 2*, 285–297.—Presents findings that BAS scores are internally consistent, stable, and yield evidence of convergent, content, discriminant, and incremental validity among U.S. college women.

Cash, T. F. (2008). *The body image workbook: An eight-step program for learning to like your looks* (2nd ed.). Oakland, CA: New Harbinger.—Offers an eight-step program including worksheets to assist people to challenge negative body perceptions, minimize body imperfections, promote body acceptance, and celebrate the body.

Frisén, A., & Holmqvist, K. (2010). What characterizes early adolescents with a positive body image? A qualitative investigation of Swedish girls and boys. *Body Image: An International Journal of Research, 7*, 205–212.—Reveals that Swedish adolescents with a positive body image (1) have a functional view of their body and accept their perceived body imperfections, (2) engage in and enjoy physical activity, and (3) minimize the importance of appearance-related comments.

Homan, K. J., & Boyatzis, C. J. (2010). The protective role of attachment to God against eating disorder risk factors: Concurrent and prospective evidence. *Eating Disorders, 18*, 239–258.—Reveals that women who reported feeling loved and accepted by God are buffered from body dissatisfaction, pressure for thinness, and thin-ideal internalization.

McCabe, M. P., Ricciardelli, L. A., & Ridge, D. (2006). "Who thinks I need a perfect body?" Perceptions and internal dialogue among adolescents about their bodies. *Sex Roles, 55*, 409–419.—Examines the nature and impact of body-related messages Australian adolescents receive and found that (1) girls receive more positive and negative body messages than boys, and (2) messages could be internalized, distorted, or deflected.

Parker, S., Nichter, M., Nichter, M., Vuckovic, N., Sims, C., & Ritenbaugh, C. (1995). Body image and weight concerns among African American and White adolescent females: Differences that make a difference. *Human Organization, 54*, 103–114.—Via qualitative and quantitative methods, notes that African American adolescent girls were more likely than White girls to have a more flexible conceptualization of beauty and define beauty in terms of grooming rather than achieving a certain thin-ideal youthful standard.

Striegel-Moore, R. H., & Cachelin, F. M. (1999). Body image concerns and disordered eating in adolescent girls: Risk and protective factors. In N. G. Johnson & M. C. Roberts (Eds.), *Beyond appearance: A new look at adolescent girls* (pp. 85–108). Washington, DC: American Psychological Association.—Suggests sociocultural, family environment, intrapersonal, and life event factors that may protect girls' resistance to unhealthy dieting and disordered eating.

Swami, V., Airs, N., Chouhan, B., Leon, M. A. P., & Towell, T. (2009). Are there ethnic differences in positive body image among female British undergraduates? *European Psychologist, 14,* 288–296.—Studies ethnic differences in levels of body appreciation and found that Hispanic women had the highest body appreciation, followed by African Caribbean, Caucasian, and South Asian women, respectively.

Tylka, T. L., & Augustus-Horvath, C. L. (2010). Fighting self-objectification in prevention and intervention contexts. In R. M. Calogero, S. Tantleff-Dunn, & J. K. Thompson (Eds.), *Self-objectification in women: Causes, consequences, and counteractions* (pp. 187–214). Washington, DC: American Psychological Association.—Discusses practical interventions to promote characteristics of positive body image in girls and women.

Williams, E. F., Cash, T. F., & Santos, M. T. (2004, November). *Positive and negative body image: Precursors, correlates, and consequences.* Paper presented at the 38th Annual Meeting of the Association for Advancement of Behavior Therapy, New Orleans, LA. Paper available from Thomas F. Cash (*tcash@odu.edu*) by request.—Reveals characteristics indicative of flourishing among women with positive body image and demonstrated the distinctiveness of positive body image from low levels of negative body image.

Wood-Barcalow, N. L., Tylka, T. L., & Augustus-Horvath, C. L. (2010). "But I like my body": Positive body image characteristics and a holistic model for young adult women. *Body Image: An International Journal of Research, 7,* 106–116.—Interviews U.S. college women with positive body image and body image experts, and articulates features and processes of positive body image, factors that form and maintain it, and the process of "protective filtering."

PART II

DEVELOPMENTAL PERSPECTIVES AND INFLUENCES

CHAPTER 8

Body Image
Development in Childhood

LINDA SMOLAK

Introduction

Body image concerns, including worrying about weight and shape, are clearly evident in adolescence. Considerable research has identified some of the risk and protective factors involved in body dissatisfaction during adolescence and adulthood. Furthermore, body dissatisfaction in early adolescence has been related to disordered eating, depression, and eating disorders (see Chapters 9 and 10). Finally, dozens of studies have examined the effectiveness of prevention of body image issues, and their negative outcomes, with adolescents and adults.

What is not obvious is what all of this has to do with children. This chapter aims to consider body image in children under 12 years old. The first of three sections describes body image in children, including developmental changes. The second section examines risk and protective factors that have been linked to body dissatisfaction among children. Finally, section three considers the prevention of body image problems with children. The empirical work used in each of these sections was overwhelmingly published after the previous edition of this volume in 2002.

Developmental Trends in Body Image

Even infants recognize that they are distinct entities within the environment. For example, 4-month-olds look and smile more at videos of other

67

babies than videos of themselves. However, it is not until about age 2 years that children have a clear sense of "me," recognizing themselves (and their characteristics) in mirrors and photos and referring to themselves as "I" or "me." Furthermore, toddlers demonstrate pride and shame, while preschoolers (ages 4–6) can compare their behavior to one other child. By about age 8, children compare themselves to many other children. Among the social comparisons they make are appearance comparisons. Not surprisingly, it is around the same time that children's self-evaluation is differentiated into four areas: academic competence, social competence, physical/athletic skills, and physical appearance. These last two self-evaluation categories are clearly components of body image. Thus, self-development, including burgeoning social comparison skills, is part of the foundation of body image.

Much of the research concerning body image in children focuses on weight and shape concerns, including interest in both thinness and muscularity. Looking at the work with preschool-age children underscores the limitations of this approach. While preschoolers are aware of the social disapproval of fat people, their own body image concerns are not focused primarily on weight and shape. They are more worried about their clothing and hair. Girls may already be more invested in appearance than boys, perhaps in part because their toys (e.g., Barbie) and the websites they play on (including the Barbie website) encourage them to focus on outfits for themselves and play characters. Girls may also be exposed to more appearance-oriented role models, including their mothers, older sisters, and television characters. Boys, on the other hand, may be more focused on action than appearance. This is reflected in their toys (including sports equipment), the male characters they see on television, and the gender role expectation that "boys will be boys." Even the action figures so often cited as exemplars of unrealistic muscularity are used in active play rather than primarily changing their outfits or hair styles.

There is some concern about body size among 5-year-olds. Many of these boys and girls wish to be bigger. This may simply reflect their desire to grow up, to be like the "big kids" they know. By age 6, however, there is clear evidence that children are beginning to be concerned about weight and shape in ways that approximate adolescent and adult concerns. Precise rates of body dissatisfaction vary with sample characteristics as well as measurement techniques. It is not uncommon to find that 40–50% of elementary school-age children (6–12 years) are dissatisfied with some element of their body size and shape. Short-term longitudinal data tend to indicate some stability in body dissatisfaction even at this age.

Gender and Culture Differences

When general or overall concerns about appearance or body shape are measured, there are typically few differences between girls and boys.

This is at least partly because these general concerns accommodate boys' concerns about muscularity as well as girls' worries about thinness. Even among preschoolers, when boys express shape concerns, they emphasize muscularity (e.g., wanting "six-pack abs"), whereas girls worry about thinness (e.g., "fat tummies"). Although these gender differences are not always as large as they are among adolescents and adults, when pressure to conform to gender roles is greater than it is during childhood, they are generally significant. These findings raise the possibility that even young children are exposed to gendered messages about ideal body shape. By school age, social comparison, including to siblings and peers, is likely to be part of this process. Much more research is needed on the specifics of this process in young children.

It is interesting that gender differences are also often evident cross culturally. For example, among fourth- to sixth-grade Czech children, 29% of boys but 14.5% of girls wanted to be larger whereas 44% of girls and 34% of boys wanted smaller bodies. On the other hand, normal-weight Chinese girls were more likely than boys (ages 6–12) to say they wanted larger bodies, though this may partly reflect the fact that boys are generally more satisfied with their bodies. Weight and shape concerns are evident in a sizeable minority of children (typically > 30%) from various countries, including children from Western and Eastern Europe, Asia, Australia, and North America.

Risk and Protective Factors

Models of the development of body dissatisfaction among children are similar to those for adolescents and adults. They tend to emphasize socio-cultural factors, particularly media, peer pressure, and parental influences. Most models have also included body size, as indexed by body mass index (BMI). Various cognitive or personality factors, including autonomy, thin-ideal internalization, social comparison, and appearance schemas, have also been in models, though these appear less frequently than do sociocultural influences and BMI.

Body Mass Index

The single most consistent risk factor for body dissatisfaction among children is BMI. As early as age 6, overweight or obese children are more dissatisfied with their weight than are other children. This relationship has been documented cross culturally. In some samples, this effect is stronger and appears earlier in girls than in boys. The correlation between body dissatisfaction and BMI increases during elementary school.

In some ways, this relationship is not surprising. Researchers have long reported that by about age 6, children have strong anti-fat biases.

Even 4-year-olds will not select "chubby" figures as their ideal, though they do not clearly express that being fat is "bad." In elementary school, children prefer average-weight children rather than overweight children as friends. Overweight boys may be judged less harshly than overweight girls. This anti-fat message may come from parental modeling or from media. Parents are even less likely than preschoolers to pick chubby body ideals for their children, although this may be less true among Latinos/ Latinas and African Americans. Older siblings may also model anti-fat bias and a preference for lean bodies.

Sociocultural Factors

Researchers have investigated a variety of sociocultural risk factors in children. These include media, toys, and peer and parental comments and modeling. Cross-sectional data routinely demonstrate concurrent relationships between sociocultural influences and a variety of forms of body image. In order to establish an influence as a risk factor, either longitudinal data demonstrating temporal precedence of the risk factor or experimental data are needed. This discussion is limited to these types of data as well as data establishing that young children are indeed exposed to the thin ideal for women and the muscular ideal for men.

Mass media (magazines, television shows, children's cartoons and animation films) and toys (video games, Barbie dolls, action figures such as GI Joe) portray the thin ideal for women and the muscular ideal for men, as well as the importance of attractiveness. Animated cartoons, for example, are three times more likely to portray overweight, compared to under- and normal-weight, characters as unattractive. In turn, unattractive cartoon characters are more likely to be portrayed as unintelligent and antisocial. Female characters are particularly likely to be attractive. Similar patterns are evident in children's videos and, to a lesser extent, in children's books.

Longitudinal findings on the effects of media on children's body image are mixed. There is evidence that in girls as young as 5–8 years old, watching appearance-focused television predicts appearance dissatisfaction. However, other data indicate no relationship between media exposure and body image in preadolescent boys or girls. Yet, reading gaming magazines predicted increases in drive for muscularity among young White, but not Black, boys (mean age = 8.77 years). It may be important that the latter study looked at a very specific form of media that emphasized body shape more than do many other media directed at children. Such differences in defining the media to be investigated may partly explain the inconsistency in the findings.

Another reason for the inconsistent findings may be the relative lack of attention to moderating and mediating factors in the media–body image relationship among children. Research with adolescents and adults has clearly implicated both moderators and mediators in this relationship. That this may also be true for children is indicated, for example, by research suggesting that media awareness may contribute to the development of appearance schemas, which in turn predicts body dissatisfaction in preadolescent girls. Appearance schemas likely mainly consist of an understanding of social standards and their implications in preschoolers. It is probably not until age 6 years or later that the appearance schemas include a self-definition element. Thus the meaning and effects of appearance schema may change during childhood.

Toys also provide children with models of what an adult body should look like. Many dolls, especially Barbie, and action figures, including GI Joe, have unrealistic body shapes. Experimental research shows that even brief interactions with Barbie can negatively impact the body satisfaction of young (5-year-old) girls. In reality, most American girls grow up with several Barbies, and Barbie is marketed internationally. Thus, it seems possible that the experimental data underestimate the power of dolls like Barbie as negative influences on girls' body image. Unfortunately, although research indicates that handling action figures lowers college men's body esteem, there are no experimental or longitudinal studies of this effect among young boys.

Peer influences may take the form either of modeling attitudes about weight and shape or making comments to a child. Peers' body dissatisfaction may predict girls' own body esteem and desire to be thin, even in early elementary school. However, as was true with media, findings concerning the effect of peer modeling during childhood are inconsistent. Appearance-related peer teasing shows prospective relationships to girls' weight esteem, despite the finding that boys are more likely to be teased than girls. Messages from best friends to lose weight may impact girls' own weight esteem. Some cross-sectional data suggest that the negative effects of peer teasing may be particularly pronounced for overweight children. Research with adolescents indicates that sibling appearance-related teasing is also linked to body dissatisfaction and this association in childhood deserves more attention.

Parents may also serve as role models or make comments about their child's appearance. However, parents may also send subtle messages about body shape, including the child's own appearance, via the food choices they make or their attempts to control their child's eating. Prospective data demonstrate that such attempts at control are associated with later disordered eating in children. The specific influence of these control efforts on body image deserves more research. Longitudinal research further suggests that comments about body shape from mothers may be more influential than those from fathers for both boys and girls. So, for example, boys whose mothers suggest they should be more muscular become more dissatisfied with their muscles.

While the longitudinal data are neither as strong nor as consistent as the cross-sectional data, they do suggest that sociocultural variables affect the development of body image in both boys and girls. This is evident very early in elementary school, by age 6.

Individual Characteristics

Measurement is always an issue when doing research with children. While advances have been made in measuring body esteem, particularly among elementary school-age children, assessment of risk and protective factors continues to be problematic. This is particularly true of the individual characteristics discussed in this section. Measures of many of these important influences were developed for use with adolescents and adults. Sometimes vocabulary demands are lowered. But it is rare for such measures to be truly validated with children, particularly young children. Given that children's conceptualizations of internal states and traits differ from those of adults, this is an important consideration.

As with adults, models of the development of body dissatisfaction during childhood typically postulate individual characteristics that moderate or mediate the relationships among sociocultural factors, BMI, and body image. These factors include internalization of the thin ideal, appearance schemas, self-esteem, and negative affect. Although theoretical models include these characteristics, few longitudinal studies have addressed such relationships.

Longitudinal data generally have not supported the prospective relationship of self-esteem to the development of weight and shape dissatisfaction. Indeed, some evidence suggests that poor body esteem may predict lowered self-esteem. There may well be a reciprocal relationship between general self-esteem and body esteem. Furthermore, it seems likely that the direction of the relationship varies at different points in development. Research addressing such issues has yet to be done.

Internalization of the thin ideal and appearance schemas both appear to be risk factors in late elementary school-age girls. Girls who are high on internalization and appearance schemas have declining body satisfaction over the course of a year. Research on boys and early elementary school children using comparable constructs is lacking and greatly needed.

Although social comparison and negative affect have been investigated as risk factors during adolescence, little work has been done with children. Interestingly, cross-sectional research suggests that social comparison may be an important factor for boys. Negative affect may be related to body esteem, including preoccupation with muscularity, in both girls and boys. Given the centrality of social comparison and negative affect in theory and research with adults, this is an area that needs immediate empirical attention.

Protective Factors

Protective factors lower the likelihood of developing a problem behavior despite the presence of risk factors. In attempting to identify protective factors, researchers seek to find unique contributors rather than simply "reversed" risk factors (e.g., low exposure to appearance teasing). At least two factors have emerged as possible protective factors during childhood.

First, the personality characteristic of autonomy may serve to protect against the declines in body satisfaction among elementary school-age girls. Autonomy refers to the ability to resist pressure from others, a characteristic that prevention programs often try to foster. The second possible protective factor is girls' actual rejection of the media-promoted thin ideal. This is not simply a relatively low score on a measure like the Sociocultural Attitudes Towards Appearance Scale. Instead, when shown a picture of an ultrathin celebrity, girls say they don't like how she looks. In cross-sectional research, girls ages 6–12 who rejected the media image had higher levels of body esteem. Again, prevention programs, particularly those focusing on media literacy, often try to encourage this type of attitude. Boys shown pictures of very muscular men showed less consistent responses to the photos than girls (to the ultrathin photos) and rarely completely accepted or rejected the portrayed ideal. The boys' reactions were not related to body esteem. Thus, it is not clear how effective media literacy focusing on muscularity would be with young boys.

Prevention

The younger the children, the more likely prevention programs for them are to be "universal." Universal prevention programs are not directed at a preselected population. The participants do not demonstrate an elevated risk for the development of body image or eating problems. The average-to-high levels of body satisfaction and body esteem that exist at the outset of such programs make it difficult to document a salutary effect of the program particularly if follow-up assessments are short term. However, these programs might actually *prevent* the development of body image problems and so are worth investigating.

Over a dozen prevention programs have been developed for children. Most of these have targeted late-elementary (≥ fourth grade) school students. Given the range in delivery techniques, material, and evaluations, it is not surprising that the studies have yielded mixed results. Nonetheless, most of the studies have reported at least some success changing body image-related attitudes (e.g., beliefs about fat), body esteem, or body change techniques. Future research might include prevention programs for younger children, identifying successful program components, and developing some programs (see Chapter 49) that focus on children with incipient body image issues.

Conclusions and Future Directions

Much progress has been made during the past decade in our understanding of body image development during childhood. For example, it is now clear that body dissatisfaction appears in a substantial minority of children by early elementary school. This is true across ethnic groups as well as cross culturally. Even in childhood, body image is gendered with boys tending to focus more on muscularity and girls on thinness, though we understand little about the process by which gender role is integrated with body image. The foundations for these attitudes are likely laid down during the preschool years when children learn to disparage fat and embrace the culturally defined body ideals.

Many factors influence the development of body image in children. BMI is particularly powerful during this stage of development, perhaps because of the strong cultural anti-fat bias. In addition, media, toys, peers, and parents may play a role. These relationships are complex, however, and are likely to be moderated or mediated by other factors. Stronger models of these possible relationships are needed, as is prospective research that can test the nature of these pathways, preferably over extended periods of time.

Most of the research on children's body image, particularly the work examining influences and outcomes, has been done with White American and Australian children. Much more work is needed with children from various ethnic groups and cultures. It is widely held that body image is culturally determined; if this is so, then we can expect substantial variation in the process of body image development across ethnic and cultural groups. This variability will aid in developing culturally sensitive prevention programs and in identifying risk and protective factors.

Finally, more research is needed on the outcomes of early body dissatisfaction. How continuous are body image problems? Research on factors that might interrupt the development of body esteem problems will also be crucial. All of this should aid in the development of more effective programs to help prevent body image problems from ever developing.

Informative Readings

Clark, L., & Tiggemann, M. (2008). Sociocultural and individual psychological predictors of body image in young girls: A prospective study. *Developmental Psychology, 44,* 1124–1134.—An unusual examination of internalization of the thin-ideal, autonomy, and appearance schemas, as well as media and peer influences.

Dohnt, H., & Tiggemann, M. (2006). The contribution of peer and media influences to the development of body satisfaction and self-esteem in young girls: A prospective study. *Developmental Psychology, 42*, 929–936.—A longitudinal evaluation of body image development among 5- to 8-year-olds.

Harrison, K., & Bond, B. (2007). Gaming magazines and the drive for muscularity in preadolescent boys: A longitudinal examination. *Body Image: An International Journal of Research, 4*, 269–277.—One of a few studies that examine media effects on boys' body image.

Holt, K., & Ricciardelli, L. (2008). Weight concerns among elementary school children: A review of prevention programs. *Body Image: An International Journal of Research, 5*, 233–243.—Emphasizes methodological issues that need to be addressed in future programs.

Klein, H., & Shiffmann, K. (2006). Messages about physical attractiveness in animated cartoons. *Body Image: An International Journal of Research, 3*, 353–363.—Content analysis indicates the presence of gendered appearance stereotypes in cartoons.

Levine, M. P., & Smolak, L. (2006). *The prevention of eating problems and eating disorders: Theory, research, and practice.* Mahwah, NJ: Erlbaum.—Contains a lengthy description of elementary and middle school prevention programs, as well as a discussion of methodological challenges in designing and implementing such programs.

Li, Y., Hu, X., Ma, W., Wu, J., & Guansheng, M. (2005). Body image perceptions among Chinese children and adolescents. *Body Image: An International Journal of Research, 2*, 91–103.—Examines gender and age differences in the development of body image in China.

McCabe, M., & Ricciardelli, L. (2005). A longitudinal study of body image and strategies to lose weight and increase muscles among children. *Applied Developmental Psychology, 26*, 559–577.—Investigates the influences of multiple factors, including both mothers and fathers, on boys' and girls' body image development.

Musher-Eizenman, D., Holub, S., Edwards-Leeper, L., Persson, A., & Goldstein, S. (2003). The narrow range of acceptable body types of preschoolers and their mothers. *Applied Developmental Psychology, 24*, 259–272.—The first in a series of studies about preschoolers' beliefs about body shape published by Musher-Eizenman and colleagues.

Smolak, L. (2004). Body image in children and adolescents: Where do we go from here? *Body Image: An International Journal of Research, 1*, 15–28.—A review of several methodological and theoretical issues in studying body image in children.

Smolak, L., & Thompson, J. K. (Eds.). (2009). *Body image, eating disorders, and obesity in youth: Assessment, prevention, and treatment* (2nd ed.). Washington, DC: American Psychological Association.—Contains several chapters that focus on children's body image—especially those by Wertheim et al., Ricciardelli et al., Anderson-Fye, Smolak, Yanover, and Thompson, and Levine and Smolak.

CHAPTER 9

Body Image Development in Adolescent Girls

ELEANOR H. WERTHEIM
SUSAN J. PAXTON

Introduction

Adolescence is an important time in an individual's life as it signals a transition from childhood to adulthood. For adolescent girls, a range of body and social changes take place during and following puberty that can strongly influence their body image. This chapter provides an overview of the nature of body image in adolescent girls, including factors related to the development of body image concerns and the implications of those concerns.

Overview of Body Image in Adolescent Girls

Body Image and Body Image Disturbances

Body image is generally viewed as a multidimensional construct, involving cognitive, affective, and behavioral elements. Body dissatisfaction involves a preference for body characteristics different from how the body is currently perceived by the person and is associated with negative affect. Body image disturbances (BID) in adolescent girls are generally focused on specific body characteristics, the most commonly studied of which (due to their association with eating disorders) involve body weight and shape dissatisfaction. However, a range of other body image concerns exist in girls, such as concern about facial characteristics, skin appearance, muscularity, fitness, and strength.

Body Size Dissatisfaction in Adolescence

Numerous studies of body image in adolescent girls have examined the proportion preferring to be thinner. Studies generally use questionnaire or interview responses assessing how an individual's perceived current body shape, size, or weight compares to how she would ideally like to be. Of girls, a substantial proportion reports wanting to be thinner than they are and this preference appears to increase as girls develop from childhood to adolescence. In their review, Wertheim, Paxton, and Blaney concluded that at preadolescence about 40–50% of girls report preferring to be thinner, and during adolescence, this increases to over 70%. These percentages far exceed the proportion that is objectively overweight using healthy weight standards. Only about 10% of girls report preferring to be larger or to weigh more and generally these girls are underweight by healthy weight standards.

In addition to understanding preferences to be thinner, it is important to understand how *important* that is to the person, since a preference without it being perceived as very important is unlikely to have an influence on an individual. Adolescent girls often think that being thinner would make them happier, healthier, and better looking. Consistent with these views, many studies find that larger girls are more likely to be dissatisfied with their body and to feel less good about themselves in general. A substantial proportion of adolescent girls also reports taking active steps to lose weight, diet, or use more extreme methods. Depending on the study, as many as one-third to over half of girls also report experimenting with, or regularly engaging in, unhealthy weight loss methods such as fasting, crash dieting, vomiting, or laxative use.

At the more extreme end, some adolescent girls undergo surgical or cosmetic procedures to address body concerns. As described in a review by Sarwer, Infield, and Crerand, a substantial number of adolescent girls reported undergoing liposuction, nose reshaping, breast alterations, facial implants, ear or eyelid surgery, hair removal, and acne treatments (see Chapter 45). Eating disorders such as anorexia nervosa (AN) and bulimia nervosa (BN) are also considered manifestations of strong body concerns (see Chapters 32–34).

Body Image across Cultures and Ethnic Groups

While the desire to be thinner has often been considered a largely Western phenomenon, there is growing evidence that a proportion of adolescent girls in non-Western cultures (such as Croatia, Iran, China, and Japan) also report wanting to be thinner and engaging in weight loss diets. Furthermore, within a particular society, ethnic differences are found (see Chapters 25–28). For example, within the United States, African American adolescent girls report a larger ideal size and less body dissatisfaction than girls from other ethnic groups, and groups such as Hmong Americans have reported high levels of body concerns.

Factors Associated with the Development of Body Dissatisfaction in Adolescent Girls

Multiple factors appear to contribute to the development of body image and body dissatisfaction. Researchers often provide evidence for what is known as the bio–psycho–social model. This model suggests that *biological* factors, such as a girl's actual physical characteristics, together with individual *psychological* characteristics, *social* influences, and *interpersonal* interactions, all influence the development of body image. Multifactorial models, including the following elements, are proposed to explain sequences of events and core factors leading to body disturbance among adolescent girls.

Biological and Physical Factors

Actual biological and physical characteristics are a fundamental element of BID. Biological characteristics and neurobiological disorders can directly result in body disorientation, distortion of body perception, or body discomfort, such as when body size changes rapidly or physical disorders involve pain. However, most BIDs are thought to develop when one's body characteristics do not fit within culturally prescribed norms about the "desirable" body size and shape or specific body features. For example, a higher weight-to-height ratio (body mass index) that does not conform to prevailing cultural beauty ideals and is stigmatized, is often associated with greater body dissatisfaction in girls. More severe acne, which develops at puberty and is generally considered unattractive, is associated with lower body esteem. Thus, particular physical characteristics set the context in which other risk factors for developing body concerns play their role.

Developmental Challenges of Puberty

Around puberty, as girls mature physically, they must adjust to a series of dramatic changes in their body. These hormone-associated changes involve commencement of menstruation as well as alterations in the size and shape of the body, including increases in fat deposits in areas such as the breasts and hips. The addition of body hair and in many youths the development of acne are other transitional features. Girls must manage these changes, adapt to menstruation, and adjust their view of self. These obvious physical changes may be viewed as a passage to adulthood with an accompanying range of emotions from joy and pride to fear or shame. Breast increases, for example, may be associated with becoming a "woman" and be a cause for enhanced body image. However, the changes can also symbolize for some girls the lack of control she has over her body and self. A shift in girls' images of who they are physically and developmentally needs to take place as they mature.

Puberty-related changes can be particularly concerning for girls who mature at a different rate from their peers. Whether girls are early or late maturers, they may compare themselves to others and worry that they do not match their peers' rate of change. This can be especially problematic because adolescence is associated with the need to fit in and be like one's peers.

Some longitudinal studies of girls in the pubertal period have suggested that girls who begin menstruating earlier than their peers, particularly if they increase their body size before their peers do, may develop greater body dissatisfaction. As girls find themselves moving farther from societal ideals that indicate that beauty involves thinness, they may develop greater body concerns and/or become more vulnerable to other forms of influence. For example, girls who have started menstruating appear to have greater similarity to their mother's drive for thinness than girls who are premenstrual, so if mothers diet strictly, the daughter may be more likely to do so.

Sociocultural and Social Influences

The role of social or sociocultural influences in determining young people's standards of beauty is well established. The culture or subculture in which one lives has norms about what is considered beautiful and how important a particular body type is considered to be. Broad social norms are communicated on a mass scale through media, which can take many forms, including television, radio, magazines, movies, and, in more recent years, the Internet. However, at least as important are the social influences from parents, peers, siblings, neighbors, schools, the medical profession, and even the shape of dolls, which can either promote unhealthy and unrealistic body ideals or encourage positive body image and self-acceptance.

A girl's immediate subculture includes a combination of these influences and when she perceives many of them promoting an ideal body type that differs from her own, she will be more likely to internalize those norms and become dissatisfied with her own body. Given that current Western ideals of beauty involve a level of thinness that is unattainable for most women, these social norms set the stage for body dissatisfaction.

The role of media influences has been supported by experimental studies in which adolescent girls are shown media images of idealized females, such as thin models. These studies have found that girls exposed to these images report immediate decreases in body satisfaction. However, not all girls are equally susceptible to these media images. For example, Durkin, Paxton, and Sorbello found that adolescent girls who believed that appearance was important and who frequently compared their body to others' were most susceptible to this sort of influence (see Chapter 12).

Parents also play a role, in that they may model relevant behaviors, such as crash dieting, which children then copy (see Chapter 13). Or parents may directly influence their daughter by making critical comments or suggesting ways to "improve" their daughter's body, such as by losing weight or dieting.

Adolescence is a developmental period in which peer groups become increasingly important and opinions of friends may begin to take precedence over those of parents. Friendship groups have been found to share body attitudes. If a girl's peer group places importance on weight and eating, she is more likely to have weight concerns herself. Friends' dieting is associated with early adolescent girls developing increased body concerns over time. One way this may come about is through appearance-related conversations concerning clothing, weight, and dieting, as well as what is known as "fat talk," in which girls describe themselves as "fat," and friends respond and compare themselves to each other.

Appearance-related teasing and critical comments about weight, body shape, or particular features have been found to negatively influence body image in girls. Similarly, adolescent girls with dermatological conditions, particularly acne, report being teased and bullied about their skin and they report lower body esteem and quality of life. Pubertal changes can be accompanied by sexual harassment and a girl's body being objectified by others. Sexual harassment can result in girls themselves surveying their own body as an object to be observed and evaluated, which is associated shame about one's body.

Individual Psychological and Cognitive Characteristics

Particular individual psychological characteristics may make some girls especially vulnerable to societal ideals and messages. Several psychological and cognitive characteristics have been particularly strongly supported by longitudinal studies (which track body image over time), and/or experimental studies of adolescent girls. These include a tendency to "internalize" the dominant societal ideals, equating thinness with beauty, and to place a high value on appearance in general or on a particular body shape. A tendency to frequently compare one's body with others (appearance comparisons) has been found to predict body concerns, as have greater appearance-related *cognitive schemas*, which are cognitive sets or thinking styles that influence how information from the world is processed. Each of these characteristics has been found to moderate the effect of exposure to idealized images of female beauty. Thus, girls scoring highly on these characteristics are most likely to report increases in concerns about their own body after viewing the idealized images.

Other individual personality characteristics have been found to be associated with body concerns, such as low self-esteem, depressed mood, general well-being, and perfectionism. However, it is not clear whether these characteristics foster body dissatisfaction versus result from or simply correlate with body concern. A 5-year study of early adolescent girls by Paxton and colleagues identified self-esteem as a risk factor for body dissatisfaction, although other studies examining a shorter time period did not find such a relationship and depressive symptoms have not been found to predict body dissatisfaction in girls (see Wertheim, Paxton, and Blaney review).

Psychological Disorders Associated with Body Image Problems

Adolescence is a time of particular risk for girls in that during this time BIDs can develop into more severe psychological disorders. The most common are AN and BN, which can be viewed as manifestations of overconcern with shape and weight. AN most commonly emerges in early or later adolescence and BN in later adolescence.

Another body image-related disorder is body dysmorphic disorder, which involves a preoccupation and distress over an imagined defect or physical anomaly. While most cases occur in adults, some cases have been reported in adolescents, and adults with the disorder often report that their symptoms arose in early or middle adolescence.

Longitudinal Research into Stability and Change in Adolescent Girls' Body Image

Longitudinal studies of adolescent girls find that body image remains fairly stable over time, and more severe body disturbances can also be maintained over many months or years. Furthermore, Wertheim, Paxton, and Blaney's review of 21 prospective studies found that in 16 studies weight and shape concerns in middle school or early high school-age girls predicted later increases in eating problems such as dieting, drive for thinness, bulimic symptoms, binge eating, compensatory behaviors, and partial syndrome BN over periods ranging from 8 months to 4 years. Similarly, while not as many studies have been done, body image concerns in girls also predicted worsening of depressive symptoms, and in some studies, general self-esteem. Therefore, once established, body dissatisfaction does not appear to go away through simple development, a finding supporting the importance of prevention programs and early intervention when problems appear.

Conclusions and Future Directions

Given the high prevalence of body concerns, their stability over time when established, and the potential negative consequences of body dissatisfaction, a deeper understanding of body image during this period is required. Further research is needed to identify particularly salient and modifiable risk and protective factors at different phases across adolescence. While risk factors are variables that increase the likelihood of body image concerns, protective factors are factors that lower the likelihood of body image concerns. Risk and protective factors can be opposite ends of one continuum such as high or low self-esteem. But protective factors can also refer to interactive factors that reduce the negative impact of a risk factor on a problem outcome. To date, there has been very little research that has specifically tried to identify factors that can protect against body image concerns in the presence of risk factors. For example, little is known about whether a supportive peer environment can protect against or moderate the negative impact of frequent exposure to appearance-focused media. Information of this kind could help inform research to identify strategies to prevent body disturbances, or to intervene at an early stage.

Long-term longitudinal studies examining relationships between body image and general well-being, psychopathology, self-esteem, and personality characteristics such as perfectionism are still needed. In addition, much of the literature to date has focused on adolescent girls' weight and shape concerns, which are certainly important; however, other forms of body image difficulties have received relatively less attention, such as concerns associated with alterations in skin appearance, nose size, height, and body hair development that can arise through physical changes in adolescence. Finally, although the number of studies examining body image in different cultures and ethnic groups has grown in recent years, further research is needed that differentiates culturally specific risk and protective factors (such as wearing traditional clothing that covers the body or embracing particular value systems) versus factors that appear to be cross-cultural.

Informative Readings

Cafri, G., Yamamiya, Y., Brannick, M., & Thompson, J. K. (2005). The influence of sociocultural factors on body image: A meta-analysis. *Clinical Psychology: Science and Practice, 12*, 421–433.—An analysis of 22 studies suggesting the importance of internalization of a thin ideal, perceived pressures to be thin, and awareness of the thin ideal in body image.

Chisuwa, N., & O'Dea, J. A. (2010). Body image and eating disorders amongst Japanese adolescents. A review of the literature. *Appetite, 54*, 5–15.—An example of a review demonstrating that body image concerns and associated disturbed eating patterns are being found in non-Western societies.

Durkin, S. J., Paxton, S. J., & Sorbello, M. (2007). An integrative model of the impact of exposure to idealized female images on adolescent girls' body satisfaction. *Journal of Applied Social Psychology, 37,* 1092–1117.—An example of a study showing how the effect of exposure to idealized media images varies depending on personal characteristics of the adolescent girl.

Kornblau, I. S., Pearson, H. C., & Radecki Breitkopf, C. (2007). Demographic, behavioral, and physical correlates of body esteem among low-income female adolescents. *Journal of Adolescent Health, 41,* 566–570.—A study of adolescent girls exemplifying studies that look at a range of characteristics associated with body esteem, including ethnicity, socioeconomic status, smoking, and acne.

Lindberg, S. M., Grabe, S., & Hyde, J. S. (2007). Gender, pubertal development, and peer sexual harassment predict objectified body consciousness in early adolescence. *Journal of Research on Adolescence, 17,* 723–742.—A description and evaluation of a model of how sexual harassment in early adolescence could be linked to body shame through a girl's experiencing "objectified body consciousness."

Magin, P., Adams, J., Heading, G., Pond, D., & Smith, W. (2008). Experiences of appearance-related teasing and bullying in skin diseases and their psychological sequelae: Results of a qualitative study. *Scandinavian Journal of Caring Sciences, 22,* 430–436.—An example of a study that has examined the presence of sociocultural pressures in body concerns in relation to non-weight-focused physical characteristics, specifically dermatological disorders.

Myers, T. A., & Crowther, J. H. (2009). Social comparison as a predictor of body dissatisfaction: A meta-analytic review. *Journal of Abnormal Psychology, 118,* 683–698.—A statistical review of 156 studies supporting the relationship between social comparison tendencies and body dissatisfaction, suggesting that the relationship is strongest in individuals who are younger and female.

Paxton, S. J., Eisenberg, M. E., & Neumark-Sztainer, D. (2006). Prospective predictors of body dissatisfaction in adolescent girls and boys: A five year longitudinal study. *Developmental Psychology, 42,* 888–899.—Example of a longitudinal study tracking body dissatisfaction starting from early and middle adolescence.

Paxton, S. J., Schutz, H. K., Wertheim, E. H., & Muir, S. L. (1999). Friendship clique and peer influences on body image concerns, dietary restraint, extreme weight-loss behaviors, and binge eating in adolescent girls. *Journal of Abnormal Psychology, 108,* 255–266.—Friendship influences are demonstrated using social network methodology in which adolescent girls report about themselves and their friends.

Price, B. (2009). Body image in adolescents: Insights and implications. *Paediatric Nursing, 21,* 38–43.—A practice-oriented review written for nurses and other health professionals to increase awareness about developmental issues related to body image, how physical illnesses may impact on body concerns in adolescence, and how to discuss these issues with adolescents and health professionals.

Rodgers, R., & Chabrol, H. (2009). Parental attitudes, body image disturbance and disordered eating amongst adolescents and young adults: A review. *European*

Eating Disorders Review, 17, 137–151.—Covers recent research on parent influences in body image concerns.

Smolak, L., & Thompson, J. K. (Eds.). (2009). *Body image, eating disorders and obesity in youth: Assessment, prevention and treatment* (2nd ed.). Washington, DC: American Psychological Association.—Provides a range of review chapters relevant to body image development in young people, including two reviews cited in this chapter (i.e., Wertheim, Paxton, & Blaney; Body image in girls, pp. 47–66, and Sarwer, Infield, & Crerand; Plastic surgery for children and adolescents, pp. 303–326).

CHAPTER 10

Body Image Development in Adolescent Boys

LINA A. RICCIARDELLI
MARITA P. McCABE

Introduction

Body image is now recognized as an important aspect of social and emotional development for adolescent boys. This is reflected by the increasing number of studies that include a focus on adolescent boys in journals such as *Body Image, Sex Roles, Journal of Youth and Adolescence, Psychology of Men and Masculinity,* and *Journal of Clinical Child and Adolescent Psychology.* In the 2001 review by Cohane and Pope, only 17 papers were identified that included preadolescent and adolescent boys ages 18 or younger. In fact, many researchers and clinicians in the 1980s and 1990s were of the view that boys did not have body image concerns or eating problems, and hence boys were often excluded or ignored.

The Nature of Boys' Body Image Concerns

Many boys display a normative preoccupation for "lean muscularity." The drive for lean muscularity is displayed among adolescents across cultures, and is a common source of boys' body image concerns, with many boys wishing to be stronger and more muscular than they currently are. In its extreme form this is manifested as reverse anorexia. Reverse anorexia is a disorder characterized by a fear of being too small, and a perception that one is small and weak, even when one is actually large and muscular. In the late 1990s it was renamed "muscle dysmorphia" and is now recognized as a subcategory of body dysmorphic disorder.

In addition to boys' concerns with muscle size and strength, many adolescent boys desire to be lean and this is becoming even more important with the rising prevalence rates of obesity. Many boys are concerned about their weight and engage in extreme and unhealthy body change strategies to lose weight. These include purging and the use of laxatives.

Other aspects of the body that boys value are synonymous with the attributes that are desirable for sporting performance. These include functional aspects of the body such as overall size, height, speed, strength, fitness, and endurance. In addition, sports are often used as a forum for competing with other boys both on the playing field and by using sport performance to make favorable social comparisons about their own body size (e.g., "the best on the field," "the strongest in the class," and "wanting to be bigger than their friends"). The emphasis on competition among males is viewed as having a strong and adaptive evolutionary function in promoting the survival of males.

We and other researchers have also found that boys often focus on the positive aspects of their body and this has been interpreted as suggesting that boys do not have body image concerns. However, this ability to refract body image concerns may also be protective and adaptive. Boys from an age of 8 years are already more likely than girls to use self-serving biases to produce and maintain an unrealistically positive view of their own abilities and attributes. Self-serving biases reflect beliefs that one is better than average on desirable traits and below average on undesirable traits.

Theory and Research

The role of three main types of factors has been investigated in the development of body image in adolescent boys. These include biological factors such as pubertal development and pubertal timing; individual factors such as self-esteem and other self-concepts, mood, and perfectionism; and sociocultural factors such as direct and indirect messages transmitted by family, friends, and the media, and the role of culture and ethnicity.

Puberty Development and Timing

Pubertal development is usually a positive experience for boys, as the majority of boys move closer to the societal ideal shape for a man. Boys add muscle and their shoulder width increases. These physical characteristics fit the "ideal" cultural messages for men's body shape and size.

Although puberty is experienced by all adolescents, the timing may differ considerably. In fact, the actual timing of puberty in relation to one's peers has been shown to be more important than pubertal development per se. From a developmental deviance perspective, experiencing pubertal development prior to one's peers is associated with feelings of alienation and depression. This has been more fully elaborated as "the off-time hypothesis," which predicts that both early- and late-maturing adolescents will manifest more social, emotional, and behavioral problems than their on-time age-mates. The off-time hypothesis has been more fully developed in the case of early-maturing girls but there is increasing evidence that it also holds for late-maturing boys. Several studies have linked late maturation in boys with less social competence, low peer popularity, more conflict with parents, more internalizing tendencies, more drinking problems, and lower school achievement.

Only one longitudinal study was located that has examined the role of pubertal timing in understanding attitudes and behaviors associated with the pursuit of muscularity. Late-maturing boys were found to be more likely to use food supplements to build up their body than early-maturing boys and this predicted an increased use of strategies to increase their muscle size.

Different Stages of Adolescence

We have also shown that many of the factors that impact on development of boys' body image are similar for both preadolescent and adolescent boys. Thus it is essential that we commence studying the development of boys' body image as early as possible (e.g., 3 years of age). We also do not yet fully understand how different phases of adolescence may mediate and/or moderate the development of boys' body image concerns. One view is that as boys enter puberty at a later age than girls, it is possible that body image and appearance concerns may develop during the later phases of adolescence in males. However, early adolescence is also a high-risk period, as boys' physical characteristics do not resemble the muscular ideal at this stage of life.

Individual Factors

Several individual variables have been found to be consistently associated with boys' weight and muscle concerns. These include negative mood, self-esteem, perfectionism, peer relationships, the use of alcohol and other drugs, and other risk-taking behaviors. However, as much of the work with boys is based on cross-sectional research it is not possible to separate causes from consequences. As a result, many of the variables that have been identified as risk factors may in fact be consequences or only correlates.

Sociocultural Messages and Social Comparisons

In-depth individual and focus group interviews conducted with adolescent boys have been invaluable as these allow body image issues to be examined more fully. For example, these have allowed us to gain access to boys' own ideas and terminology regarding their body image. In our 2000 study, we found that for approximately one-third of the boys, parents, siblings, friends, and the media were perceived to have at least some influence over boys' feeling about their body and body change strategies. Importantly, we found that feedback from mothers and female friends was viewed as having a positive impact on boys' body image, whereas feedback from fathers and male friends was viewed as more important in influencing body change methods. Moreover, contrary to the research with girls, only a few boys felt negative about their body when they compared it to others. Most boys who used social comparisons reported feeling either more positive or neutral about their body. These findings may again be due to the different ways boys use social comparisons and the way they more effectively use self-serving biases. These strategies may equip boys to ignore negative messages and assist them in evaluating their body more positively even when using social comparisons, and when confronted with peer teasing and other types of peer pressure.

Culture

In recent years there has been a growth of research on body image and related behaviors among youth from countries outside of Western countries. These include Chile in South America, Korea in Southeast Asia, and both Fiji and Tonga in the Pacific.

As with other countries, we found that boys in Chile reported less body dissatisfaction than girls. However, boys and girls were no different in the pressure they perceived to lose weight from adults in the family or from older siblings and cousins. Girls experienced more pressure to lose weight from the media than boys but boys reported more pressure from peers to lose weight than girls, and more pressure than girls from all sources to increase their muscles. The greater pressure from peers to lose weight for boys suggests that peer messages to lose weight may be more focused on leanness and body tone, which are difficult to separate from weight concerns. Lastly, we found that only one factor predicted boys' body dissatisfaction and this was the perceived pressure from adults in the family to lose weight. Family influences are known to be critical socializing forces during childhood and adolescence, and our findings highlight that the family in Chile may play an even more important role in the boys' body image development than peers and the media.

A recent study of adolescents in Korea has shown that adolescent boys had greater body dissatisfaction and engaged in more behaviors associated with disordered eating than did their age and gender cohorts in the United States. These findings parallel those from our 2007 review that showed that many adolescent boys and adult men from a range of different cultural groups displayed more body image concerns than European men from Western countries.

In another recent study we compared Indigenous and Indo-Fijian adolescents living in Fiji, and Tongans living in Tonga, with European Australians living in Australia. Consistent with the findings from Western countries, we found that girls in Fiji and Tonga reported more dissatisfaction with their weight and shape, whereas boys were more dissatisfied with their muscles. Moreover, it was the Indo-Fijian boys who evidenced the highest level of dissatisfaction with their body. This may be because Indo-Fijian boys' body build tends to be on average smaller and weaker than Indigenous Fijians. Boys who are below-average weight for their height or view themselves as underweight tend to be more negative about their body image, achievement aspirations, and overall self-concepts. In addition, we found that overweight Tongan and Fijian adolescents evidenced higher levels of body satisfaction than either Australians or Indo-Fijian adolescents. These findings are consistent with the endorsement of the large body ideal for both Tongan and Fijians, and suggest that less stigma and dissatisfaction is experienced by overweight adolescents in these communities. The findings also highlight the acceptance of a larger and more robust body size that has been traditionally endorsed by many Pacific Islanders.

Eating Attitudes and Behaviors and Body Change Strategies

There is extensive evidence that body image concerns are associated with eating attitudes and behaviors that include disordered eating, muscle-building strategies (e.g., use of steroids, protein powders, and other food supplements, and extreme exercise regimes) and body change strategies. Body dissatisfaction and other indicators of poor body image have been found to be related to dieting and other strategies to lose weight, the Eating Disorder Inventory, the Eating Attitudes Test, and strategies to increase muscles.

Future Research

More research is needed on the different factors that may impact on boys' body image development. More research is also needed to examine factors that are specific to boys, such as the role of sports. Sports for boys plays an important socializing role in promoting physical, mental, and social development during childhood and adolescence. Sports participation for boys is associated with higher self-esteem and boys more than girls view participating in sports as a way of increasing their social status and peer popularity. Also some factors, such as the media, may work differently for boys. For example, the media in some studies has been shown to have an enhancement effect for boys but not girls. However, the theoretical model underlying these findings is not well understood. Other factors that have not been well researched but which appear to be important for understanding the development of boys' body image include self-serving biases, the role of competition, gender roles (conformity and stress), and friendships and peer networks.

The majority of studies have only examined direct relationships among a set of variables. However, variables such as body mass index and pubertal timing may act as moderators or even mediators of the relationship between individual factors and/or sociocultural influences and body image concerns. For example, social comparisons have been found to be more strongly related to body dissatisfaction among boys who perceive themselves as overweight.

Prevention Research

Prevention research with adolescent boys is underrepresented in the field in comparison with adolescent girls (see Chapters 49–52). An increasing number of researchers are now including adolescent boys; however, they often do not include measures that are sufficiently sensitive to detect boys' concerns. In addition, many prevention programs include a focus on media literacy, which may not be as important for boys as it is for girls.

Our recent prevention program was specifically designed for adolescent boys. It focused on two areas that have been shown to be associated with body image concerns among boys, that is, self-esteem and peer relationships. The program consisted of five sessions that examined (1) individual differences with an emphasis on the identification of unique physical and psychological attributes; (2) communication skills, including the importance of body language, and the giving and acceptance of positive and negative feedback; (3) social skills training, initiating positive interactions, and the use of assertive communication; (4) coping skills, particularly in relation to dealing with stress and other negative feelings; and (5) consolidating the new skills via revision of previous sessions.

Our study demonstrated that the new program was not effective in changing boys' body dissatisfaction, strategies to increase muscles, use of food supplements, negative affect, and peer relations in the intervention group compared to the control group over a 12-month period. However, it raised a number of important issues that now need to be examined further:

1. Twelve months is likely to be too short a period to detect any preventative effects. A 24-month follow-up period is required in order to fully evaluate preventative effects.

2. Our program focused on early adolescents, but this may not be the most optimal period for implementing prevention programs for boys.
3. We still have a limited understanding of the development of boys' body image so we may not be targeting the most critical factors.

Conclusions

In the last 20 years, an increasing number of studies have specifically focused on the development of boys' body image. However, we have only begun to unravel how the development of body image in boys differs from that of girls. More research is needed that specifically targets boys, the broader social context, and their lived experiences.

Informative Readings

Cohane, G. H., & Pope, H. G. (2001). Body image in boys: A review of the literature. *International Journal of Eating Disorders, 29*, 373–379.—An early review of body image and the negative impact for preadolescent and adolescent boys.

Grogan, S., & Richards, H. (2002). Body image: Focus groups with boys and men. *Men and Masculinities, 4*, 219–232.—Qualitative analysis of focus groups interviews that examine British boys' and men's body image.

Halliwell, E., & Harvey, M. (2006). Examination of a sociocultural model of disordered eating among male and female adolescents. *British Journal of Health Psychology, 11*, 235–248.—An examination of sociocultural factors, including social comparisons, among adolescents from the United Kingdom.

Hargreaves, D. A., & Tiggemann, M. (2006). "Body image is for girls": A qualitative study of boys' body image. *Journal of Health Psychology, 11*, 567–576.—Qualitative analysis of Australian boys' body image using focus group interviews.

Jones, D. C., Bain, N., & King, S. (2008). Weight and muscularity concerns as longitudinal predictors of body image among early adolescent boys: A test of the dual pathway model. *Body Image: An International Journal of Research, 5*, 195–204.—Highlights the importance of examining both weight and muscularity concerns among adolescent boys.

Jung, J., Forbes, G. B., & Lee, Y. (2009). Body dissatisfaction and disordered eating among early adolescents from Korea and the U.S. *Sex Roles, 61*, 42–54.—Provides support for feminist theories that maintain that increases in body dissatisfaction among Eastern cultures is associated with rapid social changes.

McCabe, M. P., Ricciardelli, L. A., & Karantzas, G. (2010). Impact of a healthy body image program among adolescent boys on body image, negative affect, and body change strategies. *Body Image: An International Journal of Research, 7*, 117–123.—New prevention program developed for adolescent boys that targets self-esteem and peer relationships.

McCabe, M. P., Ricciardelli, L., Waqa, G., Goundar, R., & Fotu, K. (2009). Body image and change strategies among adolescent males and females from Fiji, Tonga and Australia. *Body Image: An International Journal of Research, 6,* 299–303.—Investigates body image and body change strategies among adolescents in Fiji, Tonga, and Australia.

Mellor, D., McCabe, M., Ricciardelli, L., & Merino, M. E. (2008). Body dissatisfaction and body change behaviors in Chile: The role of sociocultural factors. *Body Image: An International Journal of Research, 5,* 205–215.—Investigates body image and body change strategies among adolescents in Chile.

Ricciardelli, L. A., & McCabe, M. P. (2007). The pursuit of muscularity among adolescent boys. In J. K. Thompson & G. Cafri (Eds.), *The muscular ideal: Psychological, social and medical perspectives* (pp. 199–216). Washington, DC: American Psychological Association.—Review of the biological, individual, and sociocultural factors associated with the pursuit of muscularity.

Ricciardelli, L. A., McCabe, M. P., & Banfield, S. (2000). Body image and body change methods in adolescent boys: Role of parents, friends, and the media. *Journal of Psychosomatic Research, 49,* 189–197.—Qualitative analysis of individual interviews of adolescents boys' body image and the role of sociocultural factors.

Ricciardelli, L. A., McCabe, M. P., Mussap, A. J., & Holt, K. E. (2009). Body image in preadolescent boys. In L. Smolak & J. K. Thompson (Eds.), *Body image, eating disorders, and obesity in youth: Assessment, prevention, and treatment* (2nd ed., pp. 77–96). Washington DC: American Psychological Association.—Review of the biological, individual, and sociocultural factors associated with the development of body image concerns among preadolescent boys.

Ricciardelli, L. A., McCabe, M. P., Williams, R. J., & Thompson, J. K. (2007). The role of ethnicity and culture in body image and disordered eating among males. *Clinical Psychology Review, 27,* 582–606.—Review of body image, disordered eating, and body change strategies among preadolescent, adolescent, and adult males from various cultures including Blacks, Hispanic Americans, Asians, Native Americans, Pacific Islanders, and men from Middle Eastern countries.

Smolak, L., & Stein, J. A. (2006). The relationship of drive for muscularity to sociocultural factors, self-esteem, physical attributes, gender role, and social comparison in middle school boys. *Body Image: An International Journal of Research, 3,* 121–129.—Highlights the importance of sociocultural and individual factors and the importance of targeting boys in the middle school years.

CHAPTER 11

Body Image Development in Adulthood

SARAH GROGAN

Introduction

Much of the literature on adult men's and women's body image is based on young adults, partly because so much research has been conducted with college and university students who tend to be in their late teens and 20s. However, there is a growing literature on body image in older adults to investigate how body image develops as they move into their 40s, 50s, 60s, 70s, and beyond. Although some of the physical changes associated with aging (e.g., increases in body weight, skin wrinkling, reduction in body tone and muscularity) may take people farther away from a socially idealized slender, wrinkle-free, and toned body, studies of body satisfaction in older adults show that this does not inevitably lead to greater body dissatisfaction. In fact, there is some evidence for more positive body image as people enter their 60s and beyond, particularly for women.

After considering social pressure to maintain a youthful appearance, this chapter examines what we know about the development of body image in adulthood. This involves a discussion of evidence about how body image changes as people progress from young to mature adulthood, focusing in particular on how body satisfaction and appearance investment may change. Of course, the evidence is based on cross-sectional research that compares people in different age groups. This is certainly not the same as longitudinal research that compares the same individuals as they age. For example, people in different age groups are not from the same generation, with the particular life experiences that that would entail. Not surprisingly, no lifespan longitudinal studies of body image exist. Finally, because gender is an important predictor of body image (see

Chapters 19 and 22), the current chapter focuses separately and comparatively on women and men.

Social Pressures to Maintain a Youthful Appearance

Various researchers and social commentators have suggested that women in Western societies are expected to try to maintain a youthful appearance as they age, a pressure that is not imposed on men to the same extent, and that this fuels the cosmetic surgery industry. Many researchers have noted a double standard whereby women are judged more harshly than men in terms of physical attractiveness as they show signs of aging. Wykes and Gunter have argued that the predominant image of "woman" in contemporary Western media is of a young, conventionally attractive, usually White woman. Older women are often portrayed as asexual, lonely, and depressed; and sexual desire in older women is often a point of ridicule. When an older woman is portrayed in a sexual role, she is usually a woman who has a youthful appearance, and the director often avoids exposing her body by implying sexual activity rather than actually filming her naked or partially naked, using body doubles, or by filming from a distance.

Since the 1990s, idealized, slender, and moderately muscular young men's bodies have been depicted more frequently in advertisements for non-body-related products and in television and on film. Although it is rare to see women in their 40s and 50s in sexual roles, men in their 50s are frequently portrayed on film as attractive and sexual, and as having sexual relationships with much younger women. It is easy to think of examples of Hollywood actors who still play "love interest" roles in their 50s and 60s (e.g., Richard Gere, Harrison Ford, Pierce Brosnan, Bruce Willis, Kevin Costner), and it is not uncommon for men to be presented as lovers of women who are 20 years younger. However, men over 70 years are often portrayed as incapacitated, incompetent, pathetic, and the subject of ridicule. Bodies of men over 70 are rarely seen on film, except in roles where bodies might be expected to be exposed (e.g., as hospital patients).

Body Image and Aging in Women

Exposure to Western media where slender, youthful bodies are idealized has been linked to body weight ideals and body dissatisfaction in women. In a large-scale international study published in 2010, Swami and colleagues found that exposure to Western media predicted both preference for a thinner body type and body dissatisfaction in women. However, one of their most interesting findings was that women's body dissatisfaction was not predicted by age. This is unexpected as one would assume the disparity between the thin, toned, youthful media ideal and women's actual appearance would lead to higher levels of body dissatisfaction in older women. Other cross-sectional research has shown consistently that women do not become more dissatisfied with age, and they may even become more satisfied as they age, particularly between 60 and 85 years.

In interviews discussed in Grogan's *Body Image* book, women from 16 to 63 years reported similar levels of dissatisfaction with weight and shape. Areas of the body that presented most cause for concern did not differ by age. Women reliably reported dissatisfaction with stomach, hips, and thighs irrespective of age. Most were motivated to lose weight. The main motivator for women of all ages was being able to wear favorite clothes. Women of all ages were able to identify parts of their body that they would like to change, and almost all wanted to be a bit slimmer if possible, regardless of objective size. Other researchers have shown that women over 63 years also report some dissatisfaction with weight. Clarke's interviews with Canadian women ages 61–92 years revealed that women were dissatisfied with their weight and reported that a key motivator for weight loss was an expected positive impact on their appearance. She found that most women were dissatisfied with the weight gain they had experienced as they aged, which they linked with lack of self-control and reduced physical activity.

Although many older women may report dissatisfaction with weight, there is some evidence that fewer older women report appearance concerns than younger women. Harris and Carr, in a large-scale U.K. study published in 2001, found that relatively fewer women (33%) in the over 61 years group expressed such concerns than those in the 51–60 years group (60%) or the 18–30 years group (69%). Body satisfaction may be even higher in women in their 80s than in their 60s. In a 2009 study of body image in 148 Australian men and women, Baker and Gringart found that women ages 79 and over evaluated their appearance significantly more positively than those ages 65–71 years.

So how do we make sense of the finding that women may have equivalent or even fewer body concerns as they age despite the fact that weight gain is likely with aging? It may be that older women have body shape ideals that are different and more realistic than those of younger groups, producing a smaller discrepancy between current and ideal body shapes. In work reported in Grogan's *Body Image* book, we investigated body image role models in 16- to 49-year-old women. We found that younger women (under 30) were most likely to cite specific celebrities (actresses and models) as body image ideals. Middle-aged women (40–49) were likely to cite a family member, or no particular person. One of the interesting findings of this study was that role models tended to be age appropriate. Youthful media models became less important standards for comparison as women became older. Older women may make realistic age-based comparisons when judging their attractiveness, being concerned to "look good for their age," rather than to look like women in magazine pictures or on television, seeing body-related changes such as weight gain as an inevitable part of the aging process. Having more realistic ideals may be protective against the negative effects of observing idealized models that occur in younger women. There is still much more work to be done in this area to understand body image role models in women in older age groups.

There is also some evidence that the importance attached to appearance may be lower in older women, and that the link between body satisfaction and self-esteem may be weaker than in younger women. Body image investment may also diminish with identity development as women's identities become less closely linked with their looks and more with their role in relation to family, career, and community. Tiggemann, in a review published in 2004, suggested that appearance investment may decrease as women move into their 60s and beyond—resulting in lowered self-objectification, reduced body monitoring, and less appearance anxiety as women age. As a result, self-esteem may also be less closely linked with body satisfaction as women age. In the aforementioned Australian study, Baker and Gringart found that appearance evaluation did not predict self-esteem in women ages 65–85 years, although health evaluation and overweight preoccupation were significant predictors of self-esteem. Whereas there is evidence from qualitative research that some older women may desire to lose weight for appearance reasons, health concerns may be an additional motivator for weight loss that is more important to older women than to those in young adulthood or in their middle years.

Body Image and Aging in Men

One of the most consistent findings across body image studies is that men are generally more satisfied than women. However, there is some evidence that this gap in satisfaction shrinks as men and women move into their 60s and beyond. Janelli found that her 60- to 98-year-old men and women participants did not differ significantly on overall body dissatisfaction, and Baker and Gringart have shown that the 79- to 85-year-old women in their Australian sample were significantly *more* satisfied than the men in the same age group; the reverse pattern was found consistently in younger groups.

Research on age differences in men's body satisfaction has produced conflicting findings. Some research suggests that older men are less satisfied than younger men, some studies found no differences in satisfaction, and some found that older men have fewer body concerns than younger men. Lamb and colleagues in the 1990s found that middle-aged men (in their 50s) presented body ideals that were much slimmer than their perceived size and had a significantly larger disparity between ideal and current size than younger men (in their 20s). The older men were objectively heavier than the younger men (i.e., an average of 181 vs. 165 pounds, respectively) and selected a significantly heavier current figure. However, there were no differences in ideal size between the men in their 20s and in their 50s. This resulted in a wider gap between perceived and ideal size in the middle-aged cohort, suggesting less satisfaction in middle-aged than in younger men.

Other studies produced quite different results. Pliner and colleagues, also in the 1990s and covering a much wider age range than Lamb and colleagues (between 10 and 79 years), found that older men were just as satisfied as younger men. There is even some evidence that older men have fewer appearance concerns than men in the 19- to 21-year-old group. Harris and Carr found that the highest levels of concern for men (56%) were in the youngest (18–21 years) group, with only 24% of 51- to 60-year-olds and 21% of men over 61 years reporting appearance concerns. In a meta-analysis of 222 studies of gender differences in self-rated attractiveness and body image, Feingold and Mazzella found that men's self-rated attractiveness was higher among older groups. Reboussin and colleagues also suggest that men in the 65- to 75-year-old group were more satisfied than younger men. There is also some evidence that overweight preoccupation may reduce as men become more elderly even if they have an increase in other body concerns. Baker and Gringart found that men in the 79- to 85-year-old group showed significantly lower levels of overweight concern relative to men in the 65- to 71-year-old group, although men in the 79- to 85-year-old group scored lower on overall appearance evaluation. It is difficult to compare between studies as different researchers used varying measures and focused on different age groups. More research is needed in this area to understand more fully the nature of any differences in body satisfaction as men age.

There is some evidence that men's body image ideals may be different at varying ages. In the aforementioned study of body image role models, middle-aged men were not able to cite particular male body image role models. However, some men, in response to the open-ended question, "Who would you like to look like?" responded, "Like myself when I was younger." Perhaps middle-aged men are likely to compare their current body with their own body at a younger age rather than against bodies of other men. If this is the case, then the drop in satisfaction in the middle years would be expected, since most men (and women) gain some weight as they move into middle age. The role of these temporal comparisons is unclear, although for most people comparison between one's current body and one's body at a younger adult age would be likely to be an upward comparison. We need to know much more about body image comparison models in older men. Based on existing research, it is unclear which standards for comparison older men tend to use and how important such standards are.

Most studies suggest that adult men attach less importance to their own appearance than women at all ages. This does not appear to vary by age and is seen up to 85 years. As in studies with women, there is also good evidence for a decrease in rated importance of appearance as men move to older adulthood with studies showing a steady and consistent decline in appearance investment with age. Perceptions of health and fitness may be better predictors of self-esteem than appearance evaluation in older men. For instance, in Baker and Gringart's study, appearance evaluation did not predict self-esteem in their 65- to 85-year-old men, whereas health invest-ment and fitness evaluation were significant predictors. Physical exercise can improve perceptions of mastery of the body and can have a positive impact on men's (and women's) body image as they age, probably through increasing fitness and refocusing attention onto health, fitness, and body function and away from concern about physical appearance.

Conclusions and Future Directions

Current data suggest that women are likely to be more body dissatisfied than men between 18 and 60 years, although there may be less difference between the genders over 60 years old, and women in their 80s may be more satisfied than men in their age group. Research to date has shown that older women are at least as satisfied as younger women, despite a cul-tural focus on appearance of youthfulness, body tone, and slimness that may decline with age. This may be because women choose age-appropriate models for body image comparisons as they age and/or because appear-ance becomes less important and less strongly linked to self-esteem. Work on the impact on men's body image of aging is inconsistent, although there is some evidence for increased satisfaction between 65 and 79 years with a decrease after 79 years. There is good evidence for a decrease in the value attributed to appearance and an increase in focus on fitness and health as men age.

One of the problems in comparing different age cohorts with each other is that historical/cultural pressures and experiences vary between people raised in different social contexts. Future research in this area needs to use longitudinal studies that follow the same cohort through the various key age points. This will enable us to control more effectively for the effects of historical changes in body shape ideals on the development of both men's and women's body image through adulthood. Further work also needs to look at body image role models and how these change with age, and to consider the impact of aging on body image in the full range of ethnically diverse participants across cultures.

Informative Readings

Baker, L., & Gringart, E. (2009). Body image and self-esteem in older adulthood. *Aging and Society, 29,* 977–995.—Compares body image and self-esteem in men and women ages 65–85 years.

Cash, T. F., & Henry, P. (1995). Women's body images: The results of a national survey in the USA. *Sex Roles, 33,* 19–28.—Body image survey of 803 women from 19 to 70 years.

Clarke, L. H. (2002). Older women's perceptions of ideal body weights: The tensions between health and appearance motivations for weight loss. *Aging and Society, 22,* 751–773.—Interviews with 22 women ages 61–92 years where women discuss motivations for weight loss.

Feingold, A., & Mazzella, R. (1998). Gender differences in body image are increasing. *Psychological Science, 9,* 190–195.—Reports a meta-analysis of gender differences in attractiveness and body image including 222 studies over a 50-year period.

Grogan, S. (2008). *Body image: Understanding body dissatisfaction in men, women and children* (2nd ed.). London: Routledge.—Reviews work on body image and aging (in chapter 6), and age differences in media role models (in chapter 5).

Harris, S., & Carr, A. (2001). Prevalence of concerns about physical appearance in the general population. *British Journal of Plastic Surgery, 54,* 223–226.—Reports age differences in appearance concerns in a large sample of men and women from 18 to 61 years and over.

Janelli, L. M. (1993). Are there body image differences between older men and women? *Western Journal of Nursing Research, 15,* 327–339.—Compares satisfaction with particular body parts in a sample of men and women ages 60–98 years.

Lamb, C. S., Jackson, L., Cassiday, P., & Priest, D. (1993). Body figure preferences of men and women: A comparison of two generations. *Sex Roles, 28,* 345–358.—Compares body silhouette choices in men and women ages 20 versus 50 years.

Pliner, P., Chaiken, S., & Flett, G. (1990). Gender differences in concern with body weight and physical appearance over the life span. *Personality and Social Psychology Bulletin, 16,* 263–273.—Evaluates age differences in scores on body image measures between men and women ages 10–79 years.

Reboussin, B. A., Rejeski, W. J., Martin, K. A., Callahan, K., Dunn, A., King, A. C., et al. (2000). Correlates of satisfaction with body function and body appearance in middle- and older-aged adults: The activity counselling trial (ACT). *Psychology and Health, 15,* 239–254.—Examines correlates of body satisfaction in men and women ages 35–54 and 55–75 years.

Swami, V., Frederick, D., Aavik, T., Alcalay, L., Allik, J., Anderson, D., et al. (2010). The attractive female body weight and female body dissatisfaction in 26 countries across 10 world regions: Results of the International Body Project I. *Personality and Social Psychology Bulletin, 36,* 309–326.—Results from a survey of body image and media exposure in 7,434 participants in 26 countries across 10 world regions.

Tiggemann, M. (2004). Body image across the adult lifespan: Stability and change. *Body Image: An International Journal of Research, 1,* 29–41.—A narrative review of literature on body image in adults across the adult lifespan.

Wykes, M., & Gunter, B. (2005). *The media and body image.* London: Sage.—Reviews media representations of men's and women's bodies and the impact of these media images.

CHAPTER 12

Media Influences on Body Image

MICHAEL P. LEVINE
KELSEY CHAPMAN

Introduction

Institution of a market-based mass media in two vastly different cultures, Fiji and the Ukraine, preceded increases in internalization of the slender beauty ideal and in body dissatisfaction among adolescent girls. This correlation supports several well-established sociocultural models that link media, as well as parent and peer, influences to negative body image and disordered eating behavior (see Chapter 2).

Does exposure to mass media really "cause" negative body image in females, and perhaps in males as well? Logically, if mass media constitute a *causal risk factor*, then there will be strong empirical evidence for affirmative answers to the questions posed in the next six major headings. This chapter considers the relevant data and their implications for prevention, treatment, and research.

Are Vulnerable Audiences Exposed to Media Offering Potentially Influential Content?

Mass media, including television, magazines, video games, cinema, and the Internet, are a major part of the lives of millions of children, adolescents, and adults. These media are saturated with multiple, overlapping, and unhealthy messages about ideal body sizes and shapes in relation to pleasure, morality, gender, attractiveness, self-control, food, weight management, and power.

Body Ideals

The ideal female constructed by mass media is young, tall, thin, and White, with at least moderately large breasts. This iconic image is framed by themes that are social norms and elements of a "thinness schema," such as (1) women are naturally invested in their beauty assets; and (2) the slender beauty ideal is not an enjoyable fantasy based on digital technology but rather is normal, healthy, and achievable through personal dedication.

The male body ideal is more variable. Also tall and lean, it typically has one or two added features: well groomed and expensively, fashionably dressed; and/or exceptional ("chiseled" or "ripped") muscularity. Since the 1980s there has been a trend toward magazines and movies featuring a muscular, action-ready male body in a state of objectified undress. This development has been accompanied by increased media attention to exercise and weightlifting as paths to sexual (not romantic) prowess, and by glorification of "bulked up," dominating, hypermasculine action figures in the form of heavily marketed toys for younger boys and video game characters for older males.

Are Mass Media Experienced by Masses of People Other Than Social Scientists as a Source of Influence?

If media pressures exert a strong, straightforward influence on body ideals and social comparison processes, as emphasized by sociocultural theories, then large numbers of people will report experiencing those pressures in relation to body image. Nearly 70% of adolescent girls report that magazine images influence their conception of the "perfect body shape," and a significant minority indicates that such images generate body dissatisfaction and motivation to lose weight. A desire to look like celebrities and models is a strong predictor of weight concerns.

Internalization of the Media Body Ideals

Internalization of the slender beauty ideal, emphasizing investment in media-based models and standards of beauty, is a consistent predictor of perceived media pressure to be thin and of negative body image. Awareness and internalization of the muscular ideal negatively affects the development of some boys, but such appearance concerns are generally not integral to psychosocial development in males. If the muscular ideal is internalized, it is not as influential as internalization of the thin ideal is for females in determining body image and weight and shape management, unless there is a strong commitment to defining the self in terms of weight and/or muscularity.

Is There a Cross-Sectional Correlation between Media Exposure and Body Image?

Females

The amount of time adolescent girls spend viewing appearance-focused media (e.g., fashion and glamour magazines, soap operas, and music videos) is positively and modestly correlated with internalization of the thin ideal, drive for thinness, and body dissatisfaction. For adolescents and young adults, involvement with magazines is more influential than the amount of television watched, and the strongest correlate is internalization of the slender beauty ideal.

Males

The more a boy or young man reads magazines addressing "fashionable" young men or male health and fitness—or the more pressure he reports from these sources—the more likely he is to report lower levels of body satisfaction, to be concerned with muscularity and fitness, and to use muscle-building supplements and steroids to look bigger. These correlations are small but increase between childhood and young adulthood.

Is Media Exposure a Longitudinal Predictor of Body Image?

The few studies available suggest that for girls ages 6–13, as well as young adults, extent of media exposure predicts increases in negative body image and disordered eating. Television is more influential for children, whereas for adolescents and young adults it is magazines. However, several well-conducted longitudinal studies of media exposure and body image in adolescents have not found significant predictive relationships.

Less is known about longitudinal media effects for boys and men. Independent of body dissatisfaction, Australian boys ages 8–11 who reported feeling pressure from media to gain muscle and control their weight are more likely to report actually trying to change their bodies. White boys ages 7–10 in the United States, but not Black boys, who read more gaming magazines showed an increase in drive for muscularity 1 year later, even when important variables (e.g., body mass index) were controlled. A 1-year follow-up of a small sample of U.S. college men found that extent of exposure to an extremely popular genre of media targeting 18- to 26-year-old males, namely magazines such as *Maxim* that promote fitness and fashion within a "masculine," raunchy lifestyle, predicted objectified self-surveillance, but not appearance anxiety.

Do Controlled Experiments Demonstrate That Media Exposure Negatively Affects Body Satisfaction?

Females

Controlled exposure to the slender ideal in magazines, television, and video games tends to generate a moderately large negative effect on girls' and women's body satisfaction at the time (i.e., their "state" body dissatisfaction). Adolescent girls whose body satisfaction was most negatively affected in this way by television commercials had greater levels of characteristic (or "trait") body dissatisfaction and drive for thinness 2 years later, even when initial individual differences in trait body dissatisfaction were controlled. It is noteworthy that 20–30% of high school and college females exposed to magazine images of attractive models subsequently exhibit an *increase* in state body satisfaction.

Males

Australian boys ages 13–15 responded to presentations of the muscular ideal in television commercials with self-evaluative appearance comparisons and negative feelings, although these reactions were less prominent than those of adolescent girls—and the boys showed no significant decrease in body satisfaction. Males ages 15–27, however, consistently demonstrate increases in muscle dissatisfaction following exposure to commercials or advertisements displaying the muscular body ideal. Unlike the case for females and body/weight dissatisfaction, this effect is not greater in males already dissatisfied with their muscularity. Experimental exposure to the fashionably dressed, high-status ideal also produces a decrease in body esteem and self-esteem.

Controlled Analogue and Field Experiments: Does Resisting or Mitigating Media Effects Reduce Negative Body Image?

If media exposure is a causal risk factor, then "media literacy" techniques to reduce or eliminate negative media influences should eventually reduce or prevent negative body image. Controlled outcome studies of laboratory interventions, brief lessons in actual school settings, and longer, intensive school- or organization-based programs provide promising but inconclusive data. Current media literacy programs may be more effective for youth ages 9–14 and for young adults. There exist no well-controlled, long-term studies of whether media literacy in particular prevents development of negative body image.

Integrating the Evidence:
Some Working Conclusions

For females, media effects meet a majority of the criteria for a causal risk factor in relation to body image. Nevertheless, lack of strong, replicable longitudinal and prevention outcome data indicates that, currently, engagement with mass media is best considered a *variable* risk factor that might later prove to be a causal risk factor.

For males there are insufficient longitudinal and prevention studies to draw a meaningful conclusion about causality. A reasonable conclusion is that media influence more males more than was previously assumed. Status, style, and muscularity concerns are increasingly important themes in media for males, and exposure to these salient messages inside and outside the laboratory is significantly but modestly correlated with body dissatisfaction. Moreover, it appears that the "self versus media ideal" negative effect on state body satisfaction in controlled experiments is similar in magnitude for males and females.

Processes of Influence: Mediators and Moderators

Progress in clarifying media effects and their limitations has been accompanied by gains in understanding of major mediating and moderating factors.

Media Characteristics as Moderators

The negative impact of media images depends on conscious, that is, supraliminal perception of clear, direct, and attractive social messages. Further research is needed on the interplay between media ideals of slenderness (or muscularity) and cues for objectification of the body. Presenting attractive media images in a sexist, objectified fashion leads to an immediate and significant reduction in male as well as female body satisfaction, perhaps by priming appearance concerns related to sexual success. Conversely, presenting White adolescent girls and young women with attractive media models who are average size and/or engaged in nonlean sports requiring larger but healthy, vigorous bodies has a positive effect on viewers.

Ethnicity as a Moderating Factor

Carefully constructed media images embodying ("selling") the thin ideal are very likely to be White or light-hued females with all traces of ethnicity erased. Thus, in the United States, media effects are stronger for

White, European American females than for individuals from other ethnic backgrounds, notably African Americans and Latinas (see Chapters 25 and 27). However, female bodies of color exhibited in mainstream media are becoming thinner, and recent surveys point to increasing similarities in effects among Black and White girls, especially prior to puberty.

Person Variables as Mediators and Moderators

The negative effect of experimental presentations of media body ideals is appreciably greater in females who are heavily invested in appearance concerns and/or who are already self-conscious about their body shape. Such women tend to compare their appearance unfavorably to a spectrum of social comparison targets including peers, fashion models, celebrities, and even a thin versus a fatter, rounded vase. Women with higher levels of body dissatisfaction probably make such broad, unhealthy, and self-defeating social comparisons because their body-relevant self-schema in general is activated more readily.

For females, the following variables mediate and moderate the connection between media exposure and body dissatisfaction or negative body image: internalization of the slender beauty ideal, social comparison, and activation of appearance schema. Other processes deserving of research are self-objectification (see Chapter 6) and activation of a chronically accessible discrepancy between perception of the actual self's weight/shape and ideal weight/shape, or what one ought to weigh and look like. For example, when exposed to thin-ideal images, females who have already internalized the slender ideal will automatically access the self-ideal discrepancy. There are, apparently, fewer moderators for males, but more research is needed concerning processes defining and constraining media effects for males. Promising candidates are appearance orientation, investment in the male gender role, and propensity for social comparison.

The Internet and Body Image

The Internet is already the mass medium of the future. Yet, few studies have explored its effects on body image. Millions of people of all ages, worldwide, are involved daily with ad-driven search engines and social networking sites. Given the growing number and burgeoning popularity of celebrity and fashion sites, diet websites, and pro-eating disorder websites, it is unlikely the Internet has no effect on body image.

Pro-Eating Disorder Websites

The estimated 400+ pro-anorexia ("pro-ana") and pro-bulimia ("pro-mia") websites currently operating cater to females ages 12–24 who have an eating disorder or severe body image problems by defying psychology's and psychiatry's definition of eating disorders as highly dangerous biopsychiatric illnesses. These sites view, if not promote, eating disorders as sources of security that are integral parts of the identities and lives of visitors to the sites.

Survey-based studies suggest that pro-ana/mia sites are no more or less toxic for their intended audiences than are "pro-recovery" sites. In contrast, in two controlled laboratory studies female undergraduates who viewed a site with prototypical pro-ana/mia elements immediately reported lower social self-esteem and lower self-efficacy, perceived themselves as being heavier, and reported feeling worse relative to participants who viewed either a fashion website focusing on the female body or a neutral website. This effect was independent of dispositional levels of thin-ideal internalization and disordered eating. Pro-ana/mia websites appear to have harmful effects, but we do not know what effects these sites have on adolescent girls and young women who avidly and frequently seek them out because they already have a full-blown eating disorder.

Intervention on the Web

While the Internet is potentially a dangerous place in terms of body image, it has also become a method to deliver new interventions for body dissatisfaction. Various online, computer-assisted individual and group interventions have shown considerable promise in helping high school students and young women who are struggling with negative body image and unhealthy eating/weight management (see Chapter 50). Undoubtedly, the Internet will be an increasingly important part of prevention, treatment, and support.

Conclusions and Future Directions

More longitudinal studies with males as well as females are needed to clarify the predictive validity of media exposure, motives for media use, and the subjective experience of media influences. This research requires theoretical models of the transactional relationships between specific media content (e.g., the thinness- or muscularity-depicting features); hypothesized processes such as schema activation, social comparison, and affective processes; and media effects. These models need to situate media effects on body image within ecological (including ethnic) and developmental contexts. Further understanding of media effects also requires more attention to (1) development of valid measures of key theoretical constructs; and (2) use and impact of the Internet, and in particular such interactive "spaces" as Facebook, celebrity gossip sites, diet websites, and diet/weight management blogs.

Prevention

Although school-based media literacy programs have produced promising results (see Chapter 49), a multisystem approach is necessary to empower youth and adults to translate sociocultural research into sociocultural change. Scientist-practitioners need to create ways to combine the critical social consciousness fostered in classroom literacy programs with instruction and practice in the activism and advocacy necessary to effect lasting, positive changes in media content (see Chapters 6, 19, 51, and 52).

Clinical Work

Clinicians in all disciplines need to follow the lead of the Society for Adolescent Medicine and the American Academy of Pediatrics in making their own media literacy a priority. However bizarre or frivolous the resources of the World Wide Web (including pro-anorexia and celebrity websites, and marketing by the diet and fitness industries) may seem to clinicians, these media warrant clinical attention precisely because females at higher risk of suffering from an eating disorder are those most likely to seek out portrayals of the ideal body and instructions for attaining it. Clinical assessment of media use, motivation, social comparison, and effects in relation to body image is an important, but underdeveloped area.

Clinicians need to be a model of critical consciousness and active resistance for their patients and their families (and their own families), challenging the media's harmful effects by proactively asserting themselves in, through, and with the media. Knowing that their therapist has taken public and publicized stands to challenge the objectification of the human body and the glorification of thinness and muscularity may help patients struggling with negative body image feel empowered, validated, and hopeful.

Informative Readings

Ata, R. N., Ludden, A. B., & Lally, M. M. (2007). The effects of gender and family, friend, and media influences on eating behaviors and body image during adolescence. *Journal of Youth and Adolescence, 36,* 1024–1037.—Detailed analysis of how adolescent body image and eating are related to variables such as perceived pressures from media.

Bartlett, C. P., Vowels, C. L., & Saucier, D. A. (2008). Meta-analyses of the effects of media on men's body-image concerns. *Journal of Social and Clinical Psychology, 27,* 279–310.—Two statistical reviews demonstrating a small but significant positive relationship between exposure to muscular ideals in the media and negative body image in men.

Dittmar, H. (Ed.). (2009). Body image and eating disorders (no. 3; Special Issue).

Journal of Social and Clinical Psychology, 28(1).—Articles addressing media content, mediating and moderating processes, and body image.

Grabe, S., Ward, L. M., & Hyde, J. S. (2008). The role of the media in body image concerns among women: A meta-analysis of experimental and correlational studies. *Psychological Bulletin, 134,* 460–476.—Review of 77 studies showing that media exposure has a positive relationship with females' body dissatisfaction.

Harrison, K., & Hefner, V. (2006). Media exposure, current and future body ideals, and disordered eating among preadolescent girls: A longitudinal panel study. *Journal of Youth and Adolescence, 3,* 146–156.—One-year follow-up of over 250 preadolescent girls shows that extent of television viewing predicted a thinner postpubescent body ideal.

Jones, D. C., Vigfusdottir, T., & Lee, Y. (2004). Body image and the appearance culture among adolescent girls and boys: An examination of friend conversations, peer criticism, appearance magazines, and the internalization of appearance ideals. *Journal of Adolescent Research, 19,* 323–339.—Cross-sectional study showing that girls ages 11–14, as compared with boys, were more invested in appearance-oriented magazines, were more likely to internalize the beauty ideals in them, and had greater body dissatisfaction.

Levine, M. P., & Murnen, S. K. (2009). "Everybody knows that mass media are/ are *not* a *cause* of eating disorders": A critical review of evidence for a *causal* link between media, negative body image, and disordered eating in females. *Journal of Social and Clinical Psychology, 28,* 9–42.—Review of whether media-effects data for girls and young women meet criteria as a causal risk factor for negative body image.

Schooler, D., Ward, L. M., Merriwether, A., & Caruthers, A. (2004). Who's that girl: Television's role in the body image development of young White and Black women. *Psychology of Women Quarterly, 28,* 38–47.—Examines effects of television aimed at Black and White audiences.

Tiggemann, M. (2006). The role of media exposure in adolescent girls' body dissatisfaction and drive for thinness: Prospective results. *Journal of Social and Clinical Psychology, 25,* 523–541.—Longitudinal study of over 200 Australian girls ages 13–15 demonstrated no effects of media exposure variables.

Trampe, D., Stapel, D. A., & Siero, F. W. (2007). On models and vases: Body dissatisfaction and proneness to social comparison effects. *Journal of Personality and Social Psychology, 92* 106–118.—Set of studies showing that women who are self-conscious about their bodies are vulnerable to body dissatisfaction based on social comparison to a wide variety of targets.

Wilksch, S., & Wade, T. D. (2010). Reduction of shape and weight concern in adolescents: A 30-month controlled evaluation of a media literacy program. *Journal of the American Academy of Child and Adolescent Psychiatry, 48,* 652–661.—Evaluation of an eight-lesson media literacy program for Australian boys and girls ages 13–14.

Interpersonal and Familial Influences on the Development of Body Image

DIANE CARLSON JONES

Introduction

Body image satisfaction is an individual's evaluation of his or her physical size or shape. Although this subjective evaluation is an individual judgment based on internalized values and goals, it reflects and is shaped by experiences with others in the social world.

In this chapter, I review the literature on the influence of interpersonal experiences in the development of body image for children and adolescents. A central principle in developmental theory is that development always takes place in a context. From this principle comes the impetus for examining the interpersonal context as a force in the development of body image. Humans are fundamentally social-relational beings who strive for attachments and acceptance by others, primarily through relationships with parents and peers. These relationships are considered the core social connections that influence body image.

The relational experiences with parents and peers are also embedded in larger sociocultural contexts. From the developmental and sociocultural perspectives, beliefs, values, and norms about appearance are broadly communicated within cultures (e.g., ideal representations in media and art) and enacted in daily lives with parents and peers. The culturally based appearance values intersect with gender to distinguish appearance expectations for boys and girls (see Chapter 19). Masculine and feminine stereotypes are translated into the male appearance ideals of lean, strong, muscular bodies and into the female ideals of thin, sexualized bodies in Western cultures. Females are also more likely to be judged on appearance than are boys and, regardless of race or ethnic background, experience greater body dissatisfaction, beginning around 6–7 years old (see Chapter 8). Thus it is important to remember that although developmental and interpersonal processes are similar for boys and girls, the specific content, goals, and outcomes of appearance-related experiences with parents and peers are highly gendered.

Familial Relations and Body Image

Families provide the primary relationships in development and play a formative role in shaping attitudes and values in their children about body image. Parents express their expectations and beliefs about appearance in the lifestyle patterns they create for eating, dieting, exercise, and evaluation. They serve as models, critics, and advocates in the development of body image starting in early childhood.

Parents serve as models in multiple ways. Their expressed attitudes about appearance as well as their evaluations of their own and each others' bodies serve as models for children and adolescents to value or critique themselves and others. Exercising and dieting activities of the parents serve as behavioral examples for engaging in physical activity or restricting food intake. In married couples, there is more emphasis placed on wives to lose weight than on husbands. The impact of these types of modeling is evident early in development such that the body dissatisfaction of young girls and boys (ages 5–8 years) is related to their perceptions of mothers' body dissatisfaction. Other research indicates that parental modeling may continue to be important through adolescence, though findings are inconsistent.

The characteristics of the parent–child interactions related to appearance can make a direct contribution to body image satisfaction. Both mothers and fathers play critical roles in communicating appearance messages although there are variations among studies in the relative impact of each parent's behavior on body satisfaction. Although parents' positive messages about appearance and general support can serve as protective factors in the development of body image, most research has examined parents' explicit negative messages about appearance that have a deleterious effect on body image. When mothers and fathers put great value on appearance, stress the importance of being thin, and exert pressure on their children to lose weight, girls and boys are more likely to initiate dieting and hold negative views about their appearance and body. The concern with muscularity among boys has also been related to parental messages. Appearance criticism and teasing by mothers and fathers, whether about weight or muscularity, have consistently been related to greater body dissatisfaction, particularly in cross-sectional studies. Overall, families that emphasize appearance and put pressure on attaining appearance ideals are more likely to have children and adolescents with greater body dissatisfaction.

Parents also facilitate and manage children's access to the symbols of the societal appearance culture. Toys and media are among the major representations that are typically part of children's lives. The research tends to show that greater exposure to the stereotyped, ideal appearance images in toys and media is related to increased body dissatisfaction. It may be though that the relationship is also a reflection of the heightened value placed on appearance and traditional gender roles in some families.

It is important to note that the content of the parental modeling and messages varies across families, ethnicities, and cultural groups. For example, in studies of Black populations, there is greater acceptance of larger body sizes, less endorsement of the thin ideal, and higher body satisfaction. Still, parental modeling, messages, and managing of the access to toys and media are similar ways in which parents across cultures influence the body image of their children.

The role of siblings in the development of body image has also been investigated. The limited research suggests that siblings are likely to share similar levels of body dissatisfaction and can actively reinforce change strategies such as weight loss. Appearance teasing is also fairly common among siblings, especially by older brothers, but is more likely to occur in families in which parents tease children about appearance. When both parental and sibling behaviors and attitudes are considered in multidimensional models, it is typically parents' behavior and attitudes that best predict body dissatisfaction. These types of findings suggest that sibling experiences reflect general family dynamics rather than contribute uniquely to body image. Further research is needed that examines the effects of sibling gender, birth order, and ages of siblings within the complexities of family system dynamics.

Peer Relations and the Peer Appearance Culture

Experiences with peers represent another important social context for the development of body image. Peers have been linked to body image development in research on friendship, popularity, peer acceptance, peer teasing, and romantic partners. Children and adolescents bring to these peer interactions the values and expectations about appearance and gender they have learned in the family. They further create an appearance culture with their peers that is governed by norms and expectations that are modeled and reinforced by peers. These accumulated interpersonal experiences within the peer appearance culture thus reflect and shape individual behaviors and attitudes about body image of self and others.

Friends and Cliques

Friends and extended friendship groups known as cliques typically share similar interests and values in a variety of areas including appearance. Friends tend to have similar attitudes toward the importance of appearance and similar experiences in appearance change strategies such as dieting, disordered eating, and muscle building. These relationships are typically stronger when the assessments of body satisfaction of self and friends are completed by the same person. A more rigorous way to test the similarity of body image or related concerns is to obtain independent assessments by the nominated friends. When independent assessments of body dissatisfaction are correlated for clique members, there is less consistent evidence for the concordance of body dissatisfaction in friendship groups.

The level of endorsement of the peer appearance culture among friends does matter for body image. When friends share a heightened concern with appearance and endorse societal weight/shape ideals, then patterns of greater body dissatisfaction are evident. In cross-sectional studies of preadolescents and adolescents, appearance-oriented friends and cliques report talking more about dieting, acknowledging the importance of friends in the decision to diet, comparing their bodies more often, and teasing each other about weight and shape. In longitudinal research, perceived friend dieting is a prospective risk factor for body dissatisfaction, especially in early-adolescent girls.

Another way in which friends influence body image concerns is through conversations about appearance and body change strategies such as dieting and muscle building. The attention and reinforcement given to appearance issues in conversations with friends highlight appearance as an important attribute, support the construction of appearance norms and ideals, encourage social comparison, and facilitate evaluation of the self relative to others on physical attributes. Research verifies that preadolescent and adolescent girls and boys who report more frequent conversations with their friends about appearance also report greater body dissatisfaction. For girls, appearance conversations with friends are a prospective contributor to body dissatisfaction.

Appearance conversations can also train individuals to be highly evaluative of appearance. "Fat talk" (e.g., "I'm so fat") has been highlighted as a discourse style among White adolescent girls in which they repeatedly criticize and lament the size of their own body in the presence of peers. It has been suggested that "fat talk" solicits peer assurances (e.g., "No, you're not") and promotes group solidarity. However, the repeated experiences of verbalizing these negative self-evaluations have the potential to normalize self-disparaging discourse and internalize a critical judgmental stance toward one's own body, increasing the likelihood of body dissatisfaction. These types of conversations may be less prevalent among

Black adolescent girls who have reported more positive appearance feedback among friends and greater body satisfaction.

Positive friendship characteristics such as communication, trust, and acceptance have been studied among high school girls. They are neither correlated with body dissatisfaction nor appear to serve as protective factors. Rather negative friendship qualities (alienation and conflict) are the features that are most frequently related to body dissatisfaction. In addition, the loss of friendships can be especially problematic in early adolescence. In a longitudinal study of early-adolescent boys and girls, loss of friendships over a school year predicted decreases in body esteem but not in other dimensions of self-esteem. This finding indicates the vital impact of friendships on the developing body image.

Peer Popularity, Peer Acceptance, Peer Teasing, and Romantic Partners

Peer experiences in schools are embedded in the social hierarchy of the peer ecology. At the top of the social hierarchy are popular students who have greater access to the attention and resources of the school community. Popular students are identified by students as the most prominent source of peer appearance pressure at school presumably because "ideal" body shapes are evident in popular groups. Indeed, higher levels of popularity are associated with boys' reports of thinner, muscular figures, whereas heavier figures are related to lower levels of popularity. Among girls, smaller body shapes are a factor connected to popularity. In a recent study of older high school students, dieting behavior was most prevalent among popular boys and girls. Thus the appearance ideals and appearance change strategies that are modeled by the higher-status students presumably set the standards for individual evaluation.

Not everyone is or wants to be popular. Most children and adolescents do want to be accepted and liked by peers. Although peer-rated acceptance measures have been inconsistently related to body image satisfaction, individuals' perceptions of their acceptance by peers have been consistently related to body image among children and adolescents. Individuals who think that social acceptance is achieved by conforming to appearance ideals often engage in "if only" cognitions. For girls, these beliefs have been evaluated for being thinner ("If only I were thinner, then girls/boys would talk more to me"); for boys, the focus has been on either being thinner or being more muscular ("If only I were more muscular, then girls/boys would like me more"). When peer acceptance is perceived to be based in conformity to appearance ideals, girls and boys are at greater risk for negative body image.

Peers directly communicate their critiques of appearance via teasing. Teasing about weight is considered to be the most hurtful and least humorous form. Friends and male peers are identified as the most frequent perpetrators. Because teasing generally is deemed socially acceptable especially among friends, the effects of appearance teasing can be underestimated. Appearance teasing is not innocuous banter, but is a potent way to reinforce appearance standards and critique deviations from the norm. It frequently meets several of the criteria for bullying. It is not surprising then that in cross-sectional studies appearance teasing is consistently related to lower body satisfaction for both girls and boys regardless of ethnicity or body size. The prospective contribution of appearance teasing to body image satisfaction has not been as evident. Further research is needed to determine whether the impact of appearance teasing is indirect in its effects on body image through other potential contributors such as self-esteem or negative affect or whether the relationship between teasing and body dissatisfaction is moderated by other factors such as BMI or perceived rejection.

Body concerns are driven in part by issues of attractiveness to potential romantic partners. Body image dissatisfaction and dieting are greater for early-adolescent girls who are sexually involved with boys, especially for White adolescents. Dating does not appear to have this direct relationship to body dissatisfaction and dieting in high school girls when romantic relationships are more normative. For high school girls, the linkage between body dissatisfaction and romantic relations is based more on the importance of being popular with boys and the perceived importance of thinness to boys. If being popular with the other sex and having a romantic partner are deemed important, then adolescent girls are more likely to have negative body image.

It is true that body shape and weight are important features for attracting romantic partners for males and females. Research indicates that by adolescence, boys have internalized the sociocultural beliefs regarding attractiveness and thinness and tend to look for romantic partners based on physical appearance more so than girls do. For boys, thinness is important in making a girl appear attractive and in deciding whether to go out with her. Obese girls, but not boys, are more likely to report no dating experience than their peers. These phenomena create indirect pressure on girls to be thin and increase the likelihood of body dissatisfaction.

It is remarkable how little research is available for boys, adolescents of color, and gay, lesbian, bisexual, and transgender students. Given the importance of romantic relationships in adolescence and adulthood, this is a serious oversight that limits our understanding of the role of romantic relationships in the development of body image.

Conclusions and Future Directions

Body image satisfaction reflects the accumulation of individual experiences in relational and cultural contexts. This review provides evidence that parents and peers are powerful agents in shaping body satisfaction. The cultural body ideals are conveyed and reinforced by parents, friends, peers, and (potential) romantic partners. When the relational pressures and messages about ideal expectations for appearance are consistent in valued relationships, then children and adolescents are more likely to internalize them and experience body image dissatisfaction.

There is still much to be learned about the characteristics and dynamics of interpersonal relationships affecting body image. Distinct interpersonal relationships with parents and peers are often considered as independent contributors to body image. In the lives of individuals, these relationships are complexly interrelated, but whether the influence patterns are convergent, contradictory, or sequential is not well explicated. In the majority of cases, they are likely to converge in their impact as individuals internalize the values and messages in each interpersonal context and carry those across relationships. Alternatively, it is possible that the different relationships present distinct messages for children and adolescents. In this instance, parents or peers may provide the counterpoint for the type of experiences that individuals encounter such as when individuals with greater body mass experience teasing and rejection by peers, but have parents who are accepting. Finally, the dynamics of influence may also change across time as relationships change in their relative salience. Early in development, parental influence typically is especially powerful, whereas friends and peers tend to increase in importance during preadolescence and adolescence. This pattern too may vary by the quality of relationships, as well as cultural and ethnic values. It is clear that further research is needed to explore the complexity and patterning of convergent, contradictory, and/or the sequential influence of parents and peers on body image.

The importance of parents and peers in the development of body image points to the value of integrating the issues related to these central relations into prevention and intervention programs to improve body image satisfaction. Given the impact of families on body image development, it is surprising that there are few interventions that help families with young children and adolescents to promote healthy lifestyles and to accept a range of body types. Over a decade ago, Paxton elaborated ways to include peer relations into all levels of body image prevention and intervention. The need still exists to design and evaluate prevention and intervention programs that address parent and peer influences on body image and support body image satisfaction at all ages.

Informative Readings

Jones, D. C. (2004). Body image among adolescent girls and boys: A longitudinal study. *Developmental Psychology, 40,* 823–835.—An empirical analysis evaluating the prospective contributions of appearance conversations, teasing, and other variables to body dissatisfaction.

Jones, D. C., & Crawford, J. K. (2006). The peer appearance culture during adolescence: Gender and body mass variations. *Journal of Youth and Adolescence, 35,* 257–269.—An examination of appearance conversations, peer evaluations, and peer acceptance concerns.

Jones, D. C., Newman, J. B., & Bautista, S. (2005). A three-factor model of teasing: The influence of friendship, gender, and topic on expected emotional reactions to teasing during early adolescence. *Social Development, 14,* 421–439.—Empirical studies documenting the perceived hurtfulness of appearance teasing for boys and girls.

Lowes, J., & Tiggemann, M. (2003). Body dissatisfaction, dieting awareness, and the impact of parental influence in young children. *British Journal of Health Psychology, 8,* 135–147.—Data from interviews with young children provide evidence for maternal influence on young children's body image.

MacDonald Clarke, P., Murnen, S., & Smolak, L. (2010). Development and psychometric evaluation of a quantitative measure of "fat talk." *Body Image: An International Journal of Research, 7,* 1–7.—Describes the "fat talk" phenomenon and presents a measure that will be useful in future research.

McCabe, M. P., & Ricciardelli, L. A. (2004). Weight and shape concerns of boys and men. In J. K. Thompson (Ed.), *Handbook of eating disorders and obesity* (pp. 606–634). New York: Wiley.—Narrative literature review of factors affecting male body image at different developmental ages.

Parker, S., Nichter, M., Nichter, M., Vuckovic, N., Sims, C., & Ritenbaugh, C. (1995). Body image and weight concerns among African American and White adolescent females: Differences that make a difference. *Human Organization, 54,* 103–114.—Qualitative analyses of themes from focus groups and interviews that contrast the perceptions and concepts regarding body image, beauty, and friendship support.

Paxton, S. J. (1999). Peer relations, body image, and disordered eating in adolescent girls: Implications for prevention. In N. Piran, M. P. Levine, & C. Steiner-Adair (Eds.), *Preventing Eating Disorders: A Handbook of Interventions and Special Challenges* (pp. 134–147). Philadelphia: Brunner/Mazel.—A narrative literature review on aspects of friendships and peer relations that relate to body image with extended consideration of applications to prevention and intervention programs.

Paxton, S. J. (2005). Body dissatisfaction, dating, and importance of thinness to attractiveness in adolescent girls. *Sex Roles, 53,* 663–675.—Research describing the linkage between dating and body image satisfaction.

Paxton, S. J., Eisenberg, M. E., & Neumark-Sztainer, D. (2006). Prospective predictors of body dissatisfaction in adolescent girls and boys: A five-year longitudinal study. *Developmental Psychology, 42,* 888–899.—A longitudinal study of early and midadolescent girls and boys assessing the contributions of family, physical, peer, and psychological variables to body dissatisfaction.

Rogers, R. F., Paxton, S. J., & Chabrol, H. (2009). Effects of parental comments on body dissatisfaction and eating disturbances in young adults: A sociocultural model. *Body Image: An International Journal of Research, 6,* 171–177.—Examines the direct and mediated effects of positive and negative parental comments on body dissatisfaction.

Smolak, L., & Thompson, J. K. (2009). *Body image, eating disorders, and obesity in youth: Assessment, prevention, and treatment* (2nd ed.). Washington, DC: American Psychological Association.—Edited volume with chapters related to parental influence (Fisher et al.), body image in boys and girls (Ricciardelli et al., Wertheim et al.), and cross-cultural issues (Anderson-Fye).

Wang, S. S., Houshyar, S., & Prinstein, M. J. (2006). Adolescent girls' and boys' weight-related health behaviors and cognitions: Associations with reputation- and preference-based peer status. *Health Psychology, 25,* 658–663.—Empirical evidence supporting the relationship between body size and peer-reported popularity.

Sexual Abuse and Body Image

LINDA SMOLAK

Introduction

The relationship of sexual abuse to eating disorders has been debated for at least 30 years. Most of the focus has been on child sexual abuse (CSA). Researchers have also examined the effects of dating violence, rape, and sexual harassment on eating attitudes and behaviors. There is increasing consensus that there are important relationships among the various forms of sexual abuse and disordered eating. The core issue of the present chapter is the role of body image in these relationships.

Furthermore, other forms of body-related behaviors, most notably self-harm, are associated with CSA experiences. This relationship underscores the impact of CSA on body image. Self-harm behaviors are frequently part of borderline personality disorder (BPD) that is comorbid with eating disorders. This combination provides the opportunity to identify possible broad principles of the effects of CSA and other forms of sexual abuse on body image.

This chapter is divided into four sections. In the first, the relationships among the various forms of sexual abuse and body image are reviewed. This section includes some consideration of eating disorders and BPD. The second section delineates theoretical explanations of these relationships. The third section discusses treatment and prevention. The concluding section identifies questions for future research.

Sexual Abuse and Body Image

Feminist theorists argue that there is a continuum of sexual violence ranging from sexual and gender harassment at one end to violent rape at the

119

other. Limited research has supported this concept, indicating, for example, that sexual harassment increases women's fear of rape. Therefore, this review considers various forms of sexual abuse.

Child Sexual Abuse

Some research has found CSA to be related to negative body image during adulthood. These studies have focused mainly on women. It is noteworthy that not all studies have found this relationship. This is at least in part attributable to the typical difficulties of trying to correlate childhood experiences with adult behaviors. It also reflects methodological differences in definitions of CSA as well as differences in samples in terms of willingness and ability to disclose CSA experiences.

CSA has also been associated with eating disorders, including in a meta-analysis by Smolak and Murnen. CSA appears to be associated particularly with bulimia nervosa (BN) and binge-eating disorder (BED). The relationship to BED may partly explain the modest correlation between CSA and obesity in adulthood. Disordered eating attitudes and behaviors, as measured, for example, by the Eating Attitudes Test, have also been related to CSA. In fact, some cross-cultural studies also report this relationship.

The relationship of CSA to body dissatisfaction and eating pathology tends to be small to moderate. Other forms of childhood trauma, including physical and emotional abuse, are similarly correlated with disordered eating. In fact, in some studies, physical and emotional abuse are more strongly linked to disordered eating than CSA. Of course, a substantial portion of clients with eating disorders were not sexually abused.

Numerous reviewers have noted that CSA is not a specific predictor of disordered eating. CSA is related to a variety of disorders; BPD is one of these. Research does suggest that CSA, perhaps as mediated by negative affective states including guilt and shame, is part of one pathway to BPD, though there certainly are BPD sufferers who were not abused. This is of interest in the current chapter for two reasons. First, there is evidence that BPD is a risk factor for eating disorders. Second, and more directly, there may be body image disturbances in BPD. Though data are limited, they indicate that there is a positive correlation between BPD symptoms and body dissatisfaction, even after controlling for participants' body weight. Furthermore, clients with BPD seeking cosmetic surgery ask for more extensive surgery than those without the diagnosis. Finally, BPD is associated with a variety of self-harm behaviors, including directly injuring one's body through cutting or burning. Some theorists have argued that eating disorders are part of the constellation of self-harm behaviors. Bjärehed and Lundh have specifically reported a small-to-moderate negative correlation between self-harm behaviors and body esteem among adolescent girls but not boys. They also found that eating disorders symptoms were positively related to self-harm among girls but not boys.

Thus, there appear to be direct as well as indirect relationships between CSA and body image concerns. In addition, eating disorders (particularly BN and BED) and BPD, which both are associated with and arguably indicative of body image problems, are correlated with CSA experiences.

Other Forms of Sexual Abuse

Other forms of sexual abuse have also been linked to body image. Studies with children, adolescents, and adults have reported correlations between sexual harassment and reduced body esteem or satisfaction, especially among females (see Chapter 13). Harassment by strangers has been positively correlated with self-objectification, including body shame (see Chapter 6). Gender harassment, which includes both traditionally defined sexual harassment and negative comments or teasing about the entire gender, is extremely common among adolescents and young adults. Indeed, even bullying of girls by boys is often sexualized. Interestingly, qualitative data suggest that adolescent girls and their teachers think they see a link between eating disorders and gender teasing by boy classmates.

In an Italian sample, Faravelli and colleagues report an association between rape during adulthood and binge eating and purging. Other forms of trauma that threaten physical integrity, such as automobile accidents, were not similarly related to eating disorders.

Theoretical Explanations

Body shame is probably the most commonly cited mediator of the CSA–eating disorders relationship. Thompson and Wonderlich provide a specific description of this process. Girls who have been victims of CSA feel ashamed of and disgusted by their bodies. The girl becomes contemptuous of her body and wants to destroy it. Thus, she purges or starves herself. Less dramatically, a girl might diet to try to change her appearance. This dieting might, in turn, trigger binge eating, which can then lead to purging in order to avoid the weight gain that binges might bring. There is empirical evidence that body dissatisfaction mediates the relationship between CSA and disordered eating.

Clearly, this sense of body shame might be related to other forms of self-harm, including cutting. Severe forms of CSA may lead to a sense of the body being threatened in a way that is frightening. These emotions of shame and fear can sometimes become overwhelming. This requires an escape through a coping mechanism that is as extreme as the emotion. Self-harm is such a mechanism. It is important to emphasize that the girls and women who engage in these self-harm behaviors report their emotions as physical sensations. They are trying to regain control of their body and their relationship to it and are trying to cope with their perception of their body. Horne and Csipke suggest that self-harmers misperceive the relationship between their body and emotions in a variety of ways. These include an inability to perceive pain or other physical sensations, a dissociative sense of being disembodied as if ownership of one's body has been compromised, and a threat to physical reality. Thus, in BPD, it is not just body shame that is at work but also one's ability to accurately perceive the status of one's body.

Sansone and Sansone further suggest that such self-harm behaviors aim to restore or repair the body by reducing the physical sensations. When this mode of thinking combines with body dissatisfaction, the girl may opt to repair her body via disordered eating. This risk is particularly high when the girl lives in a family or social context that emphasizes thinness.

Piran has suggested the "disrupted embodiment through inequity" model. This model links adverse gender-based experiences with body weight and shape preoccupation as well as with disordered eating patterns. Two of the three broad types of gender-related social experiences hypothesized to contribute to the development of body dissatisfaction and disordered eating among girls and women are relevant to the current discussion. The first type is "disruption to body ownership." This includes a range of experiences that violate the experience of a rightful and safe ownership of one's body, such as the objectification and sexualization of the body, breaching of one's privacy, sexual harassment, and a range of sexual and physical violations. Piran has reported qualitative and quantitative data supporting her model, including the importance of this body-ownership component. CSA, sexual violence during adulthood, and sexual harassment all contributed to the body-ownership variable. The quantitative data include both college and community samples of women. In the second of her three types of negative gender-related experiences, Piran includes gender harassment as a contributor to "exposure to prejudicial treatment." The role of gender harassment in creating prejudicial treatment and the subsequent relationship of prejudicial treatment to disordered eating was again confirmed with college and community women.

What these theoretical models all suggest is that sexual violence makes a girl's body seem foreign to her, as if it does not belong. Sexual and gender harassment and bullying, as well as sexual violence, contribute to feelings that the body is disrespected, disgusting, or inadequate. The attempt to cope with such emotions contributes to the development of symptoms associated with eating disorders and BPD.

Treatment and Prevention

There is now substantial agreement that various forms of sexual abuse and violence contribute to the development of negative body image, at least among White American women. CSA also contributes to the development of eating disorders and BPDs, relationships that are likely mediated by body dissatisfaction. These findings have implications for both treatment and prevention.

Treatment

CSA survivors may struggle more with eating disorders treatment than other clients with eating disorders. Rodríguez, Pérez, and García investigated the relationship of CSA to treatment success in Colombian women diagnosed with eating disorders. The risk of not responding satisfactorily after 4 months of treatment was more than twice as high among CSA victims while their dropout rate was three times higher. These findings suggest that women with CSA experiences may require special forms of treatment.

It is important that women, and perhaps men, presenting with eating disorders or BPD, be evaluated for a history of CSA or other forms of sexual violence. It is possible that people with comorbid eating disorders and BPD are particularly likely candidates. It is possible that their body image issues are not solely the dissatisfaction commonly found among clients with eating disorders. Rather, they may also reflect the CSA trauma itself, including issues of ownership and safety.

Several theorists have suggested that feminist approaches, emphasizing empowerment, may be important elements of the treatment of CSA survivors. Empowerment refers to both a sense of personal control and an investment in political activism to alter the societal institutions and attitudes that foster sexual violence, as well as body image disturbances. Empowerment may allow women to feel that they have control over their body and that their body is adequate and loveable. It may help CSA survivors to feel that they have power within their own lives. Part of this process is helping the client to recognize that the context within which sexual violence, including sexual harassment, occurs contributes to the translation of CSA into eating disorders and self-harm. Research has found that empowerment, measured using a questionnaire such as the one developed by Johnson, Worell, and Chandler, is associated with more positive body image and lower disordered eating.

Prevention

Girls and women who have been victims of CSA and other forms of sexual abuse are likely to benefit from psychological evaluation and treatment. However, many, perhaps most, do not report the assault in a timely manner. Thus, as is true with unrecognized body image and eating problems, prevention programs play an important role in reducing the likelihood that serious psychiatric disorders will develop.

Piran and others have argued that feminist models can also be help-ful in developing effective prevention programs. Feminist prevention programs have two foci that are particularly relevant for girls who have been exposed to or are concerned about sexual violence (again, includ-ing sexual harassment). First, as is true of feminist treatment programs, feminist prevention programs emphasize empowerment. Programs such as Steiner-Adair and Sjostrom's *Full of Ourselves* help girls and women to feel stronger and more in control of their body. They also aim to help girls resolve threats against their body. However, feminist programs do not solely teach girls self-defense or effective coping strategies. Instead, the programs explicitly acknowledge that girls develop their behaviors within a societal context that supports sexualization, and hence sexual abuse, against them. Thus, consistent with principles of feminist empow-erment, the girls are taught not only individual coping strategies but are encouraged to engage in political activism to change objectifying and sex-ualizing social messages (see also Chapter 6).

This is the second relevant focus of feminist prevention. Feminist pre-vention seeks to actually change the context within which body image, eating, and personality problems develop. For example, Piran worked with school administrators at a national ballet school to actively address concerns that girls had about sexual and gender harassment as well as other forms of inappropriate treatment of their body. The school instituted new rules in these realms and worked to train teachers and others (includ-ing boy students) about appropriate treatment of the girls and their body. It is crucial to emphasize that these changes were made because of the girls' comments about their actual experiences. Thus, the changes became a form of empowerment.

Conclusions and Future Directions

There is solid evidence that CSA and other forms of sexual abuse contrib-ute to body image problems. Research needs to more thoroughly identify precisely what these body image problems involve in terms of percep-tions, attitudes, affect, and actions. There is reason to believe that these body image problems can translate into eating disorders as well as BPD. However, it is equally clear that sexual violence does not automatically translate into a psychiatric disorder, much less specifically into eating dis-orders or BPD. Therefore, much more research is needed to specify media-tors and moderators of the sexual violence, body image, eating disorders, and BPD relationships. Gender and ethnicity should be among the mod-erators considered. Too much of the currently available research focuses on White American girls and women.

As part of the process of identifying these developmental pathways, research delineating protective factors is arguably as important as that

concerning risk factors. For example, is empowerment a means of inter-
rupting the negative effects of CSA? Can protecting body image, via universal media literacy programs, for example (see Chapter 12), help to prevent the negative effects of CSA? Or are the body concerns of CSA victims
sufficiently unique as to require specialized programming?

In asking questions about the efficacy of various treatment and prevention approaches, researchers can help to identify some of the risk and
protective factors for the progression of sexual abuse into body image and
then eating or personality disorders. The need for such research is pressing and immediate.

Informative Readings

Bjärehed, J., & Lundh, L. (2008). Deliberate self-harm in 14-year-old adolescents:
How frequent is it, and how is it associated with psychopathology, relationship variables, and styles of emotional regulation? *Cognitive Behaviour Therapy*, 37, 26–37.—Considers the relationship between body image and self-
harm in boys and girls.

Faravelli, C., Giugni, A., Salvatori, S., & Ricca, V. (2004). Psychopathology after
rape. *American Journal of Psychiatry*, 161, 1483–1485.—Italian study demonstrating the associations between an adult trauma, rape, and eating disorders,
as well as other psychiatric disorders.

Horne, O., & Csipke, E. (2009). From feeling too little and too much, to feeling
more and less? A nonparadoxical theory of the functions of self-harm. *Qualitative Health Research*, 19, 655–667.—Includes a description of several body
image problems associated with BPD.

McGilley, B. H. (2004). Feminist perspectives on self-harm behavior and eating disorders. In J. Levitt, R. Sansone, & L. Cohn (Eds.), *Self-harm behavior and eating
disorders: Dynamics, assessment, and treatment* (pp. 75–89). New York: Brunner-
Routledge.—Considers feminist principles in the prevention and treatment
of self-harm and disordered eating.

Piran, N. (2001). Re-inhabiting the body from the inside out: Girls transform their
school environment. In D. L. Tolman & M. Brydon-Miller (Eds.), *From subjects
to subjectivities: A handbook of interpretive and participatory methods* (pp. 218–
238). New York: New York University Press.—Basis for the adverse social
experiences model and summary of a feminist prevention program.

Preti, A., Incani, E., Camboni, M. V., Petretto, D. R., & Masala, C. (2006). Sexual
abuse and eating disorder symptoms: The mediator role of body dissatisfaction. *Comprehensive Psychiatry*, 47, 475–481.—A study of young adult, Italian women documenting the mediating role of body image in links between
broadly defined sexual abuse and disordered eating.

Rodríguez, M., Pérez, V., & García, Y. (2005) Impact of traumatic experiences and
violent acts upon response to treatment of a sample of Colombian women with
eating disorders. *International Journal of Eating Disorders*, 37, 299–306.—Evaluates the impact of adult traumata on eating disorders.

Sansone, R., & Sansone, L. (2007). Childhood trauma, borderline personality, and eating disorders: A developmental cascade. *Eating Disorders, 15,* 333–346.—Theoretical model of the links among CSA and BPD and eating disorders.

Smolak, L., & Levine, M. P. (2007). Trauma, eating problems, and eating disorders. In S. Wonderlich, J. Mitchell, H. Steiger, & M. deZwaan (Eds.), *Annual review of eating disorders: Part I–2007* (pp. 113–124). New York: Radcliffe/Oxford.— Considers psychological and neurobiological factors while reviewing sexual assault–eating problems research.

Smolak, L., & Piran, N. (in press). Gender and the prevention of eating disorders. In G. McVey, B. Ferguson, M. Levine, & N. Piran (Eds.), *Improving the prevention of eating-related disorders: Collaborative research, advocacy, and policy change.* Waterloo, Ontario, Canada: Wilfred Laurier University Press.—A discussion of how gendered experiences, including sexual abuse, contribute to eating problems and their prevention.

Steiner-Adair, C., & Sjostrom, L. (2006). *Full of ourselves: A wellness program to advance girl power, health, and leadership.* New York: Teachers College Press.—A feminist-oriented body image and eating disturbance prevention program.

Thompson, K. M., & Wonderlich, S. (2004). Child sexual abuse and eating disorders. In J. K. Thompson (Ed.), *Handbook of eating disorders and obesity* (pp. 679–694). Hoboken, NJ: Wiley.—An important discussion of theoretical and empirical issues.

PART III

BODY IMAGE ASSESSMENT

CHAPTER 15

Crucial Considerations in the Assessment of Body Image

THOMAS F. CASH

Introduction

The scientific value of research on body image can only be as good as the tools employed in the measurement of this multidimensional construct. Over the past decade, there have been significant advances in the development and validation of body image assessments. The primary purpose of the present chapter is to highlight important considerations and practices for researchers, as well as clinical practitioners, in their selection and use of the available assessments. This author's intent is to provide practical guidance informed by over 30 years of experience in developing and validating body image assessments and editorial experience in evaluating body image research for publication. This chapter may be particularly helpful to newcomers to the field. The subsequent three chapters in this section of the handbook identify and discuss many of the available body image assessments.

What Do You Want to Measure?

Body Image Is Body Images

Researchers who want to measure "body image" must give careful thought to what they really mean by this term. Most often, they mean something like "how people feel about their body." So perhaps they want a measure of body image satisfaction–dissatisfaction. They might wish to assess feelings of physical self-consciousness or feelings of shame about their appearance. Maybe the desired concept isn't so much about "feelings" but is more about persons' beliefs about their appearance, such as beliefs about its attractiveness or how well it matches their personal ideals or the extent to which they appreciate their body. On the other hand, for some researchers, the need is for a measure of how people "feel" about a more specific physical characteristic, such as weight or shape or muscularity or facial features. It is essential that investigators give thought to these distinctions within the context of the specific aims of their study, because each calls for a different assessment of evaluative body image. Similarly, investigators of interventions to treat or prevent body image problems should select outcome measures that match the goals or foci of these interventions. Such measures should have supportive evidence of their ability to detect change.

While evaluative body image measurement is the focal concept of many studies, additional dimensions are essential to the understanding of body image functioning. For example, body image investment pertains to the cognitive and behavioral importance that individuals place in their physical appearance. This significant component of the body image construct is properly receiving growing attention in the scientific literature. Depending on their goals, researchers should consider not only how people evaluate their looks but also how important their looks are to them and their sense of self-worth.

In the past decade, advances in body image scholarship have produced advances in assessment, particularly the assessment of specific aspects of body image functioning that transcend simple satisfaction–dissatisfaction measurements. These tools not only include measures of body image investment but also measures of body image behaviors, thought processes, coping strategies, body image emotions in a range of situational contexts, and the impact of body image experiences on the quality of life. Following a period in which body image research focused almost exclusively on girls and women and their concerns about attainment of a thin ideal and reports of eating pathology, there has been a growth in the development of assessments for boys and men and concerns about muscularity and leanness. Furthermore, as Chapter 17 discusses, assessments using crude figural depictions of a continuum of body sizes for persons to select self-percepts and ideal percepts are gradually being replaced by more sophisticated methods, including the use of computerized digital imaging.

Trait Assessments versus State and Contextual Assessments

The majority of body image research pertains to trait dimensions—persons' general dispositions to feel, think, or act in certain ways.

However, as discussed in Chapter 5, an individual's body image experiences vary as a function of specific situational contexts. For example, a woman may report that she is dispositionally dissatisfied with her weight. However, it is unlikely that she constantly experiences this discontent or dysphoria. Perhaps when at the beach or when trying on outfits at a clothing store, she is especially cognizant of and feels extremely bothered about her weight. When going to the movies with her husband she doesn't feel particularly concerned and after exercising she actually feels rather content about her weight.

A very important area of research considers how body image experiences wax and wane. Such investigations call for state assessments—measures of how people think or feel about their body at specific points in time, especially as a function of certain situations or events. For example, state measures are essential in experimental studies of the momentary effects of exposure to media images that depict societal ideals of appearance versus exposure to control stimuli.

Another type of research that requires state measures is called ecological momentary assessment (EMA). Recently, several EMA studies of body image have been published. These studies used various electronic technologies (e.g., telephonic data entry, personal data assistant) to assess persons' momentary body image evaluations at random or quasi-random points in their daily life. For example, EMA studies by Melnyk et al. and Rudiger et al. evaluated the predictors of women's evaluative body image states and the intra-individual variability in these states assessed one or more times per day over several days. In 2008, Leahey and Crowther investigated predictors of the influences of naturally occurring appearance-focused social comparisons on women's affect, appearance esteem, and thoughts about dieting.

A variant of state assessments measures body image experiences within specified contexts rather than experiences in general. These contextual assessments serve to enhance our understanding of body image functioning beyond trait-level concepts. For example, the Body Exposure during Sexual Activities Questionnaire (BESAQ) measures physical self-consciousness and exposure avoidance during sexual intimacy. Research findings consistently confirm that this contextual body image measure surpasses trait body satisfaction–dissatisfaction in the prediction of the quality of sexual functioning (see Chapter 31).

Chapter 18 provides information on some of the state body image measures that have been used in research. In effect, these assessments use Likert-type scales or visual analogue scales to query participants about what they feel (or think) right now, at this moment. One should never use body image trait questionnaires to measure states, as they would likely lack sensitivity.

Who Is Your Target Population?

Age

One must select age-appropriate body image assessments. Unfortunately, fewer measures have been developed for children (see Chapter 16) than for adolescents and adults (see Chapter 18). The latter instruments are apt to be more complex, require higher levels of reading comprehension, and may include items that are not relevant or appropriate for children. The key is to determine whether the assessment you have in mind has actually been validated for the specific age group you are studying.

Sex and Gender

Male bodies differ from female bodies, and cultures emphasize different appearance standards or ideals for the sexes. Thus body image issues are gender influenced. Body image research has also been gender influenced, in great part because of its history in attempting to understand body image issues of girls and women who are more physically objectified and at greater risk for eating disorders in many cultures. As a result, the study of male body image is a "Johnny come lately." Some body image assessments reflect this bias and may be less useful for boys or men. Other recent assessments have been designed for men only. Researchers who wish to study and compare both sexes are well advised to be certain that the chosen assessment produces measures that are similarly reliable and valid for both sexes.

Culture

This handbook contains many chapters that speak to the influence of culture on body image. In recent years, body image research is expanding internationally, especially to non-English-speaking countries. However, most extant assessments were developed in English, within Western cultures. One cannot simply translate the existing assessment into another language and assume that it works for that culture. The translation of instruments must follow a systematic process (e.g., at minimum, forward and backward translation and reconciliation of disparities). Of course, merely translating words to equivalency does not assure that the construct has the same meaning across cultures. Because different cultures may present different issues relevant to body image, mechanical translations of questionnaires cannot capture the true meaning of the construct for a given culture. It is likely that this goal can only be accomplished with a thoughtful combination of qualitative and quantitative research. One should never force one cultural construct to represent that of another culture.

How Do You Evaluate Your Options?

The selection of a body image assessment should never be an impulsive decision based upon the judgment that "It's called a body image measure" or "It's a popular measure" or "It's got good psychometrics." Yes, it should have evidence of good reliability and validity across studies in the recently published literature, but your study's population must fall within the reasonable generalization of this literature.

A crucial test, assuming the science looks good, is for the researcher (and others) to actually read the instructions and the items for the assessments under consideration. After all, this is what the research participants will do. Does this reading reinforce the belief that this is the right assessment? I illustrate with reference to the oft-used Body Image Avoidance Questionnaire by Rosen et al. A reading of the items creates doubt about whether they really measure body image avoidance or could reflect something else entirely. The instructions simply ask that individuals rate how frequently they engage in certain behaviors, such as being inactive, wearing disliked or baggy or darker clothes, restricting food intake, and avoiding physical intimacy. Might one endorse these items for reasons that have nothing to do with body image concerns?

Caveats in the Use of Your Chosen Assessments

Administrative Considerations

Increasingly, rather than giving participants paper questionnaires to fill out, researchers administer instruments via computer (e.g., online studies). If so, it is important to be sure that the presentation of instructions, items, and response format match the established instrument and translate effectively to the screen or webpage.

In studies with multiple assessments, researchers must think carefully about the order in which these assessments are presented. Some assessments lead participants to immerse themselves in a topic that may affect their answers to subsequent questionnaires. For example, this author published an experimental study confirming that asking participants to initially report their height, weight, and desired weight in a "demographics" questionnaire worsened their body image evaluation, relative to the absence of these questions prior to the body image questionnaire. In such research, one must always think about the sequencing of assessments to avoid reactivity, whereby answering one set of questions affects answers to the next set of questions. Similarly, in experimental research to determine the momentary effects of an independent variable, asking participants to complete a pre- and posttest measure within a short period of time may be unwise, as this can be transparent and induce experimental demand.

Scoring Considerations

It is crucial that researchers closely heed developers' scoring instructions for the selected assessments. First of all, some inventories may have subscales that must be scored separately and cannot be collapsed. For example, one version of this author's Multidimensional Body-Self Relations Questionnaire (MBSRQ) has five multi-item subscales, each producing its own score. To collapse across these subscales to create a single composite score would yield a meaningless and internally inconsistent body image index. In addition, many questionnaires intentionally include items that are stated in a converse manner and must be reverse-scored (e.g., some positively worded items and some negatively worded items). Researchers should always calculate and report the internal consistency of scores derived from their own study sample. If inspection of the item-total correlations indicates negative correlations, this may signal a failure to reverse-score these items.

Researchers should follow the recommendations of the assessment's developer in deciding whether to report each participant's composite score as a mean or total of the constituent items. This author strongly prefers a mean score, because it retains the metric of the response scale and is more clearly interpretable than a summed score. Nevertheless, if a particular assessment is supposed to be sum-scored, one should do so in order that the descriptive statistics (sample or group means and standard deviations) can be compared from one study to another.

As mentioned above and in the next three chapters, body image evaluation is sometimes assessed with figural stimuli—whereby persons select a body size that they perceive to represent their actual size and a body size to convey their ideal. The derived index is the discrepancy between the scale values of these two percepts. However, the use of a signed discrepancy score (self-percept minus ideal percept) is problematic, as it may not accurately reflect the intended measurement of dissatisfaction. Imagine that stimuli have values that range from 1 (very thin) to 9 (very fat) and two participants indicate their self-percept to be a 5. One participant wishes to be thinner and reports an ideal percept of 2, receiving a discrepancy score of +3. The second participant wishes to be heavier and chooses an ideal image of 8, receiving a discrepancy score of –3. Thus, while each person perceives that he or she differs from an ideal to the same degree (i.e., 3 points away from the ideal), they receive very disparate scores. Moreover, if a study's sample contained 50% of participants like the first person and 50% like the second individual, the sample mean discrepancy score would equal 0, which incorrectly implies that on average participants perceived their bodies as congruent with their ideal. Using the proper scoring represented by an absolute value of discrepancy scores rather than signed scores, both persons would receive a 3; thus a sample mean would be 3. Other analyses could be conducted to ascertain the direction of the discrepancies. The erroneous approach to scoring typically causes greater problems in data for men than for women, because a much greater proportion of women wish to be thinner than heavier, whereas the proportions of men are closer to equivalent.

Do You Need a Novel Body Image Assessment?

Common Mistakes

Given the proliferation of body image assessments in recent years, most researchers should be able to acquire the proper assessments for their scientific work. All too often investigators create their own measure for a given study, despite the fact that a validated assessment exists. This will likely limit their study's publishability in a reputable peer-reviewed journal. A common mistake is to measure some aspect of body image with a single item, despite the fact that single-item measures are inherently unreliable. This problem is an inherent weakness of some surveys (e.g., popular magazine surveys) that attempt to capture "body image" by asking respondents one or two "homegrown" questions about how they perceive or evaluate their looks.

Another potential mistake is to modify a published assessment to make it fit one's own needs. First of all, modifying an existing assessment should never be done without consultation with its developer. Second, changing the items or instructions or response format of a validated assessment means that one cannot transfer any of the established scientific credibility of the original version to the modified version. Nevertheless, in the absence of an available instrument, thoughtful and systematic adaptation of an established one may be reasonable. For example, this author's Body Image Disturbance Questionnaire (BIDQ) instructs individuals to answer a series of questions about any aspect of their bodily appearance that gives them concern. The BIDQ's instructions may be modified to specify a physical characteristic—for example, the body part or area that they seek to change via cosmetic surgery. Similarly, the author's Body Image Quality of Life Inventory (BIQLI), which assesses the positive-to-negative effects of one's body image evaluation in general, may be adapted to focus on a specific area of body image evaluation. Again, however, such adaptations cannot be assumed to have the same psychometric properties as the original validated versions.

Patient-Reported Body Image Outcomes in Medical Research

An important area of growth in the body image literature concerns the impact of a particular appearance-altering condition (e.g., a medical condition) on persons' body image perceptions and evaluations and associated psychosocial functioning or quality of life. As medical/surgical procedures are proposed to treat these conditions, evidence-based science necessitates that their efficacy be established in controlled clinical trials, sometimes as a requirement for the governmental approval of the treatment. Critical outcome criteria are termed *patient-reported outcomes* (PROs). Established body image assessments typically won't do, because they lack sufficient focus on the treated characteristic and how it would be expected to impact the individual. Approval agencies, such as the U.S. Food and Drug Administration (FDA), have established rigorous guidelines for demonstrating treatment efficacy vis-à-vis PROs. Readers are encouraged to consult this chapter's Informative Readings regarding the FDA's guidelines and a few examples of the development of condition-specific PROs.

Conclusions

As the subsequent chapters in this section of the handbook delineate, numerous validated measures of body image variables exist. Investigators' selection of measurement tools requires thoughtful attention to the goals of the research as well as to the scientific evidence associated with available measures. Assessments must be age-, sex-, and culture-appropriate for the intended sample. Because body image is a multidimensional construct, chosen tools must produce reliable and valid scores for the particular body image dimensions that are the focus of study. The bottom line is that whereas good measures do not guarantee the fidelity of the findings, poor measures will surely undermine the internal validity of the research conclusions.

Informative Readings

Cash, T. F., Jakatdar, T. A., & Williams. E. F. (2004). The Body Image Quality of Life Inventory: Further validation with college men and women. *Body Image: An International Journal of Research, 1*, 279–287.—The second of two validation studies of the BIQLI that does not directly assess body image per se but rather the psychosocial impact of body image.

Cash, T. F., Maikkula, C. L., & Yamamiya, Y. (2004). "Baring the body in the bedroom": Body image, sexual self-schemas, and sexual functioning among college women and men. *Electronic Journal of Human Sexuality, 7.* Available at www.ejhs.org/volume7/bodyimage.html.—Describes the BESAQ, a contextual body image assessment.

Cash, T. F., Phillips, K. A., Santos, M. T., & Hrabosky, J. I. (2004). Measuring "negative body image": Validation of the Body Image Disturbance Questionnaire in a nonclinical population. *Body Image: An International Journal of Research, 1*, 363–372.—Describes the initial validation of an assessment of body image disturbance, one that may be adapted to focus on different physical attributes.

Fagien, S., Cox, S. E., Charles Finn, Y. J., Werschler, W. P., & Kowalski, J. W. (2007). Patient-reported outcomes with botulinum toxin type A treatment of glabellar rhytids: A double-blind, randomized, placebo-controlled study. *Dermatologic Surgery, 33*, S2–S9.—Illustrates the development and use of an appearance-related PRO in a clinical drug trial.

Kelly, R. E., Jr., Cash, T. F., Shamberger, R. C., Mitchell, K. K., Mellins, R. B., Lawson, M. L., et al. (2008). Surgical repair of pectus excavatum markedly improves body image and perceived ability for physical activity: A multicenter study. *Pediatrics, 122*, 1218–1222.—Illustrates the development and use of an appearance-related PRO in the evaluation of a corrective surgery procedure.

Leahey, T. M., & Crowther, J. H. (2008). An ecological momentary assessment of comparison target as a moderator of the effects of appearance-focused social comparisons. *Body Image: An International Journal of Research, 4*, 307–311.—Exemplifies EMA research that uses electronic technology to assess and study body image states in daily life.

Melnyk, S. E., Cash, T. F., & Janda, L. H. (2004). Body image ups and downs: Prediction of intra-individual level and variability of women's daily body image experiences. *Body Image: An International Journal of Research, 1*, 225–235.—Exemplifies the use of a state body image assessment within the context of daily life.

Rudiger, J. A., Cash, T. F., Roehrig, M., & Thompson, J. K. (2007). Day-to-day body-image states: Prospective predictors of intra-individual level and variability. *Body Image: An International Journal of Research, 4*, 1–9.—Exemplifies the use of a state body image assessment within the context of daily life.

Sperber, A. D. (2004). Translation and validation of study instruments for cross-cultural research. *Gastroenterology, 126*, S124–S128.—Provides procedural recommendations for the linguistic translation of questionnaires in cross-cultural research.

Thompson, J. K. (2004). The (mis)measurement of body image: Ten strategies to improve assessment for applied and research purposes. *Body Image: An International Journal of Research, 1*, 7–14.—Describes common pitfalls in body image assessments and how they may be avoided or remedied.

U.S. Food and Drug Administration. (2009, December). *Guidance for industry patient-reported outcome measures: Use in medical product development to support labeling claims.* Available at *www.fda.gov/downloads/Drugs/GuidanceCompliance-RegulatoryInformation/Guidances/UCM193282.pdf.*—A detailed document that provides very useful recommendations for the development and validation of PRO measures.

CHAPTER 16

Body Image Assessment of Children

ANDREW J. HILL

Introduction

Our children grow up in a world of unprecedented visual imagery relating to the body and physical appearance. Understanding their message does not require sophisticated verbal skills. More than ever, and younger than ever, children are drawn to make value judgments of themselves and others in terms of shape, weight, and appearance. This chapter provides an overview of how body image is measured in children under the age of 12.

Body Image Assessment of Self

Figure Rating Scales

Arrays of line drawings of human figures ranging from extremely thin to fat have been the most commonly used method of asking children about their own body shape perception and preference. Some researchers have used scales originally developed to investigate adult body image perception, whereas others have redrawn the figures to represent children. The drawings commissioned by Stunkard, Sorensen, and Schulsinger in the 1970s to allow participants to describe the typical body shape (and so weight) of their deceased parents have been the template for the more recent age-matched drawings of children.

.The figure rating scales drawn by Collins to represent preadolescents typify this type of assessment. These are separate series of male and female

138

outline figures that show an extremely thin child with ribs protruding on the extreme left and an overweight child, thickest at the waist and with a round face, on the extreme right. Collins's scales have seven figures, whereas other variants have nine. The figures between these extremes are stepped gradations in shape, although this is visual rather than based on any mathematical calculation. It follows that these scales cannot be assumed as linear, nor are the differences between adjacent pairs of figures the same. In addition, the scales for boys and girls are not identical, meaning that caution needs to be applied to interpreting sex differences in ratings.

Questions typically asked of children when using these scales are about current and ideal self: Which picture looks the most like you look? Which picture shows the way you want to look? Any difference between these two choices has been used as a measure of body shape dissatisfaction. This can be either a wish to be thinner than they currently are (conventionally a minus score) or to be heavier (a plus score). Paralleling work with adolescents and adults, some researchers have also asked children to select the ideal shape of a child of opposite sex, the ideal adult shape, and the body shape their parents would prefer. Accordingly, these scales have been used to rate children's perception of others' ideals, as well as their own.

There are interesting and important variants in figure scale presentation and use. For example, Rand and Wright produced an array of nine figures of babies (sex unspecified), to add to those of children and adults, for an evaluation of body shape ideals across all ages. To increase response resolution, colleagues and I have included a visual analogue scale (100-mm horizontal line) below the array of figures so that children can make choices that are between figures. Measured from the left-hand end of the scale, this provides a greater range of responses than one of seven or nine figure options. Pictures on individual cards presented singly in random order or spread out in front of children have been used as alternatives to the scaled arrays described above. Authors have also changed the way the figures are dressed, exchanging simple singlet or shorts for more modern clothes and hairstyle. The drawings have been further adapted to reflect the ethnicity of the children investigated.

The most radical development of this approach has been Truby and Paxton's Children's Body Image Scale (CBIS; see Figure 16.1, panel A). By using photographic images of children of known body mass index (BMI) it addresses some of the scaling issues noted above and is intended to help children identify with the images and so make better choices. Intended for use by 7- to 12-year-olds, the CBIS has had extensive psychometric investigation. For example, correlations between current self and actual BMI are good for all groups except younger boys. The scale has good test–retest reliability and the validity of body dissatisfaction scores is seen in measures of body esteem and dieting.

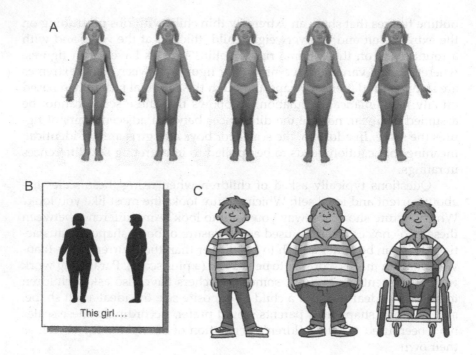

FIGURE 16.1. Examples of pictorial stimuli used in the assessment of children's body image. (A) Part of the Children's Body Image Scale for girls. From Truby and Paxton (2002). Copyright by the British Psychological Society. Reprinted with permission from the *British Journal of Clinical Psychology* and the authors. (B) Representation of an overweight girl used for attributional ratings by preadolescents (Hill & Silver, 1995). (C) Three representations of the same character, Alfie, used in storybooks with 4- to 6-year-olds (Harrison & Hill, in preparation).

There is differing opinion regarding the merits of this type of body image assessment. These scales have been criticized for lack of robust psychometric data. Relatively modest correlations between current self-ratings and actual BMI have been cited as demonstrating poor scale reliability. However, this fails to capture the most common use of these scales in children (i.e., to investigate *differences* between current and ideal perception). Overall, and collectively, figure rating scales have generated reasonably good evidence of test–retest reliability in children ages 8 and above. Their primary strengths lie in their nondependence on verbal skills, visual appeal, and ease of use.

Questionnaire Assessments

Several questionnaires measure constructs relevant to children's body image, either as the focus of the assessment or as part of a broader package. Most have been developed for adolescent or adult samples (see Chapters 17 and 18). Those with published use in preadolescent children are illustrated below.

The Body Cathexis Scale comprises a list of 15 body parts (e.g., waist, hips, thighs) and features (height, weight, body build) that participants rate on 7-point scales of satisfaction–dissatisfaction. The score reported is typically the sum or mean of these ratings. Younger, and some older, children can struggle over the quality on which they are being asked to judge their satisfaction–dissatisfaction. For example, it can be unclear whether they are being asked to make judgments of satisfaction with size, shape, function, or overall appearance.

A more frequently used assessment is Mendelson, White, and Mendelson's Body Esteem Scale, a 20-item questionnaire made up of simple statements that respondents answer by circling yes or no. The content includes statements about overall appearance, body shape and weight, and other people's opinion and behavior (parents and peers) relating to the respondent's appearance. It is therefore a general measure of appearance esteem but one that has good reliability and validity data for 7- to 12-year-olds. Several authors have used and reported adequate psychometrics with 5-year-olds. One variant has been to reduce the number of items and to use smiley-face pictures to help younger children to indicate their agreement or disagreement.

Eating disorder assessments such as the Eating Disorder Inventory (EDI-2), the Children's Eating Attitudes Test (ChEAT), the Children's Eating Disorder Examination (ChEDE), and the McKnight Risk Factor Survey (MRFS-IV) all include items or subscales relating to body image, primarily dissatisfaction. They have also been used with nonclinical groups of children, mainly girls, from the age of 9 upwards. However, their most frequent use has been with adolescents.

Susan Harter's Self-Perception Profile for Children (SPPC) measures domain-specific competence and global self-worth in children ages 8–14. One of these domains is physical appearance, or the degree to which the child is happy with the way he or she looks, likes his or her appearance, and feels he or she is good looking. It should be noted that the pictorial version designed for children from ages 4 to 7 does not include an assessment of physical appearance.

The SPPC is manualized and very widely used. It has an unusual response format designed to reduce social desirability effects in children's responses. Each question is phrased as a choice between alternative descriptions: Some kids are happy with the way they look BUT Other kids are *not* happy with the way they look. Once children select the description most like them they then decide whether it is "sort of true" or "really true" for them. The six items that make up the physical appearance scale are averaged to a scale score. Interestingly, other researchers have used a more standard response format, attaching a fixed-point scale to each of the descriptions, and claim good utility and reliability.

The SPPC also includes a separate assessment of domain importance. Of relevance here is that children are asked, in the same alternative question style, to indicate how *important* it is to be competent in these domains. Perceived importance of physical appearance, on its own and in comparison with current satisfaction, are relatively unexplored features of children's body image.

Body Image Assessment of Others

Cooley's conceptualization of the looking-glass self and Festinger's perspective on social comparison processes are reminders that self-evaluation has a social context. People draw on their perception of others and how others are treated according to appearance to evaluate their own body image and satisfaction (or otherwise). There is a long history of research into children's evaluation of and attitudes to body shape, reflecting the social value attached to thinness and interest in the development of disordered eating. This has been reignited by the rise in obesity prevalence and associated anti-fat attitudes.

Two approaches dominate children's body image assessment of others. The first has its origins in perceptions of disability, presenting children with line drawings of a child as physically normal, in a leg brace or crutches, in a wheelchair, with facial disfigurement, without a hand, or as overweight. Children are asked to choose the figure they like best, the selection is put to one side, and the question repeated to give a rank order of preference. There have been numerous studies of preadolescent children across cultures and from many different countries, the majority of which show the fat child to be chosen last. There have also been a number of variations on these line drawings, including Latner and colleagues' recent updating of the figures using 3-D modeling, realistic faces, and modern clothes.

The second approach has been to use exemplars of thin and fat body shapes to assess children's attitudes and personality attributions. Assigning adjectives to the figure preadolescents think they best describe typically shows a fat body shape to be labeled "lazy," "stupid," "sloppy," "dirty," "mean," "ugly," and "gets teased." In contrast, a thin figure more often attracts "best friend" and "has lots of friends." When a medium or average-shaped figure is included then both thin and fat figures receive fewer positive endorsements. However, fatness is consistently negatively viewed, and is especially associated with low intelligence, laziness, and social isolation.

Again, there is methodological diversity in these investigations. For example, we have used combined face-on and profile silhouettes to depict stereotypes of fatness and thinness (Figure 16.1, panel B). Others have developed cartoon drawings or used face or full-body photographs, sometimes presented with accompanying written descriptions. Fixed-point rating scales or visual analogue scales have been used to allow children to quantify their attributional judgments. And some investigators have attempted to relate personal features such as children's own weight or body dissatisfaction to these ratings.

These investigations have also been conducted with very young children. Researchers have asked 4- to 6-year-olds to associate descriptors with thin, average, or fat figures taken from Collins's figure rating scales. Combining pictures with stories is an effective way of engaging youngsters. Cramer and Steinwert, for example, combined hand-drawn pictures of a thin or fat girl or boy with short stories involving one of these characters read to 3- to 5-year-olds by the researcher. Within the story line one child was mean to another. Even 3-year-olds were more likely to choose the drawing of the fat figure as the mean character. Moreover, there was some evidence that children's relative weight affected their story-line choices, with overweight youngsters most likely to make this choice.

We have developed high-quality, color picture reading books along the lines of a popular U.K. primary school reading program in which one of the central characters is depicted as normal weight, fat, or in a wheelchair (Figure 16.1, panel C). Children ages 4–6 engage in paired reading with the researcher in their school environment and then make assessments of, and choices between, the characters. The advantage of this approach is that it is typical of the child's usual school activity. Others have used the preschool environment to show specially developed video recordings to children. Here, real-life child models were either normal weight or dressed to appear overweight. Children were individually tested, asked questions, and responded on scales anchored with smiley faces and bars of different sizes. The key to this work is the choice of assessments, procedures, and environment that are sensitive to the age of respondents.

Conclusions and Future Directions

The body image assessment of children is dominated by the use of visual representations. These have become more sophisticated in style and better matched to the age of children using them. Researchers have also become more aware of the need to collect and report information on assessment reliability and, where feasible, validity. There has been little interest in systematically comparing methods of body image assessment, so it is unclear, for example, which are the best figure rating scales to use with a specific age group.

The figures and scales described in this chapter have not been restricted to self-evaluation. They have been used to understand children's ideal body shapes as viewed by others (e.g., mothers) and to categorize the weight of children's characters on television sitcoms. There has been less concern in this age group about whether boys' body image issues are captured using assessments developed primarily for girls. More complex procedures such as self-evaluation by video technology are rarely used in preadolescent samples.

Amid the plethora of approaches available, the merits of asking simple questions should not be overlooked. Individual interviews and qualitative approaches (e.g., using some of the SPPC items as prompts) have largely unexplored value in this age group. They are especially suited to exploring children's understanding of complex constructs. Finally, the assessment of children's body image is not restricted to descriptive studies. As younger age groups increasingly become the focus of prevention programs for body dissatisfaction or obesity then body image has value as an outcome evaluation. This will provide further impetus to assessment refinement, the development of combined approaches, and evidence of psychometrics and utility.

Informative Readings

Collins, M. E. (1991). Body figure perceptions and preferences among preadolescent children. *International Journal of Eating Disorders, 10*, 199–208.—One of the most commonly used sets of female and male figure ratings scales drawn specifically for preadolescent children.

Cramer, P., & Steinwert, T. (1998). Thin is good, fat is bad: How early does it begin? *Journal of Applied Developmental Psychology, 19*, 429–451.—Use of a story with moral consequences explores how old young children are when they start to make negative associations with overweight.

Dittmar, H., Halliwell, E., & Ive, S. (2006). Does Barbie make girls want to be thin? The effect of experimental exposure to images of dolls on the body image of 5- to 8-year-old girls. *Developmental Psychology, 42*, 283–292.—Experimental study with young children using age-adapted body image assessments, including the Body Esteem Scale.

Gardner, R. M., & Brown, D. L. (2010). Body image assessment: A review of figural rating scales. *Personality and Individual Differences, 48*, 107–111.—A critical but useful review and reference source for the variety of figure rating scales that have been used with children.

Harter, S. (1993). Causes and consequences of low self-esteem in children and adolescents. In R. F. Baumeister (Ed.), *Self-esteem: The puzzle of low self-regard* (pp. 87–116). New York: Plenum.—The approach to self-esteem and its assessment that underpins Harter's Self-Perception Profile for Children.

Hill, A. J., & Silver, E. K. (1995). Fat, friendless and unhealthy: 9-year-old children's perception of body shape stereotypes. *International Journal of Obesity, 19*, 423–430.—Study of children's perception of thin and fat body shapes on attributes including health and fitness using face and profile figure drawings.

Holub, S. C. (2008). Individual differences in the anti-fat attitudes of preschool-children: The importance of perceived body size. *Body Image: An International Journal of Research, 5,* 317–321.—Study relating young children's own body size perceptions to attributions of thin, average weight, and overweight figures taken from Collins's scale.

Latner, J. D., Simmonds, M., Rosewall, J. K., & Stunkard, A. J. (2007). Assessment of obesity stigmatization in children and adolescents: Modernizing a standard measure. *Obesity, 15,* 3078–3085.—Updating and modernizing of body figures first reported on in the 1960s to investigate children's attitudes to disability.

Lehmkuhl, H. D., Nabors, L. A., & Iobst, E. (2010). Factors influencing preschool-age children's acceptance of models presented as overweight. *International Journal of Pediatric Obesity, 5,* 19–24.—Experimental study using an interview format to gather body image information, age-adapted response formats, and open-ended questions.

Mendelson, B., White, D., & Mendelson, M. (1996). Self-esteem and body esteem: Effects of gender, age, and weight. *Journal of Applied Developmental Psychology, 17,* 321–346.—Source reference for the Body Esteem Scale, a frequently used questionnaire assessment in children and adolescents.

Rand, C. S. W., & Wright, B. A. (2000). Continuity and change in the evaluation of ideal and acceptable body sizes across a wide age span. *International Journal of Eating Disorders, 28,* 90–100.—Source of body figure scales relevant to different age groups, including one of babies.

Stunkard, A. J., Sorenson, T., & Schulsinger, F. (1983). Use of the Danish adoption register for the study of obesity and thinness. In S. S. Kety, L. P. Rowland, R. L. Sidman, & S. W. Matthysse (Eds.), *Genetics of neurological and psychiatric disorders* (pp. 115–120). New York: Raven Press.—The first of the figure rating scales and the inspiration for others; although nominally adult figures they have also been used with children.

Truby, H., & Paxton, S. J. (2002). Development of the Children's Body Image Scale. *British Journal of Clinical Psychology, 41,* 185–203.—Description of a photograph-based body figure scale that should be read in conjunction with the 2008 update on psychometrics (same authors and journal).

CHAPTER 17

Perceptual Measures
of Body Image
for Adolescents and Adults

RICK M. GARDNER

Introduction

Body image is a multidimensional concept that includes perceptual, attitudinal, affective, and behavioral dimensions. Body image disturbance (BID) is commonly thought to include two components: a perceptual component and an attitudinal component. Controversy has swirled over the past 40 years regarding how best to measure the perceptual component of BID. Inconsistent findings paired with methodological shortcomings in the research led to disinterest in the topic in the early 1990s. Recent technological and methodological advances, however, have reenergized interest in this topic. This has been particularly true for the role that body size distortion plays in eating disorders. Body size distortion is defined as the difference between a person's actual size and his or her judgment of his or her body size. Several meta-analyses have confirmed that there is a relationship between body size estimation and eating pathology. Additionally, several literature reviews implicate body size overestimation to be a predictor of prior treatment failure, lack of clinical progress, early relapse following hospitalization, and poor clinical outcome in individuals with eating disorders. Further evidence also shows that body size overestimation may be a risk factor for the development of eating disorders and for relapse after apparently successful treatment of the eating disorder symptoms.

Procedures for Measuring Body Size Distortion

A variety of techniques have been developed since the early 1970s to measure how accurately individuals perceive their body size. One of the earliest was Slade and Russell's seminal 1973 study that used an apparatus referred to as the "movable caliper technique." This device had two lights mounted on tracks that participants adjusted to approximate their conceptions of their width at various body sites. The experimenter then compared these judgments to actual body site dimensions as measured by body calipers. The difference between estimated and actual widths represented the index of accuracy. Their findings indicated that individuals with anorexia nervosa (AN) overestimated their body sizes to a greater extent than did individuals without this eating disorder.

This research served as the impetus for numerous additional studies designed to examine the role that body size estimation plays in eating disorders, as well as other disorders. These techniques can be classified broadly into two categories: those for specific body sites and those for whole-image assessment. These two approaches have often been found to reflect dissimilar levels of distortion when measuring size estimations in individuals with eating disorders.

Body Site Techniques

These procedures require participants to match the width of the distance between two points to their own estimate of the width of a specific body site. Body sites typically include measurement of face, chest, waist or stomach, hips, thighs, and occasionally other body areas. Slade and Russell's 1973 study was an example of this type of procedure. A variation on the procedure called the Body Image Detection Device requires participants to adjust the width of a light beam to match the perceived size of a specific body site. Another variant called the Adjustable Light Beam involves the adjustment of four light beams projected on a wall to match the perceived size of various body sites. The Image Marking Procedure requires participants to draw or mark their perceived body size on a sheet of paper attached to a wall. These various procedures have differing levels of reliability and validity as reviewed by Stewart and Williamson.

Several researchers have developed computer-based methods of distorting body images. Participants can manipulate the width of specific body sites thereby altering body shape. Sands and his colleagues developed video distortion software that allows participants to adjust their horizontal dimensions on chest, waist, hips, thighs, and calves to measure size distortion and body dissatisfaction at these sites. Hennighausen and Remschmidt developed video-distortion software that uses silhouette drawings created from photographs of individuals' frontal and side views. The technique measures body size distortion of the body regions of lower leg, thigh, hip, waist, chest, neck, and head. Aleong and Duchesne developed similar software allowing manipulation of frontal and side views of adolescent bodies. Body sites including shoulder width, waist, hip, belly, thigh, and calf sizes can be manipulated. Finally, Harari and Furst developed software using a graphical interface that permits patients with eating disorders to adjust their body shapes. These programs provide technical sophistication in measuring distortion of body regions.

Whole-Image Techniques

In these procedures, participants view a real-life image and adjust the size of the image to make it objectively smaller or larger until it matches their view of their actual body size. Early research used an adjustable mirror that distorts the size of the whole body on both the vertical and horizontal planes. In 2002, Shafran and Fairburn developed a digital photography method for assessing the perception of body size. Here a digital photograph of an individual is projected onto a screen so that the individual can compare his or her actual reflection in a mirror to a projected image on the screen. This innovative procedure is designed to assess perception of body size as opposed to a memory for body size.

The video-distortion technique uses static images of individuals. Participants adjust the horizontal dimension of the video image of themselves to match their perceived size. Gardner and Boice have developed software that permits the distortion of whole-body images by using two psychophysical methods as described later in this chapter.

In recent years, figural drawing scales, sometimes referred to as silhouette scales, have been used to measure aspects of BID. Typically, participants match their perceived actual size selected from a varying number of line drawings representing figures or silhouettes of differing widths. Typically, the figures are presented in ascending size from very thin to very obese even though several researchers have recommended presenting the figures in random order. Body dissatisfaction is measured as the discrepancy between the figure chosen as the actual size as compared to the ideal size. Some scales are designed specifically to measure distinct body sites, differing ethnic groups, and adolescents. Stewart and Williamson provide a comprehensive review of these scales. While primarily used to measure body dissatisfaction, a few scales have been developed that also measure distortion in body size estimations. Gardner and Brown have recently reviewed the psychometric properties of these scales.

Stewart and her colleagues recently developed a software program that morphs the size of realistic illustrations of a human body from thin to obese and permits individuals to judge their current, ideal, and acceptable body size. The program allows measurement of body size distortion as well as body dissatisfaction among both men and women and can be used with both Caucasian and African American persons.

Psychophysical Techniques for Assessing Body Size

In the late 1980s, researchers began to employ sophisticated psychophysical techniques that permitted the separate measurement of the *sensory* and *nonsensory* components of body size estimation. The sensory component refers to the responses of the visual system, including the retina and visual cortex, whereas the nonsensory components, also referred to as the cognitive or affective components, reflect how the brain interprets the visual input. Previously, techniques for body size estimation had confounded these two aspects, which have been found to be largely independent measures.

All the methods used for assessing size estimation accuracy, with the exception of the Image Marking Procedure and figural drawing scales, require participants to make their judgments of body size on ascending and descending trials. Participants see an initial stimulus (video image, light beam, two separated lights, etc.) that is either too small or too large and make adjustments until it represents the size of their body. In some instances the experimenter makes the adjustments and in other situations the participant adjusts the size. Gardner and others have noted that the initial stimulus that is observed serves as an anchor that greatly influences the final size judgment. Participants who decrease an initial image that is too large (descending trials) typically reach a final judgment of their body that is too large and, similarly, when increasing a too-small image, participants reach a final judgment that is too small. These are commonly called errors of anticipation. Furthermore, the magnitude of the error differs on descending and ascending trials with the most accurate judgments made when increasing a too-small stimulus. Gardner has cautioned that the commonly used procedure of taking an average of the ascending and descending trials results in an average body size judgment that fails to represent accurately either the ascending or descending trials.

Several techniques have been developed to avoid errors of anticipation. These include the method of constant stimuli, signal detection theory, and adaptive probit estimation techniques.

Method of Constant Stimuli

One procedure used to avoid the error of anticipation employs the method of constant stimuli wherein ascending/descending trials are not used. Within the context of body image research, a range of body image sizes (typically between five and nine different values) are used repeatedly throughout testing. The images presented include those with no distortions as well as those with distortions that range from rarely detected to nearly always detected. On a given trial, one of these distortions is presented and the participant must report whether it represents an over- or underestimation. The resulting psychophysical function assumes the typical ogive (sigmoid) shape with body size estimation being the size where the participant reported 50% of the images as overestimations and 50% as underestimations. This body size estimation is known as the point of subjective equality (PSE) and represents the perceived body size that individuals judge to be subjectively equal to their actual size. A discrepancy between this perceived size and one's actual size is a measure of body size distortion. In addition, the procedure allows for the investigator to ascertain how much distortion in body size beyond the PSE is necessary before the person reliably detects the changes as a "just noticeable difference." This value is referred to as the difference threshold or difference limen (DL). The PSE reflects the attitudinal aspects of body size estimation, whereas the DL indicates the perceptual or sensory ability to detect size distortion.

Mussap and colleagues recently applied this methodology to examine body size estimations in female college students. The participants had an average PSE of 6.3%, indicating that the subjects judged an image that was 6.3% larger than their actual size as being subjectively equal to their body size. The average DL of 3% across all subjects indicated that, on average, subjects who saw their bodies distorted an average of 3% were able to detect that distortion 50% of the time. The amount of variability of the PSE values was found to be related to factors in disordered eating.

Signal Detection Theory

In 1988, Gardner and Moncrieff were the first researchers to use a signal detection theory approach to measure body size estimation. Individuals are presented with single static video images of themselves that are distorted either too wide or too thin by a set percentage or are of normal (undistorted) size. Individuals are required to state on each trial whether the image is or is not distorted. Separate measures of sensory sensitivity and response bias are found by measuring an individual's correct responses and errors. Sensory sensitivity refers to the individual's ability to detect correctly whether the image is distorted as too thin or too wide, whereas response bias measures the individual's tendency to report images as too wide or too thin. Sensory sensitivity and response bias are independent measures. Therefore, it is possible that an individual could be accurate in correctly detecting distortion in his or her image but could still have a response bias to state that his or her body is too wide or too thin.

In the first body image study using this technique, Gardner and Moncrieff found that women with AN were no more or less sensitive in their ability to detect distortions in their body size as compared with individuals without an eating disorder. However, these individuals did have a response bias or tendency to report that their image was too wide. This was the first study to document that the frequently reported perceptual size distortion in subjects with eating disorders is caused by nonsensory attitudinal factors and not by differences in sensory sensitivity. Individuals with AN often report that when they look in a mirror they "see" a fat person. This distortion is not due to any deficit in their sensory system but rather is due to a response tendency to report that images of their body are too wide. Subsequent studies by several researchers have confirmed that it is one's beliefs, attitudes, and thoughts that influence willingness to perceive one's body image as either normal or distorted. These findings could have important ramifications for clinical approaches to treating eating disorders.

Adaptive Probit Estimation

Recently, Gardner and Boice have pioneered the use of a psychophysical technique called "adaptive probit estimation" to measure the perceptual and affective aspects of body size estimations. A detailed description of this methodology is beyond the scope of this chapter, and the interested reader is referred to the informative readings at the end of the chapter. Briefly, a computer software program developed by Gardner and Boice presents a static video image of a participant that is distorted wider or thinner than his or her actual size. The subject is asked to judge whether the image is too wide or too thin. Initially, two blocks of 40 trials are presented with four images distorted ± 3.27 and ± 9.81%. Distortions are subsequently adjusted for the next six blocks of 40 trials. These adjustments are made to present four new distortion levels in each block that are centered about the calculated size of their body by participants. Following data collection, the computer program calculates an average value for the PSE and just noticeable difference (DL) values. As with the method of constant stimuli, the PSE measures the amount of body size distortion and represents the amount of distortion whereby a participant would respond that the image was distorted "too wide" 50% of the time and "too thin" 50% of the time. It thus represents the amount of distortion necessary before a respondent reported that the body size presented was subjectively equal to his or her perceived size. The DL again represents the amount of change in body size the subject required to reliably detect the change 50% of the time.

While the adaptive probit estimation technique produces the same nonsensory (PSE) and sensory (DL) values as the method of constant stimuli, it does so in a more efficient and less time-consuming fashion. Stable measurements of both values are possible after approximately 20–30 minutes of data collection. This procedure has been demonstrated to be both reliable and valid in a number of studies by Gardner and his colleagues. The software also permits investigators to use the method of adjustment whereby participants see an initial image that is too thin or too wide and can adjust the width to either the size they think they are or to the size they would like to be ideally. The software program runs on a personal computer and is available from the author.

Conclusions and Future Directions

Measurement of the perceptual aspects of body image has evolved dramatically in the past 30 years. Improved techniques for measuring body image, including psychophysical techniques that permit the separate measurement of the independent aspects of sensory and nonsensory factors, has led to a renewal of interest in this topic. Overestimation of body size has been found to be prevalent in a variety of populations and not just specific to those with eating disorders. Further development of more precise theoretical models and even more precise measurement tools promises to further advance our understanding of the role of perceptual processes in body image.

Informative Readings

Aleong, R., & Duchesne, S. (2007). Assessment of adolescent body perception: Development and characterization of a novel tool for morphing images of adolescent bodies. *Behavior Research Methods, 39,* 651–666.—Software designed specifically to measure body size and shape distortion in adolescents.

Cash, T. F., & Deagle, E. A. (1997). The nature and extent of body-image disturbances in anorexia nervosa and bulimia nervosa: A meta-analysis. *International Journal of Eating Disorders, 22,* 107–125.—A meta-analysis of studies utilizing perceptual and attitudinal measures in individuals with eating disorders.

Gardner, R. M., & Boice, R. (2004). A computer program for measuring body size distortion and body dissatisfaction. *Behavior Research Methods, Instruments, and Computers, 36,* 89–95.—Description of an available software program designed to run on PCs that uses both the adaptive probit estimation methodology and the method of adjustment to measure body size distortion and body dissatisfaction.

Gardner, R. M., & Brown, D. L. (2010). Body image assessment: A review of figural drawing scales. *Personality and Individual Differences, 48,* 107–111.—Review of psychometric properties of figural drawing scales, including those that measure body size distortion.

Gardner, R. M., Jappe, L. M., & Gardner, L. (2009). Development and validation of a new figural drawing scale for body-image assessment: The BIAS-BD. *Journal of Clinical Psychology, 65,* 113–122.—Description of a figural drawing scale that measures both body dissatisfaction and body size distortion.

Gardner, R. M., Jones, L. C., & Bokenkamp, E. D. (1995). A comparison of three psychophysical techniques for estimating body size perception. *Perceptual and Motor Skills, 80,* 1379–1390.—Comparison of method of adjustment, signal detection, and adaptive probit estimation as techniques for measuring body size estimations.

Gardner, R. M., & Moncrieff, C. (1988). Body image distortion in anorexics as a non-sensory phenomenon: A signal detection approach. *Journal of Clinical*

Psychology, 44, 101–107.—The first study utilizing signal detection theory to measure separately the sensory and nonsensory components of body image.

Harari, D., & Furst, M. (2001). A computer-based method for the assessment of body image distortions in anorexia nervosa patients. *IEEE Transactions on Information Technology in Biomedicine, 5,* 311–319.—A program specifically designed to measure body shape distortions in patients with eating disorders.

Hennighausen, K., & Remschmidt, H. (1999). The computer body image test: A procedure for the assessment of body image perception. *International Journal of Methods in Psychiatric Research, 8,* 123–128.—Describes software that permits distortion of several body sites to measure body shape distortion.

Jappe, L. M., & Gardner, R. M. (2009). Body image perception and dissatisfaction throughout phases of the female menstrual cycle. *Perceptual and Motor Skills, 108,* 74–80.—Illustrates adaptive probit estimation methodology to measure BID.

Mussap, A. J., McCabe, M. P., & Ricciardelli, L. A. (2008). Implications of accuracy, sensitivity, and variability of body size estimations to disordered eating. *Body Image: An International Journal of Research, 5,* 80–90.—An illustration of how the method of constant stimuli is used to separately measure sensory and nonsensory aspects of body size estimation.

Sands, R., Maschette, W., & Armatas, C. (2004). Measurement of body image satisfaction using computer manipulation of a digital image. *The Journal of Psychology, 138,* 325–337.—A user-friendly software program that permits morphing of the body shape and size of video images to allow measurements of body size distortion and dissatisfaction.

Sepulveda, A., Botella, J., & Antonio, L. J. (2002). Body image disturbance in eating disorders: A meta-analysis. *Psychology in Spain, 8,* 83–95.—A meta-analysis of 83 studies describing the effect sizes of body size estimations in individuals with eating disorders.

Shafran, R., & Fairburn, C. G. (2002). A new ecologically valid method to assess body size estimation and body size dissatisfaction. *International Journal of Eating Disorders, 32*(4), 458–465.—Describes a digital photography method for assessing perception of body size that assesses perception as opposed to memory for body size.

Smeets, M. A. M., Ingleby, D., Hoek, H. W., & Panhuysen, G. E. M. (1999). Body size perception in anorexia nervosa: A signal detection approach. *Journal of Psychosomatic Research, 46,* 465–477.—An illustration of how a signal detection methodology is used to measure response bias and sensory sensitivity in individuals with AN.

Stewart, T. M., Allen, H. R., Han, H., & Williamson, D. A. (2009). The development of the Body Morph Assessment version 2.0 (BMA 2.0): Tests of reliability and validity. *Body Image: An International Journal of Research, 6,* 67–74.—A software program that morphs drawings of human figures from thin to obese.

Stewart, T. M., & Williamson, D. A. (2004). Assessment of body image disturbances. In J. K. Thompson (Ed.), *Handbook of eating disorders and obesity* (pp. 495–514). Hoboken, NJ: Wiley.—Comprehensive review of body size estimation measures.

Attitudinal Assessment of Body Image for Adolescents and Adults

JESSIE E. MENZEL
ROSS KRAWCZYK
J. KEVIN THOMPSON

Introduction

Currently a wide range of measures exist that tap into peoples' perceptions of their body. Furthermore, these measures cover many facets of body image; in fact, over the past 10 years, several new measures have been developed, with many of these tapping into muscularity issues and male body image. Therefore, researchers and clinicians now have a greater selection of reliable and valid measures to use in the study of body image. This chapter summarizes the measures available for each of four major dimensions of body image—global satisfaction, and affective, cognitive, and behavioral facets—with a special section devoted to male-specific body image measures. This chapter pertains to attitudinal assessments for adolescents and adults. The reader is referred to Chapter 16 for information on body image assessment of children. Furthermore, this chapter focuses on dispositional, trait-level assessments of body image. Chapter 15 discusses the use of state-level body image measures to assess transient, momentary body image experiences.

Attitudinal body image is generally classified into four major components:

- Global subjective satisfaction or disturbance—these measures tap into one's overall evaluation of the body in terms of satisfaction.
- Affective distress regarding appearance—these measures assess one's emotions related to appearance, including stress, anxiety, or discomfort.
- Cognitive aspects of body image—these measures examine cognitions related to body image, such as appearance schemas, distorted thoughts or beliefs about one's body, and cognitive investment in appearance.
- Behavioral aspects of body image—this component of body image includes avoidance of situations or objects that evoke body image concerns and body-checking behaviors.

In contrast to the assessment of the perceptual distortion component of body image, which is an area rife with methodological perplexity (see Chapter 17), this chapter covers measures that assess a person's self-perceptions or attitudes regarding body image. As with other self-report questionnaires, there are important issues and methodological concerns to consider when selecting a measure, as discussed in Chapter 15. Table 18.1 provides a detailed summary of some of the most widely used and validated assessments available for each dimension addressed.

Global Measures of Body Image Satisfaction–Dissatisfaction

Satisfaction can be defined as a person's appreciation or favorable opinion of body components such as weight, shape, or other specific body sites. Of course, body image dissatisfaction pertains to disparaging, unfavorable opinions. Most measures of this dimension tap the bipolar continuum. Two primary methods—figural or schematic scales and questionnaires—have been used to measure this dimension of body image.

Figural Ratings

Figural drawing scales are some of the most popular and easiest to administer measures used to capture global satisfaction or dissatisfaction. The scales typically consist of contour or silhouette figures of the human body in varying shapes, weights, and sizes from very thin to obese. Individuals are typically asked to select the figure that they think best represents their current physical appearance and the figure that best represents their ideal physical appearance (usually referred to as a real–ideal or self–ideal discrepancy). Body dissatisfaction scores are obtained by calculating the discrepancy between the two figures. Figural rating scales are useful because they can be manipulated so that only one aspect of physical appearance varies among the figures such as chest size, body weight, fatness, or muscularity. Newer methods involving computer technology and anthropomorphic measurements have increased the external validity and accuracy of these measures.

Questionnaire Measures

An extensive number of questionnaire measures have been developed to help capture the many nuances and facets of body image. Questionnaire measures have helped researchers to capture the many characteristics and foci of body image disturbances (BIDs). These global measures of subjective satisfaction seem to reflect two major areas: measures that assess satisfaction–dissatisfaction with specific body sites (e.g., physical characteristic, features, or body areas) and measures that assess satisfaction–dissatisfaction with general or overall physical appearance. Measures that assess specific body sites may reflect factors (or subscales) that assess satisfaction with weight-related aspects of appearance and non-weight-related aspects of appearance. Evaluative measures of general physical appearance, on the other hand, tap into whether or not a person feels physically attractive or likes his or her "looks." Typically, these questionnaires use Likert-type response scales of the degree of satisfaction–dissatisfaction or the agreement–disagreement with item statements.

Finally, scales are available that are validated for use in assessing clinically pertinent BID. Some of these global BID measures transcend the satisfaction–dissatisfaction dimension and incorporate interrelated affective, cognitive, and behavioral dimensions of body image described in the next section. From a clinical standpoint, these assessments often assess whether a person's physical appearance plays too large a role in his or her self-evaluation and whether there exists an excessive preoccupation with or concern over physical features. Some of these scales to measure the features of BID have established community norms and cutoff points for determining clinically significant disturbance. Some of the assessments are also available in interview form and are based on the criteria from the *Diagnostic and Statistical Manual of Mental Disorders* (DSM-IV)—for example, in assessing body dysmorphic disorder (BDD) or eating pathology.

State Measures

Although the great majority of measures focus on the assessment of a dispositional or trait aspect of body image, the consideration of using a state measure is an important one for the researcher and clinician. As discussed in Chapter 15, a state measure focuses on the person's *current* body image—how he or she feels in the immediate moment. This type of index is useful for measuring the immediate effects of an experimental manipulation, or perhaps the pre–post effects of a very brief therapeutic intervention. There are currently three measures of state body image that are in wide use (see Table 18.1): the Physical Appearance State and Trait Anxiety Scale, the Body Image States Scale, and the Visual Analogue Scales.

Measures of Affective, Cognitive, and Behavioral Components of Body Image

Affective Measures

Beyond a person's perceived satisfaction or dissatisfaction with his or her body, affect also plays an important role in a person's body image. This affective component of body image includes feelings of anxiety, distress, and other emotions associated with the body. Anxiety experienced as a component of body image may be focused or directed at specific body sites or weight status in general. Anxiety and other distressing emotions can also be contextual or situational, in which a person becomes self-conscious about his or her looks, for example, in front of peers, significant others, or in public places like the beach. Shame is another salient body image emotion and is often experienced as the result of failing to meet perceived cultural ideals of appearance.

Cognitive Measures

Cognitions—beliefs, thoughts, interpretations, and attributions—comprise a very important and specific facet of body image that contributes to or maintains BID. Body image cognitions can be in the form of beliefs about appearance or appearance ideals and self-schemas about the level of importance that appearance has in a person's self-worth. Newer measures of the cognitive domain of body image have aimed to capture specific cognitive distortions related to BID.

Behavioral Measures

Self-reported behavioral measures of body image have received increasing attention, although true behavioral measures of body image are rare. While body image is traditionally thought of as an intrapsychic phenomenon, there are many behavioral manifestations of body image functioning. For example, avoidance of mirrors, public situations, or scales may be an indicator of one's anxiety surrounding his or her appearance. In contrast, increased weighing, mirror checking, and/or pinching of the skin may be an indicator of investment in or overvaluation of one's appearance. Both avoidance and checking are well-documented phenomena in the experience of individuals with eating disorders or BDD. A number of new self-report measures have been developed to assess these body image behaviors.

Body Image Measures for Males

Historically, many body image assessments have had an inherent gender bias, with item content being more relevant for women than men. Although some of the measures used to assess body image among women are applicable to men, several differences between men and women highlight the need for different assessment tools. One of the primary reasons for this is that cultural appearance ideals are not the same for men and women. As previously mentioned, women most often strive for the thin ideal, a body type characterized by very low body fat. Men, on the other hand, show a greater focus on a drive for the muscular ideal, a body type characterized by heavy musculature. Because of these differing ideals, men and women tend to emphasize different aspects of their appearance. Therefore, assessment tools often measure different constructs for men and women. For example, a questionnaire designed for women regarding overall satisfaction with appearance will likely focus on the desire to be thin. Measures of body image designed for men, however, will likely focus on relevant issues of muscularity, height, and low body fat.

Conclusions and Future Directions

This chapter reviewed a wide variety of attitudinal body image measures. It is important to note that body image measures do not all assess the same facets or dimensions, and therefore researchers and clinicians should use careful consideration when selecting measures for use. Close attention should be paid not only to the psychometric properties of the scale but also to the item content and standardization sample. Other methodological considerations are also necessary and readings are available at the end of this chapter that contain more detailed discussions of these issues. Table 18.1 is a compendium of the most commonly used and some of the newest validated assessments of various facets of the multidimensional body image construct. The table provides a practical overview of each assessment, including its description, key psychometric information, and either e-mail or website information to contact its primary author. A source citation is provided for the most relevant publications, which may be located by entering the citation into a free search engine, such as Google Scholar or Scirus, or academic subscription databases, such as PsycINFO, ScienceDirect, or Web of Science. Readers who wish to consider use of a particular assessment are strongly encouraged to seek further scientific information from the author or publication databases to determine its appropriateness for their intended research. Chapter 15 offers further helpful advice in the selection of instruments in the measurement of body image.

TABLE 18.1. Measures of Body Image Dimensions

Type and name of instrument	Reference	Description	Standardization sample and reliability	Author contact
Global satisfaction measures—Figural ratings				
Body Image Assessment	Williamson, Davis, Bennett, & Goreczny (1989)	Select from nine figures of various sizes	Sample: 659 ♀ including bulimics, binge-eaters, anorexics, control, obese subjects, and atypical eating-disordered subjects IC: n/a TR: immediately to 8 weeks (.60–93)	Donald A. Williamson, PhD *williada@pbrc.edu*
Body Image Assessment Scale—Body Dimensions	Gardner, Jappe, & Gardner (2009)	Contour drawings based on anthropomorphic body measurements; 17 female/17 male	Sample: 66 ♂ and 141 ♀ undergraduate college students IC: n/a TR: 2 weeks (.64–.88)	Rick M. Gardner, PhD *Rick.gardner@ucdenver.edu*
Contour Drawing Rating Scale	Thompson & Gray (1996)	Schematic figures, underweight to overweight; nine male/nine female	Sample: 40 ♂ and ♀ undergraduates IC: n/a TR: 1 week (.79)	James J. Gray, PhD *jgray@american.edu*
Figure Rating Scale	1. Stunkard, Sorensen, & Schulsinger (1983) 2. Thompson & Altabe (1991)	Select from nine figures varying in size from underweight to overweight	Sample 1: 125 ♂ and 204 ♀ Sample 2: 58 ♀ and 34 ♂ IC: n/a TR: 2 weeks (.71–.92)	Albert J. Stunkard, MD *stunkard@mail.med.upenn.edu*
Photographic Figure Rating Scale	Swami, Salem, Furnham, & Tovee (2008)	Photographic images of real women varying in body mass index (BMI): emaciated to obese	Sample: 208 community ♀ IC: n/a TR: 2 weeks (.88–.90)	Viren Swami, PhD *virenswami@hotmail.com*

(continued)

159

TABLE 18.1. (continued)

Type and name of instrument	Reference	Description	Standardization sample and reliability	Author contact
Quantification of Body Image Distortion	Roy & Forest (2007)	Computerized: Participants adjust a computer silhouette to best reflect perceived physical self, based on anthropomorphic measurements	Sample: 200 high school ♀, 22 teenage ♀ outpatient AN, 18 teenage ♀ inpatient AN IC: n/a TR: 4–7 days (.71)	Mathieu Roy, PhD *Mathieu.roy@umontreal.ca*
Somatomorphic Matrix	Pope, Gruber, Mangweth, Bureau, deCol, Jouvent, et al. (2000)	Computerized: 100 figures that vary on two axes: % body fat and muscularity	Sample: 200 undergraduate college ♂ IC: n/a TR: n/a	Harrison G. Pope, MD *hpope@mclean.harvard.edu*
Global satisfaction measures—questionnaires				
Body Appreciation Scale	Avalos, Tylka, & Woods (2005)	13-item measure of positive body image	Sample 1: 181 college ♀ IC: .94 Sample 2: 177 college ♀ TR: 3 weeks (.90)	Tracy Tylka, PhD *tylka.2@osu.edu*
Body Esteem Scale	Franzoi & Shields (1984)	Modification of Body Cathexis Scale with 16 new items, three-factor structure	366 ♀ and 257 ♂ undergraduates IC: females (.78–.87), males (.81–.86) TR: None given	Stephen Franzoi, PhD *franzois@marquette.edu*
Body Esteem Scale for Adolescents and Adults	Mendelson, Mendelson, & White (2001)	23 Likert scale items on three subscales: attribution, appearance, weight	Sample: 1,283–1,312 students ages 12–25 IC: (.91–.94) Sample: 95 junior college students TR: 3 months (.83–.92)	Morton J. Mendelson, PhD *mmendelson@psych.mcgill.ca*

Measure	Authors	Description	Sample/Reliability	Contact
Body Image Disturbance Questionnaire	1. Cash, Phillips, Santos, & Hrabosky (2004) 2. Cash & Grasso (2005)	Version of the Body Dysmorphic Disorder Questionnaire using continuous response format (7 scaled items)	Sample 1: 220 ♀ and 75 ♂ undergraduates IC: (.89) Sample 2: 433 ♀ and 104 ♂ undergraduates IC: (.87–90) TR: 2 weeks (.88) for 88 ♀ and 19 ♂ undergraduates	Thomas F. Cash, PhD Available for a nominal fee at *www.body-images.com*
Body Image Ideals Questionnaire	1. Cash & Szymanski (1995) 2. Szymanski & Cash (1995)	Self-ideal discrepancy and importance of ideals in 10 specific aspects of appearance and overall appearance	Sample: 192 ♂, 896 ♀ adults IC: (.76–81) TR: n/a	Thomas F. Cash, PhD Available for a nominal fee at *www.body-images.com*
Body Satisfaction Scale	Slade, Dewey, Newton, Brodie, & Kiemle (1990)	Degree of satisfaction with 16 parts (three subscales: general, head, and body)	♀ undergraduates, nursing students, volunteers, overweight subjects, anorexics, bulimics IC: (.79–89) TR: n/a	Peter D. Slade, PhD
Body Shape Questionnaire	Cooper, Taylor, Cooper, & Fairburn (1987)	34 items assessing concern with body shape	Bulimics, several control samples IC: n/a TR: n/a	Peter Cooper, PhD *p.j.cooper@reading.ac.uk*
Eating Disorder Examination Questionnaire—Shape and Weight Concerns	1. Fairburn & Beglin (1994) 2. Luce & Crowther (1999)	Measure of clinically significant shape concerns and weight concerns	Sample 1: 285 community ♀, 36 ♂ treated for AN and BN IC: n/a; TR: n/a Sample 2: 139 ♀ undergraduate students IC: (.89–.93) TR: 2 weeks (.92–94)	Christopher Fairburn, PhD *credenquiries@psych.ox.ac.uk*

(continued)

TABLE 18.1. (continued)

Type and name of instrument	Reference	Description	Standardization sample and reliability	Author contact
Eating Disorder Inventory—Body Dissatisfaction Scale	1. Garner, Olmstead, & Polivy (1983) 2. Shore & Porter (1990) 3. Wood, Becker, & Thompson (1996)	Degree of agreement with nine statements about body parts being large	Sample 1: 113 ♀ anorexics, 577 ♀ controls IC: (.91–.90) Sample 2: 195 ♂ and 414 ♀ adolescents IC: (.86–.91) Sample 3: 109 ♂ and 95 ♀ children IC: (.72–.84)	David M. Garner, PhD *www.parinc.com*
Multidimensional Body Self-Relations Questionnaire—Appearance Scales	Brown, Cash, & Mikulka (1990)	Five factors: appearance evaluation, appearance orientation, Body Areas Satisfaction Scale, overweight preoccupation, self-classified weight	Sample 1: 996 ♂, 1070 ♀ IC: AE, AO, OWP (.73–.88) Sample 2: 804 ♀, 335 ♂ IC: BASS, SCW (.70–89) Sample 3: 804 ♀, 335 ♂ college students TR: 1 month (.74–91)	Thomas F. Cash, PhD Available for a nominal fee at *www.body-images.com*
Self-Image Questionnaire for Young Adolescents—Body Image Subscale	Peterson, Schulenberg, Abromowitz, Offer, & Jarcho (1984)	Designed for 10- to 15-year-olds; 11-item body image subscale assesses positive feelings toward the body	Sample: 335 sixth-grade students, followed through the eighth grade IC: (.77–.81) TR: 1 year (.60); 2 years (.44)	Anne C. Petersen, PhD *annepete@umich.edu*

State measures

Measure	Citation	Description	Psychometrics	Contact
Body Image States Scale	Cash, Fleming, Alindogan, Steadman, & Whitehead (2002)	Six items measure state body image regarding: physical appearance, body size and shape, attractiveness, weight, personal looks, and looks compared to others	Sample: 116 college ♀ and 58 college ♂ IC: across five contexts: ♂ (.62–.84); ♀ (.77–.90) TR: ♂: (.68); ♀: (.69)	Thomas F. Cash, PhD Available for a nominal fee at *www.body-images.com*
Physical Appearance State and Trait Anxiety Scale	Reed, Thompson, Brannick, & Sacco (1991)	Eight items measure state appearance anxiety for eight different body sites	Sample: undergraduate ♀ IC: .82 TR: .87	J. Kevin Thompson, PhD *www.bodyimagedisturbance.org*
Visual Analogue Scales	Birkeland, Thompson, Herbozo, Roehrig, Cafri, & van den Berg (2005)	Two items, consisting of a horizontal 100-mm line (none to extreme) assess overall appearance dissatisfaction and physical appearance satisfaction	Sample: 73 undergraduate ♀ TR: overall appearance dissatisfaction: (.84); physical appearance satisfaction: (.80)	J. Kevin Thompson, PhD *www.bodyimagedisturbance.org*

Affective measures

Measure	Citation	Description	Psychometrics	Contact
Objectified Body Consciousness Scale—Body Shame	McKinley & Hyde (1996)	18-item measure of feelings of shame as the result of failing to meet culturally accepted ideals of beauty	Sample 1: 121 undergraduate ♀ IC: .75, TR: n/a Sample 2: 278 undergraduate ♀ and 151 middle-aged ♀ IC: (.70–.84), TR: n/a Sample 3: 103 undergraduate ♀ IC: n/a, TR: 2 weeks (.79)	Nita McKinley, PhD *mckinley@uwplatt.edu*

(continued)

163

TABLE 18.1. (continued)

Type and name of instrument	Reference	Description	Standardization sample and reliability	Author contact
Physical Appearance State and Trait Anxiety Scale	Reed, Thompson, Brannick, & Sacco (1991)	Anxiety associated with 16 body sites (eight weight relevant, eight nonweight relevant); trait and state versions available	Sample: 205 ♀ undergraduate students IC: (.82–.92) TR: 2 weeks (.87)	J. Kevin Thompson, PhD *www.bodyimagedisturbance.org*
Situational Inventory of Body Image Dysphoria	Cash (2002)	Measures frequency of negative body image emotions across 20 situational contexts	Sample 1: 1,465 ♀, 455 ♂ undergraduates IC: (.93–.96) Sample 2: 30 ♂, 118 ♀ undergraduates TR: 1 month (.81–.87)	Thomas F. Cash, PhD Available for a nominal fee at *www.body-images.com*
Cognitive measures				
Appearance Schemas Inventory—Revised	1. Cash, Melnyk, & Hrabosky (2004) 2. Cash & Grasso (2005)	20 items assess two facets of body image investment: motivational salience of appearance and self-evaluative salience of appearance	Sample 1: 135 ♂, 468 ♀ undergraduates IC: (.82–.91) Sample 2: 346 ♂, 1,567 ♀ undergraduates IC: (.77–.90) TR: subsample 2 weeks (.78–.88)	Thomas F. Cash, PhD Available for a nominal fee at *www.body-images.com*
Assessment of Body Image Cognitive Distortions	Jakatdar, Cash, & Engle (2006)	Two parallel 18-item forms assess distorted thinking about physical appearance	Sample: 263 ♀ undergraduates IC: (.93–.97) TR: n/a	Thomas F. Cash, PhD Available for a nominal fee at *www.body-images.com*

Measure	Reference	Description	Sample / Reliability	Contact
Attention to Body Shape Scale	Beebe (1995)	Seven items assess degree of focus on body shape	Sample 1: 22 ♂; 167 ♀ in three samples IC: (.70–.83) Sample 2: 22 ♂; 49 ♀ TR: (.76–87)	Dean Beebe, PhD *dean.beebe@cchmc.org*
Body Checking Cognitions Questionnaire	Mountford, Haase, & Waller (2006)	Assesses key cognitions associated with body-checking behaviors	Sample: 205 healthy adult ♀ students, 84 clinical adult ♀ IC: (.72–.87) TR: n/a	Victoria Mountford, DClinPsy *vicki.mountford@swlstg-tr.nhs.uk*
Sociocultural Attitudes Towards Appearance Questionnaire-3: General Internalization Subscale	Thompson, van den Berg, Roehrig, Guarda, & Heinberg (2004)	Nine items assess the internalization of media beauty ideals	Sample: 175 ♀ undergraduates IC: (.96) TR: n/a	J. Kevin Thompson, PhD *www.bodyimagedisturbance.org*

Behavioral measures

Measure	Reference	Description	Sample / Reliability	Contact
Body Checking Questionnaire	Reas, White, & Grilo (2002)	23-item self-report measure of body-checking behaviors covering (three factors: overall appearance, specific body parts, and idiosyncratic checking)	Sample 1: 149 ♀ undergraduates IC: (.82–92) Sample 2: 54 ♀ undergraduates TR: 2 weeks (.90–94)	Donald A. Williamson, PhD *williada@pbrc.edu*
Body Image Avoidance Questionnaire	Rosen, Srebnik, Saltzberg, & Wendt (1991)	Assesses frequency of body image-related avoidance behaviors	Sample: 145 ♀ undergraduates IC: 89 TR: 2 weeks (.87)	James C. Rosen, PhD (retired)

(continued)

TABLE 18.1. (continued)

Type and name of instrument	Reference	Description	Standardization sample and reliability	Author contact
Body Image Avoidance Scale	Engle, Cash, & Jarry (2008)	22-item measure of body image avoidance behaviors (two factors: contextual avoidance, camouflaging)	Sample: 645 ♀ undergraduate students IC: (.73–.94) TR: n/a	Thomas F. Cash, PhD Available for a nominal fee at *www.body-images.com*
Body Image Compulsive Actions Scale	Engle, Cash, & Jarry (2008)	25-measure of body image-related behaviors (two factors: appearance fixing, checking)	Sample: 645 ♀ undergraduate students IC: (.91–.93) TR: n/a	Thomas F. Cash, PhD Available for a nominal fee at *www.body-images.com*
Male body image measures				
Drive for Leanness Scale	Smolak & Murnen (2008)	Six-item measure assessing attitudes about a lean, toned body	Sample 1: 39 ♂ and 46 ♀ undergraduates TR: .69 Sample 2: 95 ♂ and 137 ♀ undergraduates IC: .83 women; .79 men	Linda Smolak, PhD *smolak@kenyon.edu*
Drive for Muscularity Attitudes Questionnaire (Cognitive)	Morrison, Morrison, Hopkins, & Rowan (2004)	Eight items assessing attitudes toward muscularity	Sample: 412 ♂ undergraduates IC: .84 TR: n/a	Todd G. Morrison, PhD *todd.morrison@usask.ca*
Drive for Muscularity Scale	McCreary, Sasse, Saucier, & Dorsch (2004)	15-item self-report measure of muscle-oriented attitudes and behaviors	Sample: 276 ♂ and 354 ♀ from high school and university settings IC: (.81–.97) TR: n/a	Donald R. McCreary, PhD *donmccreary@yahoo.ca*

166

Measure	Reference	Description	Sample	Contact
Masculine Body Ideal Distress (Affective)	Kimmel & Mahalik (2004)	Measure of distress as the result of failing to attain cultural standards of muscular physique	Sample: 154 college-aged ♂ IC: .89 TR: n/a	James R. Mahalik, PhD *mahalik@bc.edu*
Male Body Attitudes Scale (Global Satisfaction)	Tylka, Bergeron, & Schwartz (2005)	24-item measure of men's body attitudes across three dimensions: low body fat, muscularity, and height	Sample 1: 294 undergraduate ♂ IC: (.88–.93) Sample 2: 107 undergraduate ♂ TR: 2 weeks (.81–.94)	Tracy Tylka, PhD *tylka.2@osu.edu*
Male-Specific Body Checking (Behavioral)	Hildebrandt, Walker, Alfano, Delinksy, & Bannon (2010)	Measure of body checking related to the male physical ideal (four factors: global muscle checking, chest and shoulder checking, other-comparative checking, and body testing)	Sample 1: 196 ♂ and 146 ♀ undergraduates Sample 2: 27 ♂ undergraduates IC: (.93–.94) TR: 2 weeks (.68–.84)	Tom Hildebrandt, PsyD *tom.hildebrandt@mssm.edu*
Muscle Appearance Satisfaction Scale (Global and Behavioral)	Mayville, Williamson, White, Netemeyer, & Drab (2002)	19-item self-report measure assessing concern with muscular appearance (five factors: bodybuilding dependence, muscle checking, substance use, injury, and muscle satisfaction)	Sample 1: 149 ♂ undergraduate students IC: (.75–.87) Sample 2: 42 ♂ undergraduate students TR: 2 weeks (.76–.89)	Stephen Mayville, PhD *Mayo1@aol.com*
Swansea Muscularity Attitudes—Drive for Muscularity Subscale (Cognitive)	Edwards & Launder (2000)	10 items assessing desire to be muscular and bodybuilding behavior	Sample: 303 adult ♂ IC: .94 TR: n/a	Stephen Edwards, PhD *s.edwards@swansea.ac.uk*

Informative Readings

Avalos, L., Tylka, T. L., & Wood-Barcalow, N. (2005). The Body Appreciation Scale: Development and psychometric evaluation. *Body Image: An International Journal of Research, 2,* 285–297.—Describes the development of a novel measure of positive body image.

Cash, T. F. Body image assessments. Available from the author at *www.body-images.com.*—Describes 12 of the author's validated body image questionnaire assessments; materials (questionnaires, manuals, norms, scoring instructions, and/or source references) can be ordered for a nominal fee from the website.

Gardner, R. M., & Brown, D. L. (2010). Body image assessment: A review of figural drawing scales. *Personality and Individual Differences, 48,* 107–111.—A comprehensive review of all known figural drawing scales, provides psychometric information, descriptions of the scales, and discussion of methodological issues.

McCreary, D. R., Sasse, D. K., Saucier, D. M., & Dorsch, K. D. (2004). Measuring the drive for muscularity: Factorial validity of the Drive for Muscularity Scale in men and women. *Psychology of Men and Masculinity, 1,* 49–58.—A measure of satisfaction and behaviors related to muscularity; this article describes the psychometric properties of the Drive for Muscularity Scale.

McKinley, N., & Hyde, J. (1996). The Objectified Body Consciousness Scale: Development and validation. *Psychology of Women Quarterly, 20,* 181–215.—Describes a measure of self-objectification and related constructs, including the Body Shame Scale.

Stewart, T. M., & Williamson, D. A. (2004). Assessment of body image disturbances. In J. K. Thompson (Ed.), *Handbook of eating disorders and obesity* (pp. 495–514). Hoboken, NJ: Wiley.—Discusses the main theoretical frameworks underlying body image assessment and provides guidelines for selection of measurement instruments, with a focus on BID.

Thompson, J. K., & Cafri, G. (Eds.). (2007). *The muscular ideal.* Washington, DC: American Psychological Association.—Provides a broad overview of recent work on the muscularity ideal and also recommendations for selection of male body image measures and methods for assessment.

Thompson, J. K., Heinberg, L. J., Altabe, M. N., & Tantleff-Dunn, S. (1999). *Exacting beauty: Theory, assessment, and treatment of body image disturbance.* Washington, DC: American Psychological Association.—Covers multiple aspects of body image, including assessment and application of assessment to treatment selection.

Thompson, J. K., van den Berg, P., Roehrig, M., Guarda, A., & Heinberg, L. J. (2004). The Sociocultural Attitudes Towards Appearance Questionnaire-3 (SATAQ-3): Development and validation. *International Journal of Eating Disorders, 35,* 293–304.—Provides the psychometric properties for the newest edition of the SATAQ.

Tylka, T. L., Bergerson, D., & Schwartz, J. P. (2005). Development and psychometric evaluation of the Male Body Attitudes Scale (MBAS). *Body Image: An International Journal of Research, 2,* 161–175.—Provides a description of the development of the MBAS, a measure of three dimensions of male body image, and its psychometric properties.

Yanover, T., & Thompson, J. K. (2009). Assessment of body image in children and adolescents. In L. Smolak & J. K. Thompson (Eds.), *Body image, eating disorders, and obesity in youth: Assessment, prevention, and treatment* (pp. 177–192). Washington, DC: American Psychological Association.—Review of measures for assessing body image in children and adolescents and discussion of methodological issues.

PART IV

INDIVIDUAL AND CULTURAL DIFFERENCES

CHAPTER 19

Gender and Body Images

SARAH K. MURNEN

Introduction

To get an exaggerated picture of the ideal images of the female and male body, think of the Bratz doll marketed for girls, and the World Wrestling Entertainment (WWE) "action figure" aimed at boys. The Bratz doll, like her popular predecessor Barbie, is very slim, which portrays the "thin ideal" that is glorified in the mass media. The Bratz doll is more sexualized than Barbie in terms of her clothing, makeup, and pouting lips that reflect the increased sexualization expected of women in Western culture. The wrestling action figure has a massive set of muscles in his upper torso and a "six pack" of abdominal muscles. The fact that he is an action figure instead of a doll emphasizes the functionality of his body in addition to its muscularity.

These "toys" highlight some of the gendered issues associated with body image discussed in this chapter. First, research suggests that the nature of body image ideals differs for women and girls versus men and boys. Female body ideals are strongly associated with thinness, and increasingly with large breasts and other signifiers of "sexiness." Male ideals are somewhat associated with leanness, but more clearly with muscularity. There is a cultural emphasis on how women's bodies *look* versus how men's bodies *act*. Ubiquitous objectification of women and the link between appearance and social success for women mean that body image satisfaction is more strongly associated with psychological well-being for women than men, and that women spend more time and effort trying to attain a societal body ideal.

Thin, Sexy Women

The cultural depiction of the ideal woman accentuates the parts of her body that distinguish her from a man. In a typical media portrayal, the ideal woman might have long hair, long eyelashes, full lips, large breasts, a thin waist, rounded buttocks, and long legs. Increasingly, she should appear sexy, which might mean enhancing, emphasizing, and/or exposing sexualized body parts. For example, she could wear a low-cut shirt to show cleavage and stiletto heels to emphasize long legs. Victoria's Secret underwear models enact this body ideal quite well. A variety of beauty practices support the production of the ideal woman including the use of makeup and hair products, clothing that emphasizes the distinctive shape of women's bodies, efforts directed at creating and maintaining thinness, hair-removal practices, and cosmetic surgery.

Psychologists became concerned with the thinness aspect of the female body ideal starting in the late 1970s, and have researched its existence and effects. Whereas the body of the ideal woman of the 1950s was "full figured" with some fat on her hips and waist that was in proportion to her ample breasts (e.g., Marilyn Monroe), the ideal body became thinner across the 1970s, 1980s, and through the 1990s. Today the ideal woman manages to have large breasts despite her slim waist and hips (e.g., Christina Aguilera). The image is extremely unrealistic for the average American woman to attain. Barbie's body type and positioning is so improbable that if she were a real person, she would not be able to stand given her large chest and precarious, high-heeled stance.

The image of the ideal woman is portrayed prevalently in fashion magazines, and also in magazines aimed at men. Women's bodies are subjected to the "male gaze" in the media and in everyday life. In one recent study more than half of the advertisements of women found across a variety of magazines portrayed them as sex objects. Much research has shown that exposure to the thin body image ideal in the media is linked with high rates of body dissatisfaction in women, and with the development of eating-disordered attitudes (see Chapter 12). Rates of body dissatisfaction are so high among women they are described as normative. Even young girls are aware of the thin ideal and many of them report dieting behavior (see Chapters 8 and 9). In addition to media depictions, family and friends often reinforce thinness concerns. By adolescence, girls can become part of an all-female appearance subculture where much of the talk and behavior is associated with maintaining appearance (see Chapter 13). Thinness and a focus on appearance generally have become part of the expected social roles for women. Women are expected to spend time, energy, and money in pursuit of bodily perfection. Many women believe that if they look like the thin-ideal women portrayed in the media, they will have a better life. Embodying the thin ideal is associated with success in employment and romantic relationships.

Increasingly, "sexiness" is also part of the ideal image of women. The sexualization of women in the media has increased since the early 1980s, perhaps partially due to the advent of the Internet. Pornography is easily accessible, and some believe that our culture has become "pornified" in that practices and fashions that used to be portrayed only in pornography are now appearing in popular culture, such as thong underwear and stiletto heels. Women, and even adolescent girls, are being encouraged to accept a view of sex that legitimizes their role as sex objects. A sample of young women from my college indicated that there is a long list of behaviors in which most women engage to look sexy for men including (in order of importance) shaving legs, shaving armpits, wearing scents, wearing a bikini, wearing tight clothes, wearing low-cut/revealing shirts, styling hair, wearing a bra that enhances or emphasizes breasts, and shaving the genital area. In contrast, a sample of young men from the same college asked what the majority of men do to be sexy for women agreed on only two behaviors—wearing scent, and being "clean." This difference reflects the idea that women are pressured to have a "sexy" body. Young women are led by the media to believe that sexiness is empowering, but women who are sexualized are seen as less competent.

If neither the thin ideal nor the sexy ideal promotes women's competence, are there more empowering body ideals available to women and girls? There are individual groups of women and girls who experience greater body satisfaction and lower rates of eating disorders compared to others. Girls and women who participate in sports that don't emphasize leanness (e.g., basketball) are less at risk, as are Black women (see Chapter 25), lesbian women (see Chapter 24), and women who are more feminist in their attitudes. These girls and women might have different body ideal standards and/or less concern with the "male gaze." However, even these groups are not invulnerable, suggesting that cultural change on a large scale might be necessary before we see striking improvements in body satisfaction.

Muscular, Powerful Men

While the female ideal body has become more thin and sexy across time, the ideal male body has also undergone change. Going back to the action figure icon, GI Joe became more muscular across time. In the 1970s, GI Joe was quite scrawny compared to the "buff" version of the 1990s. The muscularity of *Playgirl* centerfold models and Mr. America contestants also increased across time. The ideal body for men emphasizes a "V-shape" structured by broad shoulders tapering to a thin waist with well-defined abdominal muscles (a "six pack" of abs). The ideal man is lean and muscular, and has a full head of hair. Increasingly, his chest is hairless and he is depicted shirtless. The image of actor Matthew McConaughey often portrayed in the media reflects this ideal.

In early research it was assumed that body image dissatisfaction (BID) was mainly a female problem, but then researchers took a closer look at boys and men. It was found that some boys and men want to be thinner, and a sizeable number (as many as one-third) want to be more muscular. Psychologists have developed measures of "drive for muscularity" and have found that greater concern with muscularity is associated with BID and the adoption of body change behaviors (see Chapter 22). Whereby body change behaviors in women might include dieting and aerobic exercise for weight loss, in men they might take the form of protein supplements and weightlifting.

Unlike the drive for thinness in women, the drive for muscularity in men reflects more concern about how the body functions than what it looks like. A focus on appearance is not a primary role for men, but the appearance of muscularity likely increases perceptions that a man is dominant and competitive, which are important components of masculinity. However, masculine roles can be enacted in ways that do not involve appearance. For example, a successful male corporate chief executive officer probably does not need well-developed muscles to prove his masculinity. Boys and men who have a strong drive for muscularity are more likely to agree with particular stereotypic masculine attitudes like the importance of winning and the importance of athletics, which shows that body concerns are linked with men's social roles. Athletics is a realm of influence deserving further study in that it might promote masculine values that put body image pressures on males.

Certain groups of men show more or less vulnerability to body dissatisfaction. Gay men are somewhat more dissatisfied with their bodies, and specifically want to be more muscular, compared to heterosexual men. Gay men are more likely to monitor and compare their bodies, perhaps because they are objects of the "male gaze." On the other hand, although Black men desire a larger body size than White men, they report more satisfaction with their body. Although the data are sparse, there are no other significant differences that have been found between other ethnic minority groups of men when they are compared to White men (from whom we have the most data). We are just now beginning to accumulate a sufficient number of studies that can help us understand the range of body image issues that various male groups might experience.

Gender Differences in BID

Although body ideals are disseminated for both women and men that are associated with their respective gender roles, an emphasis on appearance is promoted as more important for women than men. Thus it is not surprising that there are gender differences in rates of body dissatisfaction. Prior to the 1970s, there was no significant difference in body satisfaction among females and males. The size of the gender difference became statistically significant by the 1980s, and grew even larger by the 1990s. However, throughout the 1990s, the body dissatisfaction of both women and men increased. Other gender differences in body image-related issues include the fact that women are more likely to compare their body to those of others, are more likely to diet, and are more likely to obtain cosmetic surgery. Cosmetic surgery rates have dramatically increased in recent years, and the surgeries that women elect most often—breast augmentation, followed by liposuction—reflect their body image concerns (see Chapter 45). Further, gender differences in rates of the eating disorders anorexia nervosa and bulimia nervosa are large. On the other hand, men are more likely to report the use of protein supplements and anabolic steroids to build muscle, and to report the use of weight-bearing exercises (e.g., weight lifting) to build muscle.

Sociocultural theories can explain gender differences in body concerns (see Chapter 2). Research suggests that the same kinds of factors (e.g., parents, peers, and the media) influence female and male body dissatisfaction, but to different degrees. It is likely that the media exert a stronger influence on females than males for at least two reasons. First, there is a greater degree of objectification of women than men in the visual media. According to objectification theory, the high prevalence of objectifying images of women is believed to cultivate self-objectification in women where they start to monitor their own body and compare it to the ideal (Chapter 6). Women are likely to experience body shame given that the ideal is unrealistic. Second, appearance is more important to women's sense of self, revealed by stronger relationships between women's body satisfaction and their self-esteem. Throughout history women have been encouraged to manipulate their body to attain a societal ideal. While in the late 1800s women used corsets to create an "hourglass" body shape, today they might use extreme calorie restriction and breast implants. Feminists suggest that the persistent objectification of women exists because of women's societal subordination to men.

Conclusions and Future Directions

Both women and men are exposed to unrealistic body ideals that threaten their sense of well-being. Gender role norms promote exaggerated body image ideals that encourage a drive for thinness in women and a drive for muscularity in men. These unrealistic ideals are associated with higher levels of BID in both genders. For women, a focus on the body is an expected role all in itself. Women's and men's roles fit together in the enactment of the "heterosexual script." In this script women are stereotyped as sexual objects and men as sexual actors. Women's bodies "should" be used to attract men, so their sexiness is important, whereas men's bodies "should" project their strength and dominance. While the complementary roles of the heterosexual script might bring women and men together sexually, they promote a system through which women's inferior status as sexual objects is perpetuated.

Further, objectification is associated with women's lower status. Although researchers have recognized the high degree of objectification women experience and its effects on women's psychological functioning, we now know that men are also vulnerable to the effects of objectification. The objectification of men is increasing in the culture such that there are now beauty and skin products being marketed for the "metrosexual" man. Objectification pressures are related to the existence of capitalist consumer culture. If women and men can be encouraged to feel sufficiently dissatisfied with their body that they need to purchase products for improvement, this will benefit the fashion, diet, and beauty industries.

If it is true that gender role norms produce exaggerated and unrealistic body image ideals, then these roles need to change. Increasingly, women have more access to work roles in society, but this has not changed expectations that they focus attention on appearance. In fact, some argue that there are greater appearance pressures on women today in the dictate for "effortless perfection." We have a cultural image of the "superwoman," who achieves perfection in both work and family roles while managing to "look great." We need increased societal critique of the idea that women should be able to effortlessly balance multiple roles without support. We need to continue to evaluate the thinness role and investigate the threats posed by the increased sexualization of women. Men's roles have not changed to the extent that women's roles have, but this is necessary if the balance of power between women and men is to be changed. Men need to be encouraged to focus more on nurturing and caretaking, and less on competition and dominance. Societal promotion of minority cultures could deemphasize gendered roles and expand definitions of the ideal woman and man.

Informative Readings

Grabe, S., & Hyde, J. S. (2006). Ethnicity and body dissatisfaction among women in the United States: A meta-analysis. *Psychological Bulletin, 132*, 622–640.—Data show that most groups of women experience body dissatisfaction, although Black women experience somewhat less.

Levine, M. P., & Murnen, S. K. (2009). "Everybody knows that mass media are/are not (pick one) a cause of eating disorders": A critical review of evidence for a causal link between media, negative body image, and disordered eating in females. *Journal of Social and Clinical Psychology, 28*, 9–42.—Provides evidence for a causal link between exposure to a media thin ideal and body dissatisfaction and eating-disordered attitudes.

McKinley, N. M. (2006). Longitudinal gender differences in objectified body consciousness and weight-related attitudes and behaviors: Cultural and developmental contexts in the transition from college. *Sex Roles, 54,* 159–173.—Reveals gender differences and similarities in the experience of body dissatisfaction during college and 10 years later.

Morrison, M. A., Morrison, T. D., & Sager, C. (2004). Does body satisfaction differ between gay men and lesbian women and heterosexual men and women? A meta-analytic review. *Body Image: An International Journal of Research, 1,* 127–138.—Shows that lesbian women experience more body satisfaction than heterosexual women and gay men experience less satisfaction than heterosexual men.

Murnen, S. K., & Smolak, L. (in press). "I'd rather be a famous fashion model than a famous scientist.": The rewards and costs of internalizing sexualization. In E. Zurbriggen & T. A. Roberts (Eds.), *The sexualization of girls and girlhood.* New York: Oxford University Press.—Reviews research and theory on the implications of emphasizing "sexiness" as important for women.

Ricciardelli, L. A., McCabe, M. P., Williams, R. J., & Thompson, J. K. (2007). The role of ethnicity and culture in body image and disordered eating among males. *Clinical Psychology Review, 27,* 582–606.—Provides data and reviews theory suggesting that boys and men are also vulnerable to cultural body image ideals.

Smolak, L., & Murnen, S. K. (2007). Feminism and body image. In V. Swami & A. Furnham (Eds.), *The body beautiful* (pp. 236–258). London: Palgrave Macmillan.—Evaluates feminist explanations of women's frequent body dissatisfaction including objectification theory.

Smolak, L., & Stein, J. A. (2006). The relationship of drive for muscularity to sociocultural factors, self-esteem, physical attributes, gender role, and social comparison in middle school boys. *Body Image: An International Journal of Research, 3,* 121–129.—Shows that sociocultural theories can predict body image concerns of boys and raises concerns about the gender role in promoting a drive for muscularity in boys.

Striegel-Moore, R. H., & Bulik, C. M. (2007). Risk factors for eating disorders. *American Psychologist, 62,* 181–198.—Provides a review of eating disorder risk factors, and includes a focus on gender differences.

Tiggemann, M., Martins, Y., & Churchett, L. (2008). Beyond muscles: Unexplored parts of men's body image. *Journal of Health Psychology, 13,* 1163–1172.—Examines the influence of various issues on men's appearance satisfaction revealing that although weight and muscularity are most predictive, other factors such as body hair and penis size are important and deserve more attention.

CHAPTER 20

Obesity and Body Image in Youth

DIANNE NEUMARK-SZTAINER

Introduction

Obesity among children and adolescents has received a lot of attention in the scientific and popular literature given its high prevalence and potential consequences for physical and psychosocial health. An important question to consider is how concerned we need to be about body image issues facing overweight youth. In this chapter, the prevalence of body satisfaction among overweight youth is compared to that of nonoverweight youth. Reasons for the high prevalence of body image concerns among youth, and particularly among overweight youth, are discussed. Associations between body satisfaction and both weight-related behaviors and weight gain over time are explored to determine whether there are any potential advantages to being dissatisfied with one's body in terms of weight management. Finally, intervention ideas for working with overweight youth to improve their body image, while also improving their eating and physical activity behaviors are presented.

How Is Weight Status Determined in Youth?

Of note, between the ages of 2 and 20, in the United States, weight status is based on body mass index (BMI) percentile. The percentile for a given BMI is calculated using the Year 2000 Growth Charts from the Centers for Disease Control and Prevention (CDC). These growth charts were developed using height and weight data from children and adolescents in the

United States, collected between 1963 and 1980. Children and adolescents with BMI values above the 85th percentile but below the 95th percentile are categorized as overweight, and those whose BMI is equal to or greater than the 95th percentile are categorized as obese. The use of this terminology is fairly recent; previously the terms *at-risk for overweight* and *overweight* were used. This terminology is also somewhat controversial, in that a child could be at a high weight for height and not be overly fat. Furthermore, the term *obese* can be viewed as a derogatory term. In the current chapter, the term *obese* is used only when necessary to distinguish between the two weight categories; otherwise the term *overweight* is used whenever possible.

How Prevalent Are Body Image Concerns among Overweight Youth?

Research shows that body image concerns are higher among overweight children and adolescents than their average-weight peers. Associations between weight status and body image tend to occur across studies, regardless of participants' age, gender, or race, although strengths of association may differ. Furthermore, associations exist regardless of differences in study methodologies, including measures used to assess body image concerns.

Project EAT (Eating Among Teens) was designed to learn more about eating, activity, and weight-related topics in a population-based sample of adolescents. In Project EAT, the prevalence of body satisfaction was examined across weight status in over 4,500 adolescents. Body satisfaction was assessed with a modified version of the Body Shape Satisfaction Scale, which included 10 items assessing satisfaction with different body parts (e.g., height, weight, stomach, and hips), with five Likert response categories ranging from "very dissatisfied" to "very satisfied." Responses were categorized as low, moderate, and high based on distributions within the study population, with one-third of the population within each category. Two-thirds of the obese girls (with BMI values above the 95th percentile for age and sex) expressed low levels of body satisfaction as compared to about one-third of the average-weight girls. Among boys, about half of the obese boys expressed low body satisfaction as compared to a fifth of the average-weight boys.

In order to more fully explore the experience of being large in a thin-oriented society, and learn more about self-perceptions of overweight adolescent girls, in a different study, in-depth individual interviews were conducted with overweight African American and Caucasian adolescent girls. The girls were asked several questions about their self-image, and more specifically, their body image. The majority of girls (49 out of 50) described their body and shape in negative terms and some of their comments indicated extreme body dissatisfaction. The girls talked about wanting to get rid of their fat by cutting it off. They discussed difficulties wearing certain clothes and challenges they faced in social interactions. The girls' responses showed that being overweight was a central part of their life that negatively impacted their own body image and social interactions with others. However, nearly all of the girls had something positive to say about themselves and their lives, in spite of their extreme weight and body image concerns. The girls made positive appearance-related comments and non-appearance-related comments (e.g., about personality, talents, or involvement in activities). Thus, whereas these overweight girls faced many difficulties living in a thin-oriented society, the findings also indicated that being overweight was only one aspect, albeit a significant one, in their lives. Of note, both African American and Caucasian girls expressed concerns about their body shape and size, but African American girls were more likely than the Caucasian girls to also discuss the positive aspects of their body (e.g., their curves). These interviews demonstrated the complexities of body image issues faced by overweight youth within a society that values thinness for girls.

In summary, findings from studies on children and adolescents, using both quantitative and qualitative research methodologies, find that overweight youth are at increased risk for body image concerns. The scientific literature suggests that some groups, particularly African American girls, appear to be somewhat protected against body image concerns. However, similarities across race/ethnicity appear to be larger than differences, and overweight youth, regardless of their background, are at higher risk for body image concerns than their nonoverweight peers.

Why Are Body Image Concerns so High among Overweight Youth?

Given strong social pressures to be thin for girls, and to be lean and muscular for boys, it is hardly surprising that overweight youth tend to have higher levels of body image concerns than nonoverweight youth. Images of girls and women in the media are by and large very thin, whereas images of boys and men tend to show lean and muscular bodies with "six-pack abs." Youth are exposed to the media on an ongoing basis throughout the day. Clothes are designed for lean bodies and overweight youth often face difficulties in shopping and finding stylish clothes to fit their larger body. Thinness is often equated with beauty with larger people being perceived as less attractive than those who are thin. Furthermore, there is a lot of attention in the popular press about the importance of a thin body in terms of overall health. Finally, studies show that overweight children and adolescents are at higher risk for weight mistreatment, including being the victims of weight-related teasing. Weight-related teasing has been found to be associated with lower levels of body satisfaction and self-esteem.

In a landmark study conducted by Richardson and colleagues in 1961, 10- and 11-year-old children were shown six drawings of children and asked to rank them according to how well they liked each child. The drawings included a healthy child, an overweight child, and four children with various disabilities or disfigurements, including one child in a wheelchair and another child with a facial disfigurement. The children ranked the overweight child last on likeability. Interestingly, in 2003, Latner and Stunkard replicated this study among elementary school children and found that stigmatization of obesity by children had increased over the 40 years since the original study. In the 2003 study, the overweight child was ranked last on likeability, and was liked significantly less than in the 1961 study.

In the previously mentioned qualitative study, which included individual interviews with overweight adolescent girls, weight stigmatization experiences were explored. Nearly all of the girls participating in the interviews (48 out of 50 girls) described hurtful types of weight mistreatment. The most frequently mentioned experiences involved intentionally hurtful comments made by others (e.g., weight-related teasing, jokes, and derogatory names). Other types of weight mistreatment involved different types of comments made by others (e.g., comments that were hurtful, albeit not intentionally so), being treated differently because they were overweight (e.g., excluded from friendship groups), and having negative assumptions made about them because of their weight (e.g., regarding eating behaviors, hygiene, and personality). Girls talked about mistreatment by family members, other children, employers, and strangers. The most commonly mentioned place in which stigmatization occurred was within the school setting, followed by the home.

It has been proposed that given the higher prevalence of obesity in young people, it may now be more acceptable to be overweight, with overweight children experiencing less weight stigmatization. While further research on this issue is needed, the studies described above do not suggest that this is the case. It has also been proposed that a certain amount of body dissatisfaction among young people may be desirable in order to promote weight management and prevent obesity. This question is explored in the following section.

Body Image Concerns: Helpful or Harmful in Terms of Weight Management?

Given the high prevalence of obesity in youth and its associated health consequences, an important question relates to the impact of body image concerns on weight management behaviors and weight status over time.

Are youth with low levels of body satisfaction less likely to engage in healthy weight management behaviors, such as increased fruit and vegetable intake or regular physical activity, as compared to youth who feel good about their body? Are girls with body image concerns at increased risk for dieting, unhealthy weight control behaviors, or binge eating, which have been found to predict weight gain over time in youth?

Or, alternatively, are there advantages to having body image concerns and not being satisfied with one's body? Heinberg, Thompson, and Matzon have proposed that body image dissatisfaction (BID) is not always a negative process and that some degree of dissatisfaction may help motivate individuals at average or above-average BMIs to engage in healthy eating and exercise behaviors. They have hypothesized that the relationship between BID and healthy weight management behaviors may be illustrated by an inverted U-shaped curve. When body image distress is very low, individuals may not engage in healthy eating and exercise behaviors, even if necessary to improve health outcomes. When body image distress is very high, individuals may fail to engage in healthy weight management behaviors because of a perceived inability to make meaningful changes in their body, or they may engage in unhealthy dieting behaviors in a desperate attempt to lose weight.

In order to determine whether body image concerns are helpful or harmful in terms of weight management behaviors and outcomes, our research team conducted two separate analyses using the Project EAT 5-year longitudinal sample. In the first analysis, associations between body satisfaction and behaviors with implications for weight management were explored among 2,500 adolescent girls and boys. Among girls, lower body satisfaction at baseline predicted higher levels of dieting, unhealthy and extreme weight control behaviors, and binge eating, as well as lower levels of physical activity and fruit and vegetable intake 5 years later. After adjusting for BMI, associations between body satisfaction and dieting, extreme weight control behaviors, and physical activity remained statistically significant. In boys, lower body satisfaction predicted higher levels of dieting, healthy, unhealthy, and extreme weight control behaviors, binge eating, smoking, and lower levels of physical activity. After adjusting for BMI, associations between body satisfaction and dieting, unhealthy weight control behaviors, and binge eating remained statistically significant. Findings from this study led to the conclusion that, in general, lower body satisfaction does not serve as a motivator for engaging in healthy weight management behaviors, but rather predicts the use of behaviors that may place youth at risk for weight gain and poorer overall health.

Findings from this analysis led to a second analysis, examining associations between body satisfaction and weight gain over a 5-year period among overweight adolescent girls. The sample included 376 girls from Project EAT, who had BMIs above the 85th percentile for age and gender. Body satisfaction at baseline was divided into quartiles and changes in

BMI were examined over the study period. Statistical adjustments were made for baseline BMI and sociodemographic characteristics. The findings were quite striking and showed that overweight girls with low levels of body satisfaction at baseline increased their BMI by 3 units, as compared to an increase of only 1 unit among the girls with high levels of body satisfaction at baseline. Thus, findings suggested that body satisfaction was protective against increased BMI among overweight adolescent girls.

Findings from these two analyses suggest that lower body satisfaction may lead to poorer self-care in terms of health behaviors. Body image has many aspects and clearly more research is needed to understand associations between different aspects of body image concerns and different behaviors with implications for weight management. For example, it may be important to separate out weight dissatisfaction from global body satisfaction. Additionally, Project EAT was conducted with adolescents and less is known about associations between body image concerns and behavioral patterns with implications for weight management in younger children. Nevertheless, these findings point to the importance of helping young people of all sizes develop a positive sense of their body. They serve to guide recommendations for helping overweight children to feel better about their body and engage in behaviors likely to be helpful, and not harmful, for weight management, as discussed in the next section.

What Can Be Done to Help Overweight Youth Feel Better about Their Body?

Given that body dissatisfaction is prevalent among overweight youth, associated with a number of negative outcomes, not helpful in motivating youth to engage in healthy weight management behaviors, and predictive of weight gain over time, it is important to help overweight youth feel better about their body. Since there is real concern about the health-related consequences of obesity, there is a delicate balance that needs to happen here. It can be helpful to guide young people toward thinking in terms of "taking care of the body one has and nurturing this body toward good health" rather than "changing a body that one doesn't like since it doesn't conform to societal ideals of beauty." It may be appropriate to use similar language with overweight children as might be used with nonoverweight children, that is, where the focus would not be on "fixing" the body but rather on "healthy eating and physical activity to promote overall health." Ideas for helping young people, who are overweight or at risk for becoming overweight, feel better about their body and choose to take care of their body through healthier eating and physical activity behaviors within home, clinic, and school settings are briefly presented below.

Parents of overweight children may be concerned about their children's weight and encourage them to diet. However, research suggests that this type of encouragement will not be helpful and may backfire and lead to weight gain over time. Given that overweight children may be facing difficulties outside of their home environment (e.g., weight teasing and other social pressures), it is crucial to provide a home environment in which children feel safe, loved, and accepted for who they are. Weight-related derogatory comments should not be allowed at home. In order to help children engage in healthier eating and physical activity behaviors, parents should strive for a home environment that makes it easy for children to engage in these behaviors. Parents should be encouraged to "do more and talk less." Doing things to help children engage in healthier behaviors, such as serving healthy family meals and limiting television watching may be more helpful, and less harmful, than talking about weight-related topics.

Health care providers are similarly likely to be concerned about the health of the overweight children seen in their practices. Health care providers should assume that these children have experienced weight-related mistreatment and are at high risk for body image concerns. An empathetic approach to discussing body image and weight issues, which takes into account the sensitivity of these topics, is important. Pediatricians and health care providers play an important role in the lives of families and just letting a child know that he or she should not accept weight teasing or harassment may be helpful.

Finally, interventions aimed at obesity prevention are being implemented within school settings. Within such programs, it is crucial to direct attention toward a broad spectrum of weight-related problems, including body image concerns and unhealthy dieting practices. Our research team developed the New Moves program to prevent weight-related problems among high school girls at risk for obesity. The underlying philosophy of New Moves is to help girls feel better about themselves so that they will want to take care of themselves and their body through healthy eating, physical activity, and positive self-talk. Although New Moves did not lead to changes in weight status, it was successful in leading to improvements in body image, self-esteem, and weight-related behaviors. Further work is needed to develop interventions for children and adolescents, particularly those at risk for obesity, to help with healthy weight management and the promotion of positive self-perceptions.

Conclusions and Future Directions

In summary, body image concerns are high among overweight children and adolescents. Social pressures to be thin and weight mistreatment by other children, family members, and others contribute to the high prevalence of body image concerns and low self-esteem among overweight children. Ironically, low levels of body satisfaction do not appear to be successful in motivating young people to engage in healthy weight management behaviors and in preventing weight gain over time. Rather, body image concerns appear to lead to the use of unhealthy weight control practices. Thus, it is important to develop interventions for the home, clinic, and school that help children feel better about their body while providing them with supportive environments and skills to make it easier for them to engage in healthy eating and physical activity behaviors. Further research is needed to more fully elucidate the connection between body image concerns and behavioral patterns among youth. Likewise, further work is needed to develop interventions that are effective in promoting a positive body image and healthy eating and physical activity behaviors among young people, including both those who are nonoverweight and overweight.

Informative Readings

Barlow, S. E. (2007). Expert Committee. Expert committee recommendations regarding the prevention, assessment, and treatment of child and adolescent overweight and obesity: Summary report. *Pediatrics, 120,* S164–S192. Guidelines particularly for health care providers that include emphasis on addressing social influences.

Kuczmarski, R. J., Ogden, C. L., Guo, S. S., Grummer-Strawn, L. M., Flegal, K. M., Mei, Z., et al. (2002). 2000 CDC Growth Charts for the United States: Methods and development. *Vital Health Stat, 11,* 1–190.—Provides information on height and weight for children and adolescents in the United States.

Kutchman, E., Lawhun, S., Laheta, J., & Heinberg, L. (2009). Proximal causes and behaviors associated with pediatric obesity. In L. Smolak & J. K. Thompson (Eds.), *Body image, eating disorders, and obesity in youth: Assessment, prevention, and treatment* (2nd ed., pp. 157–175). Washington, DC: American Psychological Association.—Reviews factors contributing to the development and maintenance of obesity among children.

Latner, J. D., & Stunkard, A. J. (2003). Getting worse: The stigmatization of obese children. *Obesity Research, 11,* 452–456.—A replication of an early study on weight stigmatization by Richardson et al. (1961).

Neumark-Sztainer, D. (2005). *"I'm, like, SO fat!": Helping your teen make healthy choices about eating and exercise in a weight-obsessed world.* New York: Guilford Press.—Provides suggestions for parents on how to help their children have a healthy body image and engage in healthy eating and physical activity behaviors.

Neumark-Sztainer, D. (2009). Preventing obesity and eating disorders in adolescents: What can health care providers do? *Journal of Adolescent Health, 44,* 206–213.—Provides recommendations for health care providers concerned about obesity, eating disorders, and other weight-related problems among youth.

Neumark-Sztainer, D., Friend, S. E., Flattum, C. F., Hannan, P. J., Story, M. T.,

Bauer, K. W., et al. (2010). New Moves: Preventing weight-related problems in adolescent girls: A group-randomized study. *American Journal of Preventive Medicine, 39,* 421–432.—A school-based program aimed at improving body image and other weight-related issues among girls.

Neumark-Sztainer, D., Paxton, S. J., Hannan, P. J., Haines, J., & Story, M. (2006). Does body satisfaction matter? Five-year longitudinal associations between body satisfaction and health behaviors in adolescent females and males. *Journal of Adolescent Health, 39,* 244–251.—Examines 5-year longitudinal associations between body satisfaction and behaviors with implications for weight management in a large population-based sample of adolescent girls and boys.

Neumark-Sztainer, D., Story, M., & Faibisch, L. (1998). Perceived stigmatization among overweight African American and Caucasian adolescent girls. *Journal of Adolescent Health, 23,* 264–270.—A qualitative study exploring weight-related stigmatization experiences among overweight adolescent girls.

Neumark-Sztainer, D., Story, M., Faibisch, L., Ohlson, J., & Adamiak, M. (1999). Issues of self-image among overweight African American and Caucasian adolescent girls: A qualitative study. *Journal of Nutrition Education, 31,* 311–320.—A qualitative study exploring body image and self-image among 50 overweight adolescent girls.

Neumark-Sztainer, D., Story, M., Hannan, P. J., Perry, C. L., & Irving, L. M. (2002). Weight-related concerns and behaviors among overweight and non-overweight adolescents: Implications for preventing weight-related disorders. *Archives of Pediatrics and Adolescent Medicine, 156,* 171–178.—An examination of body dissatisfaction and weight control behaviors across weight status in a large population-based sample of adolescents.

Neumark-Sztainer, D., Wall, M., Story, M., & van den Berg, P. (2008). Accurate parental classification of their overweight adolescents' weight status: Does it matter? *Pediatrics, 121,* e1495–e1502.—Examines parental perceptions of their overweight children's weight status, parental encouragement of children to diet, and weight changes over time.

Puhl, R. M., & Latner, J. D. (2007). Stigma, obesity, and the health of the nation's children. *Psychological Bulletin, 133,* 557–580.—Review of issues facing overweight children and the stigmatization that they face.

Richardson, S. A., Goodman, N., Hastorf, A. H., & Dornbusch, S. M. (1961). Cultural uniformity in reaction to physical disabilities. *American Sociological Review, 26,* 241–247.—Early landmark study showing how children perceive overweight children negatively.

van den Berg, P., & Neumark-Sztainer, D. (2007). Fat 'n happy 5 years later: Is it bad for overweight girls to like their bodies? *Journal of Adolescent Health, 41,* 415–417.—Examines associations between body satisfaction and weight gain over time among overweight adolescent girls.

CHAPTER 21

Obesity and Body Image in Adulthood

JANET D. LATNER
REBECCA E. WILSON

Introduction

A common attitude is that overweight persons deserve to feel ashamed of their weight and body. Profound societal stigma against obese people feeds this view. Evidence that obesity is related to chronic disease and shortened lifespan provides a major justification of weight bias. Essentially, the popular view is that obesity is unhealthy, and people who are obese should be dissatisfied with their size so that they will be motivated to lose weight.

However, as discussed in this chapter, poor body image does not appear to facilitate weight control. Rather, research indicates that negative body image may in fact contribute to obesity-related health problems. Overweight and obese people who are content with their weight experience fewer physically and mentally unhealthy days than those who are weight dissatisfied. Moreover, percentage of desired weight loss predicts unhealthy days more strongly than does body mass index (BMI; kg/m^2). Overweight Whites and women have a poorer body image than other overweight groups and experience more BMI-associated morbidity and mortality at lower BMIs. Possible pathways between body image and poorer health include stress and behavioral changes related to body image distress (e.g., unhealthy weight control behaviors and fewer healthy behaviors). Research also suggests that weight and shape concerns and body dissatisfaction may mediate associations between obesity and psychosocial impairment. Thus, poor body image can have negative health consequences in obese individuals.

It should be noted that psychosocial functioning is, perhaps unexpectedly, not very impaired in unselected obesity samples. People with obesity make up a very heterogeneous group, and although obese people generally report poorer body image than nonobese people, it is more useful to consider how body image differs within the obese population. Some studies have failed to find a relationship between degree of obesity and body image dissatisfaction (BID). There may be thresholds at which an individual's level of body dissatisfaction shifts, and that within these thresholds, body image remains relatively stable. Conversely, other studies have found a positive association between BMI and BID, generally in overweight and obese men and in nonclinical samples.

Risk Factors for Body Image Difficulties

Weight Bias and Stigmatization

Individuals with obesity experience frequent bias and discrimination for their weight in employment, health care, educational, and interpersonal settings. Experiences of being stigmatized for body weight are more frequent among more obese adults; individuals with a BMI of 40 or greater are subject to significantly more stigmatizing situations than those with a BMI under 40. Weight bias can have an adverse impact on numerous physical and psychological outcomes, including body image.

In adults from both clinical and nonclinical samples, a history of being stigmatized for being overweight is associated with negative body image. Research by Annis and colleagues demonstrates that currently overweight adult women who report more experiences of weight stigmatization also report greater body dissatisfaction and distress, as well as more dysfunctional investment in their appearance. These relationships exist for stigmatization that took place in childhood, adolescence, or adulthood. However, stigmatizing experiences were not related to body image for women who were previously but no longer overweight. Greater weight stigmatization has also been shown to correlate with more body image distress among overweight men and women. Stigmatization experience remains strongly correlated with body image distress (and other psychopathology) even when controlling for weight, suggesting that poorer body image is not merely a function of weight but is related directly to stigmatization. Among adult women with binge-eating disorder (BED; see Chapter 34), a childhood history of weight-related teasing may be a particularly strong predictor of body dissatisfaction. However, among obese women seeking weight loss treatment who are non-BED, weight-related teasing that occurred in adulthood was an even stronger predictor of body image distress than childhood teasing. (For more discussion of the effects of weight-related teasing on body image in youth, see Chapters 13 and 20).

Unlike members of other stigmatized groups, overweight and obese individuals do not have more favorable attitudes toward their in-group (other overweight or obese persons). Instead, they hold anti-fat attitudes that are just as negative as those of nonoverweight individuals. Internalized weight bias (IWB), the extent to which overweight and obese individuals endorse negative stereotypes about obesity and apply these stereotypes to themselves, is an important predictor of body dissatisfaction. In non-treatment-seeking adults, IWB significantly predicts body dissatisfaction, whereas BMI and anti-fat attitudes (toward other overweight persons) do not. IWB is also associated with more negative appearance evaluation and stronger investment in appearance among overweight and obese individuals seeking behavioral weight loss treatment. Both IWB and appearance evaluation improve following treatment, and changes in these variables over the course of treatment are significantly correlated with each other. Greater IWB is also associated with greater shape and weight concerns among patients with BED.

Gender and Ethnicity

Overweight women are more likely to consider themselves overweight and to be less body satisfied than overweight men, even at lower BMI levels. Overweight women also report poorer psychological functioning than men at similar weights. In part, this may reflect differences in sociocultural body ideals. In many countries, this ideal for women emphasizes thinness, whereas for men it also involves muscularity, and the range of culturally acceptable sizes for men may be broader. When assessing desired body size, a substantial proportion of men endorse wanting to be larger. Overweight men who label themselves overweight are more body satisfied than normal-weight men who consider themselves overweight. In women, the opposite is true: Overweight women who label themselves overweight are unhappier with their body than normal-weight women who consider themselves overweight.

Consistent with differences in sociocultural body ideals, various studies have found that overweight women report more weight-based discrimination than overweight men. (A few studies have not found this difference, perhaps due to differences in sample selection and definitions of weight-based discrimination.) These gender differences in reported weight-based discrimination and psychological functioning may be most evident among overweight and moderately obese men and women, and the gender differences diminish among those with a BMI of 35 or more. Among obese persons seeking BED treatment, women report greater body image distress than men.

Rates of obesity differ among ethnic groups, yet levels of body dissatisfaction often do not correspond to these varying rates. This may reflect differences in sociocultural ideals. For example, Black women may demonstrate a greater acceptance of adiposity (see Chapter 25). Black women, who have a higher obesity risk than other groups, have moderately less body dissatisfaction than White women. This difference may be most pronounced during young adulthood. Black women report more favorable evaluations of both their weight and appearance than White women. These differences have not remained constant over time; over the past 20 years, the gap between Black and White women has increased for overall appearance satisfaction, whereas it has narrowed for weight. While it is possible that Black women have become more weight dissatisfied, it is also possible that White women have become less dissatisfied. The smaller gap in body weight evaluation may reflect a general improvement in body satisfaction and overweight preoccupation, a longitudinal trend found in both Black and White college-age women.

Similarly, among Pacific Islanders, where rates of obesity are high, obesity tends to be viewed as more acceptable, positive, and healthy. Obese Samoans, for example, are often satisfied with their body and are not trying to lose weight. On the other hand, despite a low prevalence of obesity, many Asian American girls and women report body dissatisfaction; their levels of body dissatisfaction are similar to those among Whites.

Binge-Eating Disorder

Individuals with BED are typically overweight or obese and engage in regular binge eating. This specific group of overweight and obese individuals is more likely to have disturbances in body image than overweight and obese individuals without BED. In fact, the level of body dissatisfaction in BED is as severe as in other eating disorders, anorexia nervosa and bulimia nervosa, even when controlling for body weight. However, unlike other eating disorders, body image concern is not a diagnostic criterion for BED. More frequent binge eating, but not greater obesity, is associated with more negative body image in this population.

Overvaluation of shape or weight, common across many patients with eating disorders, occurs when a person judges his or her shape or weight to be extremely important to self-evaluation, often more important than other major sources of self-esteem such as being a parent, friend, or worker. One reason that shape and weight overvaluation may be clinically significant in obese individuals with BED (as well as in other eating disorders) is that it is resistant to change and reflects core beliefs. About 55–60% of individuals with BED place supreme importance on their shape and weight. This group has higher levels of eating disturbances, mood disturbances, and health care utilization than those with BED who do not overvalue their shape and weight. Although body dissatisfaction is not part of the DSM-IV diagnostic criteria for BED, determining which patients with BED overvalue their weight and shape may help clinicians identify those with more severe syndromes and may assist with treatment planning. (Chapter 34 provides a more detailed discussion of body image in BED.)

Body Image Distortion

The findings on body image distortion in obesity are mixed. In different studies, obese samples have been found to accurately assess body size, overestimate body size, underestimate body size, and fall into a normally distributed pattern of both over- and underestimation. The incongruity between these results can be attributed to methodological and sampling differences between studies. As described in Chapter 17, methods of assessing body size perception vary widely on a number of factors that significantly impact results (such as size of images, phrasing of instructions, focus on whole body or body parts, etc.).

Additional concerns specific to studying body image estimation in an obese population include the use of figural scales, which typically do not provide adequate coverage of obese bodies or bodies with various somatic distributions of weight. Actual images of the participant are generally considered superior for assessing body image distortion. However, taking photographs of overweight and obese participants who are instructed to wear form-fitting clothing may be a stressful experience in itself, triggering weight-related concerns for some. Factors such as anxious mood can influence size estimation. Finally, participant groups vary widely across studies, with samples drawn from the general community, universities, weight loss programs, inpatient weight loss treatment programs, and bariatric surgery clinics. These samples differ systematically on variables such as body dissatisfaction, age, socioeconomic status, psychopathology, health-related quality of life, and weight change histories, making it difficult to generalize and compare results across studies.

Despite methodological differences and mixed findings across studies, the pattern of results suggests that obese individuals overestimate their body size and do so more than nonoverweight individuals. A study of lean and obese participants used three methods of assessing perceived body size, allowing comparisons between methods. In digital morphing tasks, all participants overestimated their body size, but the obese participants did so to a greater degree. When the image was converted into outline form, the same pattern emerged but overestimation was less. Using figural stimuli, only the obese participants overestimated their body size.

As noted above, some studies found that obese participants underestimated their body size. One hypothesis is that underestimation of body size reflects a sense of self-efficacy. In one study in which underestimation was found, participants were experiencing rapid weight loss that may have increased their sense of self-efficacy regarding weight control. In other studies, participants assessed before and after weight loss treatment overestimated body size pretreatment and estimated more accurately posttreatment. Additionally, women who dropped out of treatment overestimated their size more than completers, perhaps indicating less self-efficacy. Underestimation also occurred in a community sample with relatively positive weight attitudes.

Treatment, Weight Change, and Body Image

For overweight and obese individuals with poor body image, there are two broad categories of psychological treatment: weight loss treatments, which have typically neglected body image as a treatment target, and body image treatments, which have typically not included weight loss as a target of treatment. Obese individuals in behavioral weight loss treatments also show improved body satisfaction after treatment, even if only a modest amount of weight is lost. The amount of weight lost is not strongly correlated with the degree of body image improvement. However, participants in weight loss treatments typically regain weight after treatment ends, and some evidence suggests that with regaining, body image begins to revert back toward baseline levels, though some improvement remains. (Chapter 42 discusses this topic in further detail.)

Cognitive-behavioral therapy for body image in obese individuals does not produce weight loss but does improve body satisfaction, self-esteem, and mental health (see Chapter 47). Similarly, "nondieting" and "health-at-every-size" interventions, which help obese clients develop healthier lifestyles and better self-outlook without an emphasis on weight, have been shown to improve body image without weight loss. Bacon and colleagues compared outcomes between standard behavioral weight loss treatment and a treatment designed to promote body acceptance, healthy nondiet eating, activity, and social support. Participants in weight loss treatment initially lost more weight, but they regained it by 2-year follow-up and sustained fewer positive health-risk indicator changes than health-at-every-size participants, who showed improved body image and health-risk indicators at follow-up. Further studies are needed to test the long-term effects of these programs in obese samples and the effects of combining these types of treatment with standard behavior modification for weight loss.

Some research has also examined body image among formerly overweight individuals who have lost weight. Annis and colleagues found that both formerly overweight women and currently overweight women reported comparable body image concerns, including overweight preoccupation and dysfunctional appearance investment. Body image concerns were higher in these two groups than in women who had never been overweight. The phenomenon of remaining body image concerns in formerly overweight individuals has been termed "phantom fat." On the other hand, some studies have shown similar body satisfaction in formerly overweight individuals and average-weight controls, and more research is needed on "phantom fat." Related to this phenomenon is another subgroup of individuals who consider themselves overweight when they are not, a phenomenon termed "thinking fat." Compared to nonoverweight individuals who do not consider themselves overweight, nonoverweight men and women who perceive themselves to be overweight display more negative evaluations of their appearance, fitness, and health, and more effort to diet and improve their appearance. This self-perceived overweight group is largely similar to those who are actually overweight, suggesting that not only is obesity associated with body image concerns (in certain individuals and circumstances), but so is merely self-perceived overweight status.

Heinberg and colleagues suggested the possibility of a curvilinear relationship between body dissatisfaction and healthy weight control behaviors (e.g., moderate exercise and healthy eating). They argued that people who have very low levels of body dissatisfaction may lack motivation to engage in weight control behaviors, whereas a very high level of dissatisfaction may lead to increased use of unhealthy weight control behaviors or less engagement in healthy behaviors due to feeling overwhelmed by the discrepancy between their current and desired weight. Several studies have examined body image as a predictor of weight loss in behavioral treatment. Using different assessment methods, studies have shown inconsistent findings. However, the bulk of evidence suggests that more positive attitudes toward the body predict greater weight loss, and conversely, that significant BID may interfere with successful treatment outcome. Reductions in body image avoidance behaviors may predict better maintenance of weight loss.

Conclusions and Future Directions

Body dissatisfaction is not universal in obesity. However, certain subsets of the overweight and obese population are at greater risk of body image concerns. These include individuals with BED or those with a history of weight-related discrimination. There are numerous difficulties in measuring body image distortion in obese samples, but the pattern of findings suggests that obese participants overestimate their body size more than nonobese participants. Weight change may be related to changes in body satisfaction in overweight and obese individuals, and different types of treatment can improve body dissatisfaction with or without weight loss. Body dissatisfaction may also hinder progress in weight loss treatment.

More research is needed on treatments to relieve the distress and impairment associated with body image concerns in obese individuals.

Informative Readings

Annis, N. M., Cash, T. F., & Hrabosky, J. I. (2004). Body image and psychosocial differences among stable average weight, currently overweight, and formerly overweight women: The role of stigmatizing experiences. *Body Image: An International Journal of Research, 1,* 155–167.—A comparison of women who were currently, formerly, or never overweight on measures of body image, well-being, and stigmatizing experiences throughout their lifetime.

Bacon, L., Stern, J. S., Van Loan, M. D., & Keim, N. L. (2005). Size acceptance and intuitive eating improves health for obese, female chronic dieters. *Journal of the American Dietetic Association, 105,* 929–936.—A comparison of "health-at-every-size" treatment with behavioral weight loss treatment.

Dalle Grave, R., Cuzzolaro, M., Simona, C., Tomasi, F., Temperilli, F., & Marchesini, G. (2007). The effect of obesity management on body image in patients seeking treatment at medical centers. *Obesity, 15,* 2320–2327.—An investigation of the body image effects of weight loss treatment administered to a large group of obese patients at medical centers.

Durso, L. E., & Latner, J. D. (2008). Understanding self-directed stigma: Development of the Weight Bias Internalization Scale. *Obesity, 16*(Suppl. 2), S80–S86.—The development of a measure of internalized weight bias and examination of its psychological correlates, including body image, among overweight and obese individuals.

Friedman, K. E., Reichmann, S. K., Costanzo, P. R., & Musante, G. J. (2002). Body image partially mediates the relationship between obesity and psychological distress. *Obesity, 10,* 33–41.—Examines interrelations between BMI, body image, depression, and self-esteem in obese participants in a residential weight loss program.

Grilo, C. M., Crosby, R. D., Masheb, R. M., White, M. A., Peterson, C. B., Wonderlich, S. A., et al. (2009). Overvaluation of shape and weight in binge eating disorder, bulimia nervosa, and subthreshold bulimia nervosa. *Behaviour Research and Therapy, 47,* 692–696.—A comparison of eating-related psychopathology among women with BED with and without shape and weight overvaluation, women with full-criteria bulimia nervosa, and women with subthreshold bulimia nervosa.

Heinberg, L. J., Thompson, J. K., & Matzon, J. L. (2001). Body image dissatisfaction as a motivator for healthy lifestyle change: Is some distress beneficial? In R. H. Striegel-Moore & L. Smolak (Eds.), *Eating disorders: Innovative directions in research and practice* (pp. 215–232). Washington, DC: American Psychological Association.—Proposes that body dissatisfaction and healthy weight control behavior might be represented by an inverted U-shaped curve.

Johnstone, A. M., Stewart, A. D., Benson, P. J., Kalafati, M., Rectenwald, L., & Horgan, G. (2008). Assessment of body image in obesity using a digital morphing technique. *Journal of Human Nutrition and Dietetics, 21,* 256–267.—Assesses perceived body size using a digital morphing technique with two variations: one with participants' photograph, and one with an outline based on the photograph.

Mond, J. M., Rodgers, B., Hay, P. J., Darby, A., Owen, C., Baune, B. T., & Kennedy, R. L. (2007). Obesity and impairment in psychosocial functioning in women: The mediating role of eating disorder features. *Obesity, 15,* 2769–2779.—Weight and shape concerns accounted for all of the variance found between obesity and functional impairment.

Puhl, R. M., & Heuer, C. A. (2009). The stigma of obesity: A review and update. *Obesity, 17,* 941–964.—A comprehensive review of recent research on the types and consequences of stigma faced by obese individuals.

Sarwer, D. B, Thompson, J. K., & Cash, T. F. (2005). Body image and obesity in adulthood. *Psychiatric Clinics of North America, 28,* 69–87.—A review of research on BID and obesity, covering in detail the assessment of body image.

Schwartz, M. B., & Brownell, K. B. (2004). Body image and obesity. *Body Image: An International Journal of Research, 1,* 43–56.—A review of the literature on the relationship between obesity and poor body image, and the risk factors and treatments associated with this relationship.

Body Image and Muscularity

DONALD R. McCREARY

Introduction

Research examining men's body image has tended to suggest that they have fairly positive body image perceptions: they traditionally account for a small proportion of those with eating disorders, they typically report a much higher level of general satisfaction with their body, and they also report less dissatisfaction with their degree of body fat (even when they are objectively overweight). This led many to conclude that men were relatively free of the body image concerns that seem to plague women and girls. However, approximately 10 years ago, more and more researchers began to realize that asking men about their weight or body fat percentage was not the most appropriate way to assess their general body image. That is, whereas the social standard for bodily attractiveness for women is based on a thin ideal and focuses on adiposity and the distribution of that body fat, the social standard for men is focused on the muscular ideal (i.e., the addition of lean muscle mass and its distribution), leading many boys and men to develop a drive for muscularity. The focus of this chapter is to provide a general overview of the main research findings from this nascent area of body image research.

Drive for Muscularity and Psychological Well-Being

The importance of studying muscularity concerns, especially in men and boys, stems from the findings linking the drive for muscularity (i.e., the extent to which they have internalized the muscular ideal as their ideal body shape) with adverse psychological states. In one of the first studies of the drive for muscularity, Doris Sasse and I showed that scores on the Drive for Muscularity Scale were correlated with lower levels of self-esteem and higher levels of depression in adolescent boys, but not in adolescent girls. Since then, researchers have replicated and extended these findings, showing that the desire to be more muscular is also associated with increased levels of general body dissatisfaction, negative affect, and social physique anxiety, as well as poorer sexual self-efficacy.

People with a higher drive for muscularity are also at a greater risk for abusing anabolic–androgenic steroids and other supplements that purport to enhance muscularity and physical bulk (e.g., androstenedione, protein powder). The issues around steroid and supplement use may be an indication of muscle dysmorphia, an aspect of body dysmorphic disorder wherein people (typically men) perceive themselves as skinny, weak, and not muscular even though they are objectively the opposite (see Chapter 35).

Psychosocial Correlates of the Drive for Muscularity

Several studies have examined psychological and social factors associated with the drive for muscularity. From a psychological perspective, most attention has been paid to personality and individual-difference factors. Other emerging areas include the extent to which people engage in social comparison, the impact of parental and peer comments or teasing, and the role of demographic factors like ethnicity and sexual orientation.

Personality and Individual-Difference Factors

Given the relative newness of the research area, the focus on personality and individual differences is limited, but growing. Since weight training can be very self-focused, one area of interest has been the association between the drive for muscularity and narcissism. However, findings have been mixed, with only some research showing a significant positive correlation. Researchers have also found that men with a high drive for muscularity tend to report higher levels of neuroticism and perfectionism, as well as a greater orientation to both their physical fitness and their general appearance.

There is an expanding body of research exploring the relationship between the drive for muscularity and men's degree of masculinity. However, because masculinity is a multidimensional, higher-order construct, researchers measure it using several related but distinct constructs. Using a variety of these constructs, researchers have shown that the drive for muscularity is associated with higher levels of unmitigated agency (i.e., gender-typed personality traits assessing one's tendency to focus on the self to the exclusion of others), believing or engaging more often in male gender-stereotypic behaviors, experiencing elevated levels of masculine gender role stress (i.e., stress associated with feeling one is not meeting society's expectations for men) and gender role conflict (especially associated with work–family conflict and concerns around success, power, and competition), and a greater desire to conform to the male gender role norms focused on the importance of winning.

More recently, researchers have begun to explore the relationship between the drive for muscularity and self-objectification (see Chapter 6). Researchers in this area have demonstrated positive correlations between self-objectification and the drive for muscularity; however, some are questioning the extent to which current measures of objectification adequately assess the construct in men.

Interpersonal Factors

The most frequently studied interpersonal aspects of the drive for muscularity are social comparison and body-related comments and teasing from one's peers and family. With regard to social comparison, men and boys with a higher degree of the drive for muscularity more often compare their general physical appearance, as well as their degree of muscularity, to those of other men and boys. Social comparison and the drive for muscularity have also been shown to correlate positively with men's internalization of an athletic body as the ideal.

A second area of research interest has been the role that parent and peer comments, as well as peer teasing, play on boys' body dissatisfaction and a desire to become muscular. When parents and peers make comments about a boy's lack of muscularity, the boys report higher levels of both general body dissatisfaction and dissatisfaction with their muscles. These types of comments are also associated with boys' increased use of nutritional and pharmacological (e.g., anabolic–androgenic steroids) strategies to increase their muscle mass. Longitudinal research has shown that muscle-related comments from parents may be especially salient to teenage boys as comments from them, but not their peers, are predictive of increased use of muscle-enhancing supplements over time. However, this is not meant to diminish the fact that both conversations with, and comments from, peers of both genders are associated with increases in these aspects of body dissatisfaction in adolescent boys. Similar findings have been shown for body-related teasing.

Demographic Factors

The most common demographic variables studied in relation to the drive for muscularity are sexual orientation and ethnicity. Sexual orientation is of interest because of the higher degree of focus on the body within the gay community. Research with gay men, however, has not demonstrated consistent findings. Although some researchers note that a large portion of gay men report muscle-related dissatisfaction, when comparisons are made between gay and heterosexual men, differences between the two groups are not always found. When there are significant differences, the effect sizes tend to be small, suggesting that both groups have internalized the muscular ideal to a similar degree.

The relationship between ethnicity and the drive for muscularity has not been studied thoroughly, with most muscularity research having been conducted within the mostly White, North American college student population. However, what research there is (e.g., men from Ghana, Kenya, Samoa, Ukraine) suggests that the desire to be more muscular is common in many cultures (though less so in Taiwan), and may be influenced by the level of Western-based visual media saturation. An examination of behaviors to increase muscle size among Malaysian, Indian, and Chinese boys showed that all three groups engaged in these behaviors more than same-aged girls from their cultures, but that these behaviors were less prevalent among Chinese boys. Studies of racial/ethnic differences among North American college students suggest that Hispanic males are more likely than Whites to abuse anabolic–androgenic steroids, suggesting that this group might have a greater drive for muscularity. Why this might be is not known.

Media Influences on the Drive for Muscularity

There is convincing evidence that the male body is being presented by the media in a more objectified manner than it has been in the past. There appear to be two different categories into which these images fall. The first is the hypermuscular figure commonly marketed to boys and young men, often in the form of action figures or characters in video games, comic books, and action-oriented movies. These men are often presented in such a hypermuscular way that their size is actually physically impossible for human males to achieve. The second category is the moderately muscular but lean (i.e., low body fat) male used mostly to sell fashion and related products. These images can be found on billboards and television, and in magazines and movies.

The research examining the impact of viewing these images on boys' and men's drive for muscularity suggests that there is not a simple dose–response effect between the two. Laboratory studies where men are shown objectified fashion images of male models sometimes show a postintervention increase in body dissatisfaction, but findings such as these do not appear consistently. For example, the more images the participant sees, the more likely the experimental manipulation is effective at influencing the dependent variable. Additionally, video images may have a greater effect than still images. Quasi-experimental studies that examine naturally occurring media exposure and body image suggest that people who read more health- and fitness-oriented magazines have a higher drive for muscularity and more body dissatisfaction. Longitudinal research suggests that young, White boys (approximately 8–10 years old) who read gaming magazines portraying hypermuscular men have a higher drive for muscularity 1 year later, after controlling for their baseline muscularity score. But it is not just images that can evoke an increase in body dissatisfaction or an increase in the drive for muscularity; just manipulating hypermuscular children's toys in simulated play can adversely impact young men's body esteem.

Drive for Muscularity in Women

In the same way that men can be adversely affected by the thin ideal, women can display a drive for muscularity. However, women are only rarely included in research examining the drive for muscularity. Compared to boys and men, girls and women typically report lower levels of the drive for muscularity, but their scores are significantly different from zero. Whether gender moderates the association between muscularity concerns and adverse outcomes or correlates, however, depends on the variables being studied. For example, the association between the drive for muscularity and both male- and female-typed personality traits and behaviors are the same for men and women, as is the relationship between the drive for muscularity, social comparison, and social physique anxiety. But in a longitudinal study of adolescent muscle preoccupation, the outcome was predicted by self-esteem, negative affect, and peer relations for girls, but only perfectionism for boys. This, however, does not mean that the drive for muscularity is the same for all women. Female athletes, especially those for whom muscularity is a requirement to be competitive, may have a different relationship with the drive for muscularity compared to other women.

Unanswered Questions

Study of the muscularity-related aspects of body image is relatively new and, as such, there are many unanswered questions that future research needs to address. One of the most important issues is measurement related. Self-report measures such as the Drive for Muscularity Scale assess attitudes and behaviors associated with wanting to become more muscular. However, silhouette measures can capture important aspects of self-perception (e.g., shape, distribution of muscle). The problem tends to be that many silhouette measures assess only adiposity or muscularity. But because muscle lies under body fat, these types of measures do not provide a realistic portrayal of many men's (or women's) bodies. Silhouette measures should incorporate both adiposity and muscularity into the same silhouettes. While there are some measures that do this, retest-reliability issues tend to be an issue for the most face-valid measures. New assessment tools (such as computer programs that allow for the manipulation of images to make them bigger or smaller) also need to incorporate both dimensions into people's assessment options. Thus, the field needs a broader array of measures to assess a wide range of muscularity issues.

A second issue is the distinction men make between muscularity and low body fat, as well as the extent to which muscularity concerns are more salient than adiposity concerns. Many assume that men are aiming for a low percentage of body fat combined with a high degree of muscularity, and that both muscularity and adiposity concerns are equally salient. This is not always the case. Researchers have shown that self-ideal discrepancies vary more strongly on the muscularity dimension and less consistently on the body fat dimension. Also, muscularity discrepancies tend to be related to adverse outcomes in men, whereas discrepancies in body fat are associated with very few problems. In addition, studies of men's weight perceptions have shown that many normal-weight men perceive themselves as underweight, whereas many overweight men see themselves as normal weight and also report higher levels of life satisfaction and health. Thus, researchers need to begin examining how men integrate their desire to be muscular with their desire to maximize the display of that muscularity with a low amount of body fat. For example, do men just want to be big (i.e., not the proverbial "90-pound weakling") and would prefer to be muscular but will take bulk in any form?

Finally, how do factors related to the life-course influence men's perceptions of muscularity? For example, do muscularity concerns change as men age? To date, most research has been conducted on young adults, adolescents, and older children. What about adults in their later years? Is muscularity as salient then as it appears to be in younger men? If not, at what point do muscularity concerns begin to decline, and for what reasons? Drummond addresses some of these issues in an interesting series of interviews with older men. While much of the study was focused on the relationship between the body and masculinity, there are plenty of indications that muscularity salience declines with age. However, this was a small sample and there may be important individual differences that this single study has not tapped into.

Another example of a life-course influence on muscularity would be illness. In many instances, the expression or treatment of severe or chronic illness can lead to a loss of physical bulk, including muscle mass. Does this change influence the drive for muscularity or its relationship to indices of mental health (e.g., depression, anxiety)? Do these factors vary as a function of the type of illness or the person who is ill?

Conclusions

In conclusion, the study of body image and the impact the muscular ideal has on both boys and men and girls and women is a nascent area of study. To date, research has focused on the adverse effects of the drive for muscularity, as well as on individual differences (e.g., personality, interpersonal, and demographic factors) and media influences. The study of the muscular ideal, however, should not be focused on men and boys only. It is important to examine muscularity concerns in women and girls as well. Given the newness of the topic, there are many potential directions for future researchers, three of which were addressed in this chapter.

Informative Readings

Cafri, G., Thompson, J. K., Ricciardelli, L., McCabe, M., Smolak, L., & Yesalis, C. (2005). Pursuit of the muscular ideal: Physical and psychological consequences and putative risk factors. *Clinical Psychology Review, 25,* 215–239.— An excellent review of the psychological and social risk factors associated with the use of supplements to increase muscle mass.

Davis, C., Karvinen, K., & McCreary, D. R. (2005). Personality correlates of a drive for muscularity in young men. *Personality and Individual Differences, 39,* 349–359.—Examines the relationship between personality factors and the drive for muscularity in a sample of men.

Drummond, M. J. N. (2003). Retired men, retired bodies. *International Journal of Men's Health, 3,* 183–199.—This qualitative examination of how older men view their bodies provides many insights as to whether muscularity has a role to play in older men's lives.

Harrison, K., & Bond, B. J. (2007). Gaming magazines and the drive for muscularity in preadolescent boys: A longitudinal examination. *Body Image: An International Journal of Research, 4,* 269–277.—Shows that the drive for muscularity is salient even in preteenage boys and that hypermuscular media exposure is correlated with an increase in the drive for muscularity over a year-long period.

Jones, D. C., & Crawford, J. K. (2006). The peer appearance culture during adolescence: Gender and body mass variations. *Journal of Youth and Adolescence, 34,* 257–269.—Examines the role of peer comments and teasing in adolescent boys and girls, highlighting that boys are often teased about their body, especially about their lack of muscularity.

Krane, V., Choi, P. Y. L., Baird, S. M., Aimar, C. M., & Kauer, K. J. (2004). Living the paradox: Female athletes negotiate femininity and muscularity. *Sex Roles, 50,* 315–329.—Qualitative study exploring how female athletes walk the proverbial line between two opposing social norms (i.e., the athlete and the woman) and how this affects the way they view themselves outside the athletic domain.

Lavine, H., Sweeney, D., & Wagner, S. H. (1999). Depicting women as sex objects in television advertising: Effects on body dissatisfaction. *Personality and Social Psychology Bulletin, 25,* 1049–1058.—Examines the effects of viewing objectified images of women on both women's and men's self-perceptions, showing that when men view images of women the men want to become bigger and more muscular.

McCreary, D. R., & Sasse, D. K. (2000). Exploring the drive for muscularity in adolescent boys and girls. *Journal of American College Health, 48,* 297–304.—Describes the development and initial validation of the commonly used Drive for Muscularity Scale, as well as showing that the drive for muscularity is associated with adverse psychological outcomes for adolescent boys, but not adolescent girls.

McCreary, D. R., Saucier, D. M., & Courtenay, W. H. (2005). The drive for muscularity and masculinity: Testing the associations among gender role traits, behaviors, attitudes, and conflict. *Psychology of Men and Masculinity, 6,* 83–94.—Shows that only certain aspects of masculinity are uniquely associated with the desire to be more muscular and that the same aspects of masculinity tend to predict the drive for muscularity in women.

Olivardia, R., Pope, H. G., Borowiecki, J. J., & Cohane, G. H. (2004). Biceps and body image: The relationship between muscularity and self-esteem, depression, and eating disorder symptoms. *Psychology of Men and Masculinity, 5,* 112–120.—Shows that men's self versus actual muscle discrepancy was more strongly associated with higher levels of depression and lower self-esteem than their weight discrepancies.

Ricciardelli, L. A., McCabe, M. P., Williams, R. J., & Thompson, J. K. (2007). The role of ethnicity and culture in body image and disordered eating among males. *Clinical Psychology Review, 27,* 582–606.—An excellent starting point for anyone wanting to get an initial overview of the area, as it reviews the body image literature for both muscular and thin-ideal outcomes in a wide variety of ethnic groups.

Thompson, J. K., & Cafri, G. (2007). *The muscular ideal: Psychological, social and medical perspectives.* Washington, DC: American Psychological Association.—The first published volume to provide an extensive overview of the muscular ideal and its wide-ranging implications for men and women.

CHAPTER 23

Body Image and Athleticism

TRENT A. PETRIE
CHRISTY GREENLEAF

Introduction

Sport, by its very nature, is a physical endeavor. Athletes spend countless hours in physical training to achieve the highest level of conditioning and skill. In all sports, what athletes can do with their body (e.g., balance on a beam, kick a soccer ball) is related directly to their success. Thus, athletes train with coaches and teammates to increase their strength, quickness, explosiveness, flexibility, and stamina, and to develop technical skills specific to their sport. Through this training, and the development of a lean, toned, and muscular physique, athletes also accrue indirect (appearance-related) performance. For example, in some sports, how athletes appear aesthetically to judges can influence the outcome of the performance.

Given the body's centrality in sport, it is not surprising that athletes are highly aware of their body's functionality and appearance. It also is not surprising that research consistently has found that male and female athletes, particularly at the more competitive levels of sports, report a more positive body image than nonathletes. This difference is likely due to multiple factors, including the fact that athletes more closely resemble societal body ideals because of their high levels of physical training and fitness.

Why is it then that so many athletes, who are body satisfied, still want to lose weight, gain muscle, or change their physique in some way, and have slightly higher levels of eating pathology than nonathletes? Meta-analyses and recent research with collegiate and elite athletes have found that male and female athletes (1) do experience disordered eating symptoms, though subclinical rates are much higher than clinical, and (2) rely primarily on exercise, strength training, and restrictions in food intake to alter their physique. Similar to nonathletes, body dissatisfaction is also related directly to disordered eating and may be a primary risk factor. As discussed later in the chapter, this paradox (fewer body image concerns yet greater risk of disordered eating) may be best understood by considering the weight, body, appearance, and performance pressures that are specific to the sport environment.

Social versus Athletic Body Ideals

Because of their level of physical activity and fitness, athletes' physiques often are similar to societal body ideals (i.e., lean, toned, and muscular), which may enhance their body image satisfaction. For men in particular, a muscular body with "six-pack abs," defined arms, and a large, V-shaped upper body communicates strength, competence, confidence, power, and independence, all of which provide social and athletic advantages. Socially, a muscular body, along with these psychological attributes, is commonly thought to define masculinity. And, a masculine man generally is viewed as more physically attractive and desirous to the other sex and as more capable and competent professionally. In sports, male athletes' physiques are visible indicators of power, competence, and ability, and may provide a psychological edge over opponents. Because of what their body conveys, male athletes have long been idealized in the media as representing the societal body ideal. Development of a lean, toned, and muscular body, however, requires dedication and hard work and may take years to achieve, if ever at all. For many reasons, some male athletes still may view their physique as lacking because (1) their immediate comparison group includes other sport performers whose body also closely approximates or exceeds the ideal, (2) they are pressured by coaches to achieve a certain body ideal, and (3) they are highly competitive and driven to succeed. In a study of male athletes across various sports, the athletes perceived themselves to be less muscular than what they considered ideal for their sport and than what they thought would be most attractive to women. Thus, even though their body is similar to the male societal ideal, athletes still may see themselves as lacking in leanness and muscularity and falling short, both socially and athletically.

Although female athletes' bodies also approximate the lean, societal ideal, they still may experience a conflict between how their body can perform athletically and how they feel about their bodily size, shape, and appearance in social situations. Indeed, qualitative research with female athletes indicates that body image is strongly influenced by the context. For example, within sport performance environments, female athletes appreciate, value, and feel proud of their muscles and the physical functionality of their body; their strength gives them confidence to compete at their best in their chosen sport. Yet, in social situations outside of sports, female athletes may feel self-conscious about and uncomfortable with their body size and muscles, particularly when their physique is disparate from the societal ideal. This perceived conflict between social and athletic body images likely occurs because of the incongruence between the physical performance advantages of strength and power that go along with having a muscular body and the societal expectation that attractive women are lean and toned, but not "too" toned and definitely not "too" muscular. Thus, female athletes must constantly negotiate the conflicting demands of their sport environment and the larger society.

Societal versus Sport Pressures

Like nonathletes, male and female athletes are exposed to all the general societal pressures that exist regarding body size, shape, weight, muscularity, and appearance. These pressures and ideals, over time, may be internalized, and body dissatisfaction results from self-comparisons with this ideal (as detailed in several other chapters in this volume). But unlike nonathletes, male and female athletes are also subjected to unique pressures in sport environments, particularly at the more competitive levels.

The nature of sports and the physical demands of training and competing place athletes' bodies in the spotlight to be commented on and evaluated by teammates, coaches, judges, and themselves. Type of sport, perceived performance advantages, uniforms, and the level at which athletes compete may also influence how they feel about their body and contribute to heightened body awareness and body image disturbances. Moreover, sport pressures can have a direct impact on athletes' behavioral efforts to control their body size, shape, and weight. For example, in a series of studies with male and female athletes from different collegiate sports, Petrie and colleagues found an association between sport pressures and athletes' dissatisfaction with their body size and shape. Further, their body image concerns were related to eating pathology and the use of unhealthy weight control behaviors, particularly excessive exercising and restrictive dieting.

The type and nature of specific sports may contribute to perceived "ideal" body shapes and assumed performance advantages associated with specific physiques. For example, the "ideal" body for an offensive lineman in football or a men's soccer player is very different from the "ideal" body of a figure skater or a cross-country runner. Whereas the lineman's performance is thought to be improved by having a strong and massive physique, a figure skater's or a cross-country runner's ideal body is perceived to be small and lean. Athletes are well aware of the sport "body ideals" that are portrayed in the media and communicated by coaches, teammates, and parents. Athletes whose bodies do not match the sport ideal generally are body dissatisfied and experience considerable internal and external pressure to change their physique, for both appearance and performance reasons. In a study of figure skaters, those who had a body consistent with the sports' thin, petite ideal were satisfied with their level of body fat and reported high levels of sport competence. In a separate study, track athletes were found to be more body dissatisfied than a group of martial artists. The researchers concluded that the track athletes were under tremendous pressure to attain and/or maintain a very lean physique in order to improve their athletic performances. The martial artists, however, did not experience such pressures and thus were more satisfied with their bodies.

In aesthetic and judged sports, athletes are evaluated on their physical performance and skill, *and* their appearance. Figure skaters', synchronized swimmers', and gymnasts' physiques, as well as their physical attractiveness, influence judges' evaluations and scoring of their performances. In these types of sports, athletes (especially girls and women) experience strong pressures to restrict their food intake in order to achieve the leaner ideal of their sport and have a body that closely aligns with judges' expectations/ideals, which generally translates into higher scores and better performance outcomes. Athletes who experience body- and weight-related pressures associated with being judged as part of their performance success, then, are likely to be at increased risk for using pathogenic weight control behaviors and may experience negative psychological and physical consequences as a result.

Practice and competition uniforms, which in some sports are body hugging and/or revealing, may influence how both male and female athletes' feel about and relate to their body. The limited research on this issue shows that athletes identify their sport attire as one important source of body image pressure. For example, male and female athletes in sports such as swimming, diving, track and field, and gymnastics report feeling self-conscious about their physique and believing their body is being evaluated because of the revealing nature of their uniform. Female athletes, in particular, may experience their body as fat or "too big" or may feel sexually objectified because of uniforms that leave little to the imagination. Such experiences may lead to greater body image concerns, more psychological distress, increased eating pathology, and poorer athletic performances.

Another source of body image pressures comes from significant others, such as parents, teammates, and coaches, who send messages about weight, body size and shape, and appearance. These messages sometimes may be positive, such as when a teammate comments on the performance gains that have resulted from extra time spent on physical conditioning or a parent is supportive of a healthy, nutritional approach to weight loss. However, most comments are negative and can contribute to athletes engaging in unhealthy eating and exercise behaviors in order to lose weight and please their coach. For example, in studies with collegiate athletes, Petrie and colleagues found that those who were eating disordered or symptomatic reported more weight pressures from their coach, parents, friends, and teammates than those who were asymptomatic. Muscat and Long found that 58% of the female athletes identified a significant other who had made negative body-related comments about them. These comments came from family (42%), friends (33%), and coaches/trainers (25%), and were focused primarily on the athletes' appearance and need to lose weight. Further, most (70%) critical comments were made in public venues, such as at family dinners or at practices in front of teammates.

Male athletes are also pressured by significant others, both directly and indirectly, to gain weight and increase strength/muscularity, ostensibly to improve their sport performances. Coaches and teammates may comment on athletes' lack of muscularity or tease them about not being strong enough. Galli and Reel found that 70% of male athletes said they experience pressure from coaches to attain an ideal body for their sport. Because of such pressures, athletes may resort to unhealthy behaviors, such as binge eating or ingesting muscle-gain supplements (e.g., anabolic steroids), in hopes of increasing muscle mass/strength and weight. (See Chapter 36 for a review of body image and appearance- and performance-enhancing substance use.)

Finally, athletes' competitive level appears to be associated with their body satisfaction. Meta-analytic research suggests that collegiate athletes have more positive body image than recreational athletes. Because high-level athletes spend considerable time in physical training, their bodies are likely to be lean and toned, and similar to the societal ideals. Recreational athletes, however, do much less physical training. Thus, they are unlikely to accrue the same physical or appearance benefits as higher-level competitors. Being a competitive athlete also may have indirect effects on body image. Highly competitive athletes may experience more psychosocial benefits associated with being physically active and fit, including high self-esteem, physical competence, and low levels of anxiety and depression, than recreational athletes. Athletes with high levels of "psychological well-being" also have a stronger, more positive body image.

Conclusions and Future Directions

Research on and interventions with athletes, the sports environment, body image, and disordered eating continue to develop. Several directions for future research and interventions are especially significant, however. First a more complete understanding of the relative influence of body dissatisfaction and pressures within the sports environment on disordered eating is needed. Although athletes are more body satisfied than nonathletes,

athletes particularly at more competitive levels experience disordered eating at rates slightly higher than nonathletes. Are the beneficial effects of being body satisfied overwhelmed by pressures within the sports environment? Do personality factors common among athletes, such as perfectionism, exacerbate the deleterious effects of body dissatisfaction and thus increase risk for disordered eating? Future research with athletes should entail a multivariate, within-subjects approach to understand the complex and likely interactive effects of psychological, social, and environmental variables on the development of body image concerns and disordered eating. Theoretical models developed specifically for athletes, such as one proposed by Petrie and Greenleaf, may guide such research.

Second, given the complex nature of female athletes' body image and the potential discrepancy between their sport performance and appearance ideals, research must address how they balance these two competing demands. How do athletes from sports, particularly those in which the sport-ideal differs from the societal ideal, feel about themselves when they are not performing? What happens to their body image when they are no longer competing and experiencing that source of esteem and competence?

Third, because less is known about male than female athletes' body image, research needs to focus on this group. Male athletes experience pressure to gain strength and body mass, yet be lean. So, on what behaviors do men rely to achieve this dual ideal? To what extent do they experience a drive for muscularity relative to a drive for thinness/leanness? (See Chapter 22 on body image and muscularity.) Of the societal and sport-specific pressures that exist, what is their relative influence on body image concerns?

Fourth, although research has established associations between societal and sport-specific pressures and body image concerns, and between body dissatisfaction and eating disorder symptomatology, the temporal relationships among these variables is unknown. In addition, the extent to which body image is stable during a competitive sport season or across athletes' careers is unknown. Thus, future research needs to utilize prospective designs to establish temporal relationships. For example, does exposure to a weight- and appearance-focused sports environment, where coaches and teammates make critical comments about body size and shape, and communicate a need to lose (or gain) weight, lead athletes over time to become more conscious of and dissatisfied with their physique?

Fifth, if body image is a precursor to the development of disordered eating, then research needs to test interventions designed to improve body image in athletes. Research by Smith and Petrie suggests that targeted, short-term interventions that teach athletes how to think differently about themselves and their body and to eschew general societal messages about weight and appearance hold promise for improving the body image of female athletes and, ultimately, decreasing disordered eating.

Last, to the extent that sport-specific pressures play a strong role in the development of body image concerns and disordered eating, interventions need to address these messages in particular. Professionals who work with sport teams may need to intervene directly with coaches and athletes to create more positive, performance-focused (as opposed to body-focused) environments. Interventions need to disentangle the idea that weight loss (or gain) leads directly to improved performance. Instead, coaches can focus on developing athletes' strength, stamina, skills, strategies, and mental toughness as ways to improve their performance.

Informative Readings

Brannan, M., Petrie, T. A., Greenleaf, C., Reel, J., & Carter, J. (2009). The relationship between body dissatisfaction and bulimic symptoms in female collegiate athletes. *Journal of Clinical Sport Psychology, 3*, 103–126.—Results demonstrate that body dissatisfaction is directly related to bulimic symptoms, as moderated by different types of perfectionism, exercising for appearance/attractiveness, and self-esteem.

Galli, N., & Reel, J. J. (2009). Adonis or Hephaestus? Exploring body image in male athletes. *Psychology of Men and Masculinity, 10*, 95–108.—Qualitative evidence that male athletes have conflicting feelings about their body, feeling both proud and critical.

Hausenblas, H. A., & Symons Downs, D. (2001). Comparison of body image between athletes and nonathletes: A meta-analytic review. *Journal of Applied Sport Psychology, 13*, 323–339.—Meta-analysis of 78 studies concluding that athletes have more positive body image than nonathletes.

Kerr, G., Berman, E., & De Souza, M. J. (2006). Disordered eating in women's gymnastics: Perspectives of athletes, coaches, parents, and judges. *Journal of Applied Sport Psychology, 18*, 28–43.—Reveals that gymnasts who received critical comments about their body and weight and were instructed to lose weight had more problematic eating behaviors.

Krane, V., Choi, P. Y. L., Baird, S. M., Aimar, C. M., & Kauer, K. J. (2004). Living the paradox: Female athletes negotiate femininity and muscularity. *Sex Roles, 50*, 315–329.—Shows that female athletes experience conflict between their athletic bodies and socially idealized feminine bodies.

Muscat, A. C., & Long, B. C. (2008). Critical comments about body shape and weight: Disordered eating of female athletes and sport participants. *Journal of Applied Sport Psychology, 20*, 1–24.—Reveals associations between critical body and weight comments and problematic eating behaviors and negative emotions.

Petrie, T. A., & Greenleaf, C. (2007). Eating disorders in sport: From theory to research to intervention. In G. Tenenbaum & R. Eklund (Eds.), *Handbook of sport psychology* (pp. 352–378). Hoboken, NJ: Wiley.—Provides a theoretical model of the development of body image concerns and disordered eating among male and female athletes.

Petrie, T. A., Greenleaf, C., Reel, J., & Carter, J. (2008). Prevalence of eating disorders and disordered eating behaviors among male collegiate athletes. *Psychology of Men and Masculinity, 9*, 267–277.—Reveals that although most athletes are asymptomatic, a substantial minority experience subclinical disordered eating and male athletes use exercise as their most frequent way to manage their weight and appearance.

Petrie, T. A., Greenleaf, C., Reel, J., & Carter, J. (2009). An examination of psychosocial correlates of eating disorders among female collegiate athletes. *Research Quarterly for Exercise and Sport, 80*, 621–632.—Reveals direct, positive relationships between level of eating pathology and general and sport-specific weight pressures, internalization, body image concerns, and negative mood state.

Smith, A., & Petrie, T. A. (2008). Reducing the risk of disordered eating among female athletes: A test of alternative interventions. *Journal of Applied Sport Psychology, 20*, 392–407.—Demonstrates that a short-term, cognitive dissonance-based intervention led to improvements in athletes' level of internalization, body image, and depression.

Thompson, R., & Sherman, R. (2010). *Eating disorders in sport*. New York: Routledge.—Reviews the current state of eating disorders and body image among athletes and offers advice on their identification, management, and treatment.

CHAPTER 24

Gay and Lesbian Body Images

TODD G. MORRISON
JESSICA M. McCUTCHEON

Introduction: The Comparative Research Tradition

In 2004, Morrison and associates conducted a meta-analytic review of 27 studies that examined body satisfaction among different sexual orientations (i.e., heterosexual and gay men, heterosexual and lesbian women). Their findings indicated that, even controlling for differences in weight status, heterosexual men evidenced greater body satisfaction than gay men. For lesbian and heterosexual women, the overall difference in satisfaction was negligible, with weight status failing to emerge as a moderator variable. To account for these differences, the authors used the prevailing explanations that gay male subculture possesses narrow parameters in terms of what constitutes an "acceptable" body, and disseminates the message that value within the gay community is contingent upon physical appearance. The absence of a difference between lesbian and heterosexual women was explained in terms of females, regardless of sexual orientation, being socialized to accord value based on how they look, with eventual identification as lesbian and immersion in lesbian subculture being insufficient buffers against the "beauty imperative." Morrison and associates acknowledged that these explanations were speculative and that studies focusing specifically on gay and lesbian communities and the messages they transmit vis-à-vis the body were needed.

Since the publication of that meta-analysis, studies on gay and lesbian body image have remained primarily comparative in nature. Individuals, categorized as gay, lesbian, or heterosexual—typically on the basis of single-item measures of sexual orientation—are given various scales to complete, and then compared statistically. This approach has often resulted in the accumulation of discordant findings. However, the trends appear to be that gay men continue to experience, or at least may be more willing to report, greater levels of dissatisfaction than their heterosexual counterparts, and that lesbian and heterosexual women are more similar than dissimilar in terms of their body image. Peplau and associates' large-scale survey constitutes a recent example of this type of research.

Unfortunately, comparative studies do not (1) particularize how gay and lesbian individuals come to understand their own body, (2) capture the variability that exists within broad categories such as "gay" and "lesbian," or (3) delineate the ways that intersecting identities (e.g., lesbian athlete) potentially influence body image. Finally, an issue that pervades research in this area is the elision of bisexual men and women. This group is either unmentioned or, when included as participants, amalgamated with gay and lesbian individuals. Drawing upon available literature, this chapter details some of the ways in which these gaps in understanding are being, or can be, addressed.

Sexual Minorities' Understanding of Their Body

Gay men and lesbian women's perceptions of self are shaped by the broader social context in which they live, a context that affords heterosexual individuals more privilege than their homosexual counterparts. One framework that is used to understand how sexual minorities' body image may be influenced by dominant culture is entitled minority stress theory. According to this theory, gay men and lesbian women experience chronic social stress due to (1) discriminatory events (i.e., typically negative behaviors directed toward individuals because they are, or are believed to be, gay or lesbian), (2) perceived stigma (i.e., individuals' expectations that they will experience stereotyping, prejudice, and discrimination on account of being gay or lesbian), and (3) internalized homonegativity (i.e., individuals' acceptance of society's negative messages about sexual minority persons). Collectively, discrimination, perceived stigma, and internalized homonegativity are unique stressors that, operating in conjunction with the generic stressors of everyday life, compromise the physical and psychological well-being of gay men and lesbian women. For instance, Kimmel and Mahalik found that gay men who had been the victim of an antigay attack (discrimination), expected rejection and discrimination due to their homosexuality (perceived stigma), and were uncomfortable about being gay (internalized homonegativity) reported greater distress at "failing" to achieve a muscular, ostensibly more masculine physique. Other researchers, focusing more narrowly on internalized homonegativity, have documented that this stressor is positively associated with body shame, symptoms of disordered eating, body surveillance (i.e., focusing on how the body looks rather than how it feels), and overall satisfaction with one's body and specific body features (e.g., muscle tone).

To date, few published studies have applied minority stress theory to the topic of lesbian women's body image. Research is needed to address this gap. As well, this theory does not specify the role that gay and lesbian culture plays in shaping sexual minorities' attitudes toward the self. Focusing on lesbian women, Kelly asserts that body image perception is influenced by two often conflicting sets of "oppressive mandates"—one set emanating from the dominant culture, and the other from the lesbian community. Lesbian women who were "femme-identified" (i.e., they embodied dominant culture's expectations of how a woman should look) avoided the stigma of being labeled as lesbian, but reported less acceptance from other lesbian women. The converse was true for those who identified as androgynous or "butch" (i.e., they embodied dominant culture's expectations of how a man should look).

Heterogeneity of Gay and Lesbian Communities

The terms *gay* and *lesbian* do not reflect monolithic social groupings but encompass myriad subgroups, each of which may view the body in different ways. To date, this issue has received insufficient scrutiny, with the scant research available being qualitative in nature. Gough and Flanders interviewed 10 self-identified "bears" (i.e., "mature gay or bisexual men with hairy bodies and facial hair who are heavy-set," p. 236) to investigate their personal experience of being overweight, and whether they believed involvement in the "bear" community affected their body image. Analysis of the transcripts revealed that interviewees reported experiencing anti-fat prejudice and discrimination from heterosexual and mainstream gay communities, which contributed to poor body image. Embracing the "bear" label and becoming involved with a community where larger, nonmuscular physiques are eroticized and celebrated, rather than demonized, was viewed as instrumental in changing how they saw themselves physically.

Subgroups based on body shape and dress exist among lesbian populations—for example, butch, femme, and androgynous. The latter denotes women that are typically skinny, lack curves, and dress in "boyish" clothes. Unfortunately, there is little published research investigating differences among these groups in terms of body image.

Age is another factor that contributes to heterogeneity within gay and lesbian communities, and often intersects with other identities. "Bears" tend to be older in contrast to "twinks," who are typically thin, young, and hairless. Few researchers have investigated the aging process and body image in sexual minorities. The limited work that has been done uses qualitative methods, and suggests that gay men idealize and eroticize the bodies of young men and denigrate the bodies of those in middle (40–64 years) and late (65+ years) adulthood. Longitudinal research with gay, lesbian, and bisexual individuals is needed to determine whether body image changes across the lifespan and, if so, whether these changes are positive or negative. Factors that contribute to, or compromise, favorable body image as one ages also need to be identified.

Intersectionality

Individuals are never simply "gay" or "lesbian"; rather, they occupy multiple identities simultaneously, each of which may be stigmatized to varying degrees and, depending on context, rendered more or less salient at a given point in time. Researchers are now arguing for the consideration of various points of stigmatization to achieve a fuller understanding of an individual's bodily experience. It is not until an individual's multiple identities are considered together that a complete picture emerges of his or her body's discrepancy from the hegemonic construction of the ideal body (i.e., heterosexual, able, and male).

Despite the need to assess body image holistically, few studies have considered intersectionality. In an effort to start addressing this limitation, Filiault and Drummond examined body image dissatisfaction in gay sportsmen. By considering the intersection of two identities (namely, gay man and athlete), which may be viewed as contradictory (i.e., the latter is compatible with hegemonic masculinity, whereas the former is not), the researchers noted differences between the male sporting body and the gay body. Participants tended to regard the ideal gay body as artificial and "functionally useless" because it was created for the purpose of achieving a specific aesthetic. In contrast, they saw their own body, the fitness of which was attributable to playing sports, as "functional" and "natural" and thus inherently masculine.

Bisexual Men and Women

The omission of bisexual individuals in body image research constitutes a notable gap. In one of the few published studies to treat gay and bisexual men as distinct groups, Ryan and associates examined body image investment in sexual minority men 40 years of age or older. Results indicated that gay and bisexual participants did not differ in their level of body image investment, and that the correlations between investment and other variables such as hypermasculinity were similar for both groups. Because body image evaluation was not measured, it is unknown whether similar null findings would emerge for body image satisfaction. Finally, the scope of this study was quite narrow: it did not focus on key issues such as bisexual men's perceptions of the appearance expectations that emanate from gay and straight communities, and whether they believe their body image changes when they have same-sex versus other-sex partners.

Unfortunately, we are unaware of any published research—qualitative or quantitative—that examines these questions.

Slightly more research has been conducted with bisexual women. For instance, Zamboni and colleagues investigated the association between bisexual and lesbian women's body image and sexual functioning. They found that participants who reported more positive body image also were more comfortable with their sexual orientation, had stronger safer-sex self-efficacy, and reported an increased level of sexual satisfaction. The researchers posit that a positive body image and increased comfort with one's sexual orientation may be independently influenced by bisexual and lesbian women's rejection of heterosexual conventions.

Bisexual women must navigate between hegemonic and nonhegemonic cultures, with the salience of these cultures changing as a function of their relationship status. However, unlike their lesbian counterparts, bisexual women may lack clear societal guidelines to help them interpret their visual identities. As bisexual individuals are not tied exclusively to the norms of gay and lesbian culture or to those set by the larger heterosexual hegemony, these shifts from one culture to another may affect bisexual body image in ways that are currently unknown.

Conclusions and Future Directions

Avenues for inquiry have been embedded in the previous sections of this chapter—often by articulating the types of research that have *not* been conducted. In this final section, we outline particular topics that we encourage researchers to pursue. As well, methodologies that have been underutilized in the study of sexual minorities' body image are briefly discussed.

Most of the research we have summarized focuses on muscularity, weight, and overall body dissatisfaction. While these elements are important, they do not capture the full scope of body image. Recognizing that there is more to the male body than musculature and fat, Martins and colleagues investigated gay men's satisfaction with their body weight, height, muscularity, hirsuteness, and penis size. Gay participants indicated that *all* body parts were important in terms of their perception of physical attractiveness; however, of greatest concern were "excessive" body hair and "insufficient" muscularity. In another study, Martins and colleagues compared the body hair removal practices of gay versus heterosexual men. They found that body hair concerns and practices were similar across the two groups, with the majority of men regularly removing body hair to improve their appearance. Noteworthy, too, is Drummond and Filiault's qualitative inquiry on gay men's perceptions of penis size. The interviewees appeared to support the cultural notion that "bigger is better" and saw the size of men's genitalia as related to the construction of masculinity.

We recommend that researchers continue to investigate body image as a multifaceted construct. As well, it is imperative that psychometrically sound indices of body image investment and body image evaluation are employed.

Many researchers contend that gay male culture emphasizes appearance and use this "fact" to explain why gay men are at risk for negative body image evaluation and intensified body image investment. Similar arguments may be forwarded to account for lesbian women's diminished susceptibility to poor body image. However, despite widespread belief in this "fact," few content analyses of gay and lesbian media and their depictions of the body have been conducted. Further, the studies that have been done tend to focus on magazines—a medium that now possesses limited relevance. We encourage researchers to content analyze diverse media (e.g., programs offered by gay and lesbian television channels; websites that target, and are popular with, sexual minorities; and gay, lesbian, and bisexual pornography). Such work would further our understanding of the kinds of messages these media disseminate about the body.

On a related note, documenting that cultural artifacts such as media depict a given body type as "ideal" does not explain why specific groups evidence poorer body image than other groups. Experimental research is needed. However, we are unaware of any methodologically sound experiments that have been conducted focusing on the influence of sexual minority media.

Finally, researchers should examine the "strategies of resistance" that gay, lesbian, and bisexual individuals may employ to counter the hegemonic messages about the body that are (potentially) disseminated within their subcultures. For example, Whitesel discusses how some gay men in online fat communities use technology as a form of social protest by "superimposing fat onto idealized bodies in homoerotic media" (p. 95). The author also notes that "body positive" versions of popular advertisements may be employed in which an ideal muscular body is replaced with one that is more "realistic." Qualitative research may uncover other strategies that sexual minorities utilize in their efforts to possess a favorable body image.

Informative Readings

Drummond, M. J. N., & Filiault, S. M. (2007). The long and the short of it: Gay men's perceptions of penis size. *Gay and Lesbian Issues and Psychology Review*, 3, 121–129.—Examines gay men's perceptions of their penis size, an area of the body that receives little empirical attention from social scientists.

Filiault, S. M., & Drummond, M. J. N. (2008). Athletes and body image: Interviews with gay sportsmen. *Qualitative Research in Psychology*, 5, 311–333.—Considers intersectionality from interviews with openly gay tennis players. Reveals that diverse social identities can provide contradictory messages about the body.

Gough, B., & Flanders, G. (2009). Celebrating "obese" bodies: Gay "bears" talk about weight, body image and health. *International Journal of Men's Health, 8,* 235–253.—Explores "bears'" body image and how they saw it changing as a function of involvement in the "bear" community.

Kelly, L. (2007). Lesbian body image perceptions: The context of body silence. *Qualitative Health Research, 17,* 873–883.—Exhibits the need to consider subgroups (in this case, femme vs. butch) and the appearance-related mandates of lesbian culture.

Kimmel, S. B., & Mahalik, J. R. (2005). Body image concerns of gay men: The roles of minority stress and conformity to masculine norms. *Journal of Consulting and Clinical Psychology, 73,* 1185–1190.—Summarizes a web-based survey of 357 American gay men and applies minority stress theory to the domain of gay men's body image.

Martins, Y., Tiggemann, M., & Churchett, L. (2008). Hair today, gone tomorrow: A comparison of body hair removal practices in gay and heterosexual men. *Body Image: An International Journal of Research, 5,* 312–316.—Examines gay and heterosexual men's engagement in body hair removal practices.

Martins, Y., Tiggemann, M., & Churchett, L. (2008). The shape of things to come: Gay men's satisfaction with specific body parts. *Psychology of Men and Masculinity, 9,* 248–256.—Incorporates head hair, body hair, and penis size satisfaction into the analysis of gay men's body image.

Morrison, M. A., Morrison, T. G., & Sager, C.-L. (2004). Does body satisfaction differ between gay men and lesbian women and heterosexual men and women? A meta-analytic review. *Body Image: An International Journal of Research, 1,* 127–138.—Summarizes the comparative research that has been conducted from 1983 to 2003 on the dimension of body satisfaction.

Peplau, L. A., Frederick, D. A., Yee, C., Maisel, N., Lever, J., & Ghavami, N. (2009). Body image satisfaction in heterosexual, gay, and lesbian adults. *Archives of Sexual Behavior, 38,* 713–725.—A current example of comparative research, an approach that has been dominant in the study of sexual minorities' body image.

Ryan, T. A., Morrison, T. G., & McDermott, D. T. (2010). Body image investment among gay and bisexual men over the age of 40: A test of social comparison theory and threatened masculinity theory. *Gay and Lesbian Issues and Psychology Review, 6,* 4–19.—Compares gay and bisexual men on indices of body image investment.

Whitesel, J. (2007). Fatvertising: Refiguring fat gay men in cyperspace. *Limina.* Available at *www.limina.arts.uwa.edu.au/_data/page/59120/Whitesel.pdf.*—Delineates ways in which gay men, who fall outside the boundaries of acceptability in terms of body size, may use technology as a form of protest.

Zamboni, B. D., Robinson, B. E., & Bockting, W. O. (2007). Body image and sexual functioning among bisexual women. *Journal of Bisexuality, 6,* 7–26.—Uses the sexual health model to explore the relationship between body image and aspects of sexual functioning in bisexual women.

CHAPTER 25

African American Body Images

DEBRA L. FRANKO
JAMES P. ROEHRIG

Introduction

Body image in African American girls and women is an intriguing area of study in part due to the well-documented finding that Black women tend to have larger bodies and more positive body image. This association between higher weight and body satisfaction stands in contrast to that of the dominant culture and encourages creative thinking about the role of culture, ethnicity, and race in the development and presentation of body image issues. This chapter highlights relevant research published over the last 10 years examining these questions. Before beginning this review, it is important to note that the terms *culture*, *race*, and *ethnicity* are neither monolithic nor discrete variables, but instead ones that are highly nuanced. The words *African American*, *Black*, and *Caucasian* have a number of meanings and can differ widely in linguistic, historical, and generational connotations. Moreover, given the literature in this area, *Black* is a more appropriate term as samples vary in origin (e.g., African American, Caribbean American). With the recognition that a variety of terms are used when discussing race and ethnicity, *Black* and *White* are used throughout this chapter for consistency.

Body Image in Blacks

Many Black individuals celebrate a larger body ideal, often have higher body weight, and may be affected by cultural and socioeconomic factors that influence body image. Research consistently indicates that relative to White women, Black women are more likely to be comfortable with their bodies at higher weights, generally have higher self-esteem, and define attractiveness in ways that go well beyond body shape and size. That said, studies find that body dissatisfaction in Black women does exist, and may be particularly pronounced at the higher end of the weight spectrum. The presence of eating disorders in Black samples, including bulimia nervosa and particularly binge-eating disorder, suggests that for some Black girls and women, body image issues may play a role in the development of eating pathology. Understanding potential ethnic differences in body image has important implications for the development of culturally relevant prevention and treatment programs.

Body Image in Black Girls and Adolescents

To date, research has consistently found that Black girls, relative to other ethnic groups, have higher body satisfaction and less drive for thinness. Studies have shown this effect in populations as young as 8 years old. Additionally, Black girls are more likely to feel good about their body when they are at higher weights. There is some evidence to suggest that preadolescent Black girls may wish to gain weight and girls at higher weights consider themselves attractive and desirable to boys. In a large prospective study examining body dissatisfaction among adolescents, being Black predicted less of an increase in body dissatisfaction from middle to late adolescence but not from early to middle adolescence, for girls. The authors explain that this may be related to the fact that the larger body size ideal held by Black girls is more similar to the shape of young women in this later developmental period rather than earlier in adolescence. However, two smaller studies suggest that this relationship is perhaps more complicated. In a study of preadolescent Black girls (ages 8–10), those with a body mass index (BMI) at or above the 85th percentile were more likely to have greater body image discrepancy, as measured by the difference between ideal and actual size estimated by silhouette drawings. Further, girls above the 85th percentile were four times more likely to participate in dieting behaviors.

Body Image in Black Women

Studies of Black women, both college age and older, continue to find higher body satisfaction relative to White women. In a meta-analysis of 98 studies published between 1960 and 2004, both White and Hispanic women consistently reported greater body dissatisfaction than Black women. However, the average differences between the Black and White samples in the studies indicated that the difference was relatively small. The authors concluded that their review challenges the current thinking in regard to body dissatisfaction, given the order of magnitude of difference found across studies. In a second review, Roberts and colleagues reported that Blacks were more likely than Whites to have a positive body image, with the largest differences being found in early adulthood. Although there was a trend suggesting that ethnic differences have decreased over time, this tendency was found only on weight-focused measures and stood in contrast to the findings on more global body image measures, where the Black–White difference actually increased.

In a large online survey-based study of women ages 25–45, Black women selected a smaller body silhouette than White women to represent their current size, even after controlling for BMI. Indeed, literature has indicated that Black women may perceive themselves as smaller than they are. In sum, a number of studies continue to support the conclusion that Black women, relative to women from other ethnic and racial groups (including those from other minority groups), evidence lower body dissatisfaction, in spite of often higher body weight.

Body Image in Black Boys and Men

Although much less is known about body dissatisfaction in boys and men relative to girls and women, a number of studies have investigated this question in recent years. Ricciardelli and colleagues reported that in studies of preadolescents, adolescents, and adults, Black males indicated a preference for a larger body size and reported more positive body image than White males. Results from several studies suggest this may be related to greater pride in one's body and a stronger investment in physical appearance. Despite these findings, the literature also indicates that Black males are more likely to engage in extreme weight loss behaviors (e.g., chronic dieting, use of diet pills, laxatives, diuretics, and vomiting) and binge eating. These seemingly paradoxical reports may reflect Black men's willingness to engage in these behaviors to achieve a more muscular physique; however, this issue has not been investigated to date.

Factors Influencing Body Image

Body Mass Index

Blacks in the United States are disproportionately more likely to be overweight or obese than Whites. This trend is especially pronounced for Black women, who are more than twice as likely to be obese as White women. A longitudinal study found that 66% of Black women who were overweight in their early 20s were obese by their mid-30s. However, the association between higher BMI and body satisfaction tends to weaken as women approach the 85th percentile for BMI. A study of 509 Black first-year students at a historically Black university found that 75% of overweight and more than 90% of obese women preferred a smaller ideal body image. Some data suggest that overweight and obese Black women, as well as adolescent girls, underestimate or misperceive their body weight and shape. Although not conclusive, these findings suggest that Black women have a higher tolerance for variation in BMI but this could be due to inter-ethnic differences in how weight is perceived.

Socioeconomic Status

The work of Flynn and Fitzgibbon remains the most comprehensive examination of socioeconomic status (SES) and body image across ethnic groups. Their conclusions that lower-SES Black women tend to have a higher BMI, larger ideal body size, and greater body satisfaction than higher-SES Black or White women appear to be consistent with findings from more recent studies. Data examining this question with Black girls and adolescents have been inconsistent, with some studies finding an influence of SES and others reporting none. This may be due to methodological differences, including how SES is defined as well as small sample sizes. As pointed out by Grabe and Hyde, although studies of body image should include the role of SES, given its documented relationship with body size, obesity, and the importance of the social context, most investigations have not included this variable.

Media Representation and Internalization

The media have long been a source of concern in the body image literature because internalization of media thin ideals has been linked to multiple negative health outcomes. Black women have been shown to be just as susceptible to self-objectification as White women, though studies find that young Black women respond differently to and are differentially affected by media images when compared to White women. Researchers have noted that Black adolescents are regularly exposed to rap videos that emphasize the physical appearance and sexuality of Black women. A community sample of over 500 Black adolescent females found that increased exposure and perception of Black sexual stereotypes in rap music predicted more negative body image. In contrast, in one study of college women, viewing television programs with predominantly Black casts predicted a healthier body image, whereas mainstream television viewing was unrelated to body image.

A study conducting in-depth interviews with 60 ninth- and tenth-grade White and Black girls helps to clarify the effects of media images. Black girls did not identify with "White" media images and did not believe that their family and friends compared them to these images. White girls, although they did not see the images as realistic, believed that family members, peers, and especially boys, would evaluate them in comparison to these images. Taken together, these studies suggest that the influence of the media may affect Black and White adolescent girls differentially and may play some role in explaining the disparate degrees of body satisfaction in these groups. Whether media influences continue to affect the body image concerns of older Black women remains to be investigated.

Other-Sex Preferences

Recent investigations into the beauty standard preferences of Black men have suggested that other-sex preferences may influence women's perception of the ideal body image. In a comparison of Black and White men's body size preferences, Black men tended to prefer more curvaceous figures with a lower waist-to-hip ratio. However, some authors have suggested that Black and White men's other-sex preferences concerning body image may be converging. A recent study revealed that even though Black men still preferred a lower waist-to-hip ratio, both White and Black men chose figures that were at or below normal weight as their ideals.

Depression

Depression has emerged as an important variable affecting body image. A 1-year longitudinal study of Black female adolescents revealed that individuals who were depressed were twice as likely to report a negative body image. Similarly, a 5-year examination of predictors of adolescent body dissatisfaction showed depression to be associated with poor body image across ethnicities. Depressive affect has further been linked to body image concern in a community sample of Black and Hispanic women, suggesting that depression is an important area for assessment in relation to body image.

Familial and Peer Influences

Maternal and familial influences may translate into positive body image attitudes that Black adolescent girls take into and share with their peer networks. Granberg and colleagues found that *both* family racial socialization (defined as educating children about various aspects of being Black, including history, meaning, and significance) and the density of Blacks in the neighborhood reduced the negative influences of being overweight for adolescent Black girls. The family context may equip Black girls with protective skills to resist dominant cultural messages that equate thinness with positive attributes such as intelligence, potential for success, and competence.

Parker and her colleagues concluded that rather than using thinness as a standard for beauty, Black girls emphasized making what they had work for them. Black girls reported receiving more positive than negative feedback about their looks from their friends and family. Further, Black girls described themselves as being very supportive of each other, as compared to White girls who expressed competitiveness and envy regarding body-related issues. A recent study of Black female college students revealed an inverse relationship between ethnic identity and internalization of mainstream beauty ideals. Greater comfort with and even idealization of fuller figures occurs among Black girls, as compared to White girls, despite being on average heavier than Whites.

Research and Clinical Implications

Implications for Research

Although a few studies have examined social, cultural, and familial aspects that may influence body image, this work has focused primarily on obesity and weight-related concerns and less so on body image. Research exploring body image in younger Black girls is a priority, as is further study to determine whether culturally specific treatments are better suited than existing interventions for Black girls and women who struggle with eating disorders. In terms of research methodology, designs that utilize a combination of quantitative methods and qualitative methods would be useful in order to fully understand the complexities of body image in diverse groups. Areas for future inquiry include the development and evaluation of culturally appropriate assessment instruments and, as described by Roberts and colleagues, a broadening of the study of psychological and cultural factors that are likely to play a role in body image concerns.

Implications for Practice

Although Black women and men tend to embrace a larger body ideal and have a more positive body image than other groups, many studies indicate that eating disorders, with associated body dissatisfaction, do appear in this group. The current edition of the DSM-IV does not sufficiently underscore that the presentation of eating disorders symptoms may differ across race and ethnicity and it is hoped that the DSM-5 will do so. Several studies indicate that clinicians are less likely to ask about eating disorder symptoms in Blacks, relative to other groups. Evidence from adult samples suggests that even if clinicians are able to effectively recognize, assess, and diagnose eating disorders and related body image concerns, ethnic minority individuals may still be less likely to seek help for reasons that include financial difficulties, lack of health insurance, not believing that others can help, fear of being labeled, lack of or unawareness of resources, feelings of shame, and fear of discrimination. The complex combination of higher rates of obesity and lower body dissatisfaction in Black individuals makes clinical work complicated, challenging clinicians to focus on healthy weight goals at the same time as encouraging the maintenance of body and self-esteem. Moreover, if Black parents are more accepting of higher weights and less likely to seek help for overweight children and adolescents, this poses difficult questions for mental health and primary care practitioners alike. Findings documenting these observations might be extrapolated to examine whether ethnic minority families would be less likely to identify or seek treatment for eating disturbances, and if so, whether and how clinicians can respond with culturally sensitive care.

Conclusions

Although rates of body dissatisfaction in Black girls and women continue to be lower relative to Whites, recent studies have shown some inconsistencies in this literature, with some reviews suggesting this gap is getting larger, and others indicating it is smaller than previously reported in the literature. Factors that influence the development of body image have been identified, and further work is needed to translate these findings into more nuanced theories of the development of body image in Black girls and women.

Informative Readings

Cash, T., Morrow, J., Hrabosky, J., & Perry, A. (2004). How has body image changed? A cross-sectional investigation of college women and men from 1983 to 2001. *Journal of Consulting and Clinical Psychology, 72,* 1081–1089.—A cross-sectional study of body image dissatisfaction in college-age men and women from 22 studies conducted from 1983 to 2001 at one university.

Edwards George, J. B., & Franko, D. L. (2010). Cultural issues in eating pathology and body image among children and adolescents. *Journal of Pediatric Psychology, 35,* 231–242.—Concludes that eating disturbances and body dissatisfaction occur to some degree in African American, Latino/Latinas, Asian American, and Native American children and adolescents, with substantial variability across studies.

Flynn, K. J., & Fitzgibbon, M. (1998). Body images and obesity risk among Black females: A review of the literature. *Annals of Behavioral Medicine, 20,* 13–24.—A review of over 30 articles, with an examination of the role of SES and other factors.

Franko, D. L. (2007). Race, ethnicity, and eating disorders: Considerations for DSM-V. *International Journal of Eating Disorders, 40,* S31–S34.—A commentary examining three epidemiological studies of eating disorders across race, gender, and culture, and the implications of these data for the revision of diagnostic criteria in the DSM-5.

Grabe, S., & Hyde, J. S. (2006). Ethnicity and body dissatisfaction among women in the United States: A meta-analysis. *Psychological Bulletin, 132,* 622–640.—A comprehensive review of 98 studies comparing body dissatisfaction among women of different ethnicities.

Granberg, E. M., Simons, L. G., & Simons, R. L. (2009). Body size and social self-image among adolescent African American girls: The moderating influence of family racial socialization. *Youth and Society, 41,* 256–277.—A longitudinal study of 400 girls in Georgia and Iowa designed to examine contextual variables that impact body and self-esteem through adolescence.

Kronenfeld, L. W., Reba-Harrelson, L., Von Holle, A., Reyes, M. L., & Bulik, C. M. (2010). Ethnic and racial differences in body-size perception and satisfaction. *Body Image: An International Journal of Research, 7,* 131–136.—A survey-based study providing comparative data on preferred figure silhouette preferences and BMI among women from different racial and ethnic groups.

Paxton, S. J., Eisenberg, M. E., & Neumark-Sztainer, D. (2006). Prospective predictors of body dissatisfaction in adolescent girls and boys: A five-year longitudinal study. *Developmental Psychology, 42,* 888–899.—A longitudinal study evaluating potential risk factors for increased body dissatisfaction among adolescent girls and boys followed for 5 years.

Ricciardelli, L. A., McCabe, M. P., Williams, R. J., & Thompson, J. K. (2007). The role of ethnicity and culture in body image and disordered eating among males. *Clinical Psychology Review, 27,* 582–606.—A review presenting data from multiple studies on body image, disordered eating, and body change strategies among men from a broad range of cultural groups.

Roberts, A., Cash, T. F., Feingold, A., & Johnson, B. T. (2006). Are Black–White differences in females' body dissatisfaction decreasing? A meta-analytic review. *Journal of Consulting and Clinical Psychology, 74,* 1121–1131.—A meta-analysis of 35 studies published between 1984 and 2004 of differences in body dissatisfaction between Black and White women over time.

Schooler, D., Ward, L. M., Merriwether, A., & Caruthers, A. (2004). Who's that girl: Television's role in the body image development of young White and Black women. *Psychology of Women Quarterly, 28,* 38–47.—An investigation of the associations among television viewing and body image in relation to mainstream or Black-oriented television programs in a sample of Black and White college women.

Stockton, M. B., Lanctot, J. Q., McClanahan, B. S., Klesges, L. M., Klesges, R. C., Kumanyika, S., et al. (2009). Self-perception and body image associations with body mass index among 8–10-year-old African American girls. *Journal of Pediatric Psychology, 34,* 1144–1154.—Examines relationships among BMI, self-perceptions, and body image discrepancies among 303 preadolescent African American girls.

CHAPTER 26

Asian American Body Images

KATHLEEN Y. KAWAMURA

Introduction

The term *Asian American* is often used as an ethnic description of a person of Asian descent who is a resident of the United States. The Asian American population includes people of East Asian (e.g., Chinese, Japanese, and Koreans), Southeast Asian (e.g., Filipinos, Vietnamese, Cambodians, and Hmong), and South Asian (e.g., Asian Indians, Pakistanis, and Nepalese) descent. Some of the information presented in this chapter may be generalizable to Asians living in Asia and to Pacific Islanders (e.g., Hawaiians, Samoans, and Guamanians), but the focus is on the body image experiences of Asian Americans specifically. Despite the wide range of ethnic groups in the Asian American population, there exist similarities between some of the subgroups in terms of traditional cultural values, Asian ideals of beauty, and status as an ethnic minority group. This chapter discusses ways in which these common factors may impact body image development and delineates ways in which intragroup differences in acculturation and ethnic identity may also influence the body image experiences of Asian Americans.

Factors Influencing Asian American Body Images

Traditional Asian Values

Many Asian Americans, whether third-generation Japanese Americans or more recent Hmong immigrants, continue to be influenced by traditional Asian values common to several Asian American subgroups. For example, most Asian cultures are collectivistic in nature. Collectivistic cultures emphasize values that promote interpersonal harmony within the family or the community, and there is often pressure to act in a manner that does not reflect poorly on the group. Some Asian Americans feel the added responsibility of not only representing their families but Asian Americans in general, especially if they are one of few Asian Americans in their community. Collectivistic cultures also value conformity, and thus physical appearances that deviate too far from the norm are often met with disapproval. For Asian American women, collective pressure may be applied to maintaining perfect physical appearances so as to not bring shame or embarrassment to the family. In addition, some Asian American families view a married daughter as a sign of social success, and thus, physical appearance also takes on importance as a factor that may influence marital prospects.

To preserve group harmony, many Asian cultures promote modesty and restraint of strong negative emotions so as to not make others feel inferior or uncomfortable. In relation to body image, it is possible that Asian Americans are merely reluctant to acknowledge publicly any sense of pride regarding their physical appearance because of the importance of maintaining modesty. Similarly, the emphasis on the restraint of strong negative emotions may inhibit Asian Americans who are experiencing extreme body dissatisfaction from disclosing this information to others, including mental health professionals. Therefore, Asian Americans may appear to be "middle of the road" (neither extremely satisfied nor extremely dissatisfied) regarding their appearance—which may or may not be an accurate representation of their actual body image experiences.

Filial piety is a cultural value common in collectivistic cultures and includes duty to respect and honor one's parents. Accordingly, Asian American families tend to be characterized by parental involvement and control, which are qualities of authoritarian parenting styles. In European American populations, authoritarian parenting styles have been implicated in the development of psychological distress, including body image dissatisfaction (BID), but this may not necessarily be the case for Asian Americans. For Asian American families, where parental control is the desired norm and is experienced as an extension of parental love and concern, these factors may actually contribute to the development of healthy high standards. Thus, whether parental control and criticism leads to BID, may be related to whether the child perceives this as occurring within the context of parental support versus parental disappointment.

For some Asian Americans, religious values are significant cultural factors. In their chapter on Asian American body images, Kawamura and Rice identified studies that have shown a relationship between adherence to the Muslim religion and body dissatisfaction. Researchers have hypothesized that in the Hindu and Muslim religions, certain practices involving fasting and dietary restrictions may trigger eating disorder symptoms for those already experiencing BID. Reddy and Crowther argue that it is cultural conflict experienced by Muslim South Asian women living in western countries, rather than the religious practices per se, that may be the primary contributors to the development of eating disorders. In contrast, Kawamura and Rice discuss how values consistent with Islam, Buddhism, and Hinduism and practices such as those in meditation, yoga, and tai chi, which tend to focus on physical, emotional, and spiritual well-being, may actually promote a positive body image.

Asian and Asian American Ideals of Beauty

Some Asian cultures, such as those in Korea, China, and Japan, have traditionally viewed plumpness as a sign of prosperity, good health, or beauty, but this no longer seems to be the case among young women in industrialized Asia. Indeed, in their study on body image across cultures, Jung and Forbes found that Korean and Chinese women showed even higher levels of body dissatisfaction and disordered eating than women in the United States. These findings are consistent with studies reviewed by the researchers that have consistently found high levels of body dissatisfaction in Korean samples. It appears as if in parts of Asia, the ideals of thinness have become more extreme than those in the United States. Regarding body size dissatisfaction and eating disorder symptoms of Asian American compared to European American women, research reviews by both Cummins and Lehman and by Smart have indicated conflicting and inconclusive results.

Less is known about the body image attitudes of Asian and Asian American men. In their review of the few studies on the body image experiences of men, Kawamura and Rice found inconsistent results, with some showing similar levels of body size dissatisfaction among Asian American and European American men and others showing Asian American men being more likely to desire a larger body than their current size. The authors describe how some Asian American men may have a more flexible notion of masculinity based in martial arts, which values coordination, stamina, and vitality (body function) versus muscularity (body appearance). Martial arts may also promote a positive body image by encouraging Asian American men to embrace their natural body type while also connecting them to their traditional culture. For Asian American men, masculinity may also be manifested through means other than through the physical body. For example, Yang, Gray, and Pope found that Taiwanese men were less concerned with muscularity than European American men, and the researchers hypothesized that for men in Taiwan, where traditional male roles are still more common, intellect and social standing may be more important than the male body as signs of masculinity. This may also be true for Asian American men who subscribe to traditional gender roles.

For Asians, especially those from central Asian countries such as

Korea, Japan, and China, common physical features often include the epicanthic eyefold, a broad, flat nose, and yellowish skin pigmentation. Some theorists interpret the idealization of a double eyelid, or eye fold, and a narrow sculpted nose as attempts to achieve Western standards of beauty. Kawamura and Rice describe how in metropolitan areas of Korea, plastic surgery to create an eyefold is not uncommon, and in Japan, glues and tapes to create an eyelid crease are sold. Accordingly, Mintz and Kashubeck found that Asian American women report being less satisfied than European American women with their eyes and faces. The researchers hypothesized that an unattainable Western ideal of beauty contributes to dissatisfaction with racial features and low self-esteem among Asian American women. Not surprisingly, according to the American Society of Plastic Surgeons, the most requested plastic surgery procedures by Asian Americans were nose reshaping, eyelid surgery, and breast augmentation.

Unlike with the eyes and nose, the idealization of White skin is not thought to be solely a reflection of Western ideals. For centuries, some Asian cultures, such as in Japan, China, and Korea, have viewed White skin as a sign of femininity, purity, and upper-social-class status, while dark skin was seen as a product of the field labor of the lower class. In some countries, such as India, White skin has also been associated with colonial power. In many areas of modern Asia, White skin continues to be valued—as can be seen in advertisements for skin whiteners and cosmetics that purport to provide a whiter appearance. Messages regarding skin color for Asian Americans may be complicated in that light skin is valued as a sign of beauty in Asian countries, White skin is valued as a sign of social power in Western countries, and tanned skin is valued as a sign of health and vitality in the United States.

Experiences with Racism and Negative Stereotypes

Being a physically distinct ethnic minority group, Asian Americans may have a heightened awareness of racial characteristics that separate them from the dominant group. Even third- or fourth-generation Asian Americans are often perceived to be foreigners and are vulnerable to discriminatory practices. The media perpetuate racism toward Asian Americans in that, until recently, portrayals of Asian characters were primarily negative or stereotyped. Asian American women are subjected to both racist and sexist stereotypes of being exotic, passive, or sexual objects, whereas Asian American men are often portrayed as dangerous, asexual, or perpetual foreigners. Experiences with racism may lead to low self-esteem, internalized racism, and denigration of one's own physical appearance.

Several studies have shown a high incidence of dissatisfaction with racial features among Asian Americans. In their 1998 review of studies on the self-concept of Asian Americans, Lee and Zhan found that when compared to other ethnic minority groups, Asian American youth were the most dissatisfied with their physical appearance and were most likely to prefer to be White if they could choose to do so. Asian American college students also reported feeling less socially accepted because of their racial features. In Kaw's interviews with Asian American women who had undergone eyelid or nasal surgeries, the women expressed hopes that these physical alterations would not only enhance their beauty but also elevate their social status. Lastly, Reddy and Crowther found that ethnic teasing was related to body dissatisfaction in South Asian women.

Acculturation and Ethnic Identity

Acculturation is the process by which individuals integrate the customs, attitudes, and habits associated with their traditional cultures with those of the dominant culture. Theorists have hypothesized that acculturation to "American" culture would be accompanied by the adoption of Western body image ideals and increased BID; however, literature reviews by both Smart and by Kawamura and Rice found no consistent relationship between acculturation and BID among Asian Americans. This may be due to the fact that many studies utilized an acculturation scale that measures acculturation on a continuum rather than examining specific components of acculturation that may be more relevant to body image, such as ethnic identity and adherence to western versus traditional values.

Both Jung and Forbes and Jackson, Keel, and Lee suggest that it is not so much exposure to Western culture as it is the conflict between traditional and Western values, especially regarding shifting gender roles that comes with Westernization, that is the primary contributor to the development of eating disorders. Both groups of researchers examined Korean women specifically and found that South Korean women and immigrants from South Korea had higher levels of eating disorder symptoms than both European American and Korean American women. It may be that women of countries undergoing Westernization and rapid social change are vulnerable to stress, which can contribute to the development of eating disorders. In their study of the body images of South Asian women, Reddy and Crowther also found that cultural conflict regarding gender role expectations, rather than acculturation, was a more important factor in the development of body dissatisfaction and maladaptive eating attitudes.

Ethnic identity also plays a large role in the development of Asian Americans' sense of self. Phinney describes fluid stages of ethnic identity that appear to change across situations and time. An unexamined ethnic identity characterizes young children or recent immigrants who have had little exposure to the dominant culture and have not yet experienced their ethnicity as requiring reflection. Whether individuals feel positively, negatively, or neutrally about their racial characteristics would be based primarily on the attitudes of the family or the community. As exposure to racism increases, some individuals may respond by rejecting their traditional culture, which might include denigration of physical characteristics associated with being Asian. The inability to eradicate salient racial characteristics may lead to internalized racism, low self-esteem, and negative body image. Others may respond to racism with anger and may immerse themselves in their traditional culture. For these individuals, ethnic characteristics may be a celebrated source of pride. An "achieved" ethnic identity occurs when there is an acceptance of both positive and negative features associated with both traditional and dominant cultures. This stage would likely be associated with the most stable, positive, body image attitudes.

Conclusions and Implications for Future Research and Clinical Practice

Despite evidence of body dissatisfaction and eating disorders in Asian American populations, few empirical investigations have been conducted to expand the understanding of the development of Asian American body images. This lacuna may be due to the fact that Asian Americans are often characterized as the "model minority group" that suffers from few psychological problems. Furthermore, the smaller body size of Asian American women may have been mistakenly assumed to protect them from body size dissatisfaction. Dissatisfaction with physical features other than body size, such as facial features, and the body image experiences of Asian American men have also been largely ignored.

Additional empirical investigations comparing Asians, Asian Americans, and European Americans, especially those examining specific Asian subgroups, might provide further insight into the influence of Asian versus American values on the body image development of Asian Americans. In addition, rather than just making comparisons, specific cultural factors such as those described in this chapter should be investigated to help explain what might contribute to these differences. Measures of body image that have been normed primarily on European American samples should also be interpreted with caution.

Clinicians who work with Asian Americans will find it helpful to explore with their clients the potential impact of the various factors discussed throughout this chapter, as they are likely to influence aspects of psychological functioning beyond that of body image. In her article on treating Asian American women with eating disorders, Smart describes how the straightforward, solution-focused style of cognitive behavioral therapy appears to be a good match for Asian American clients but adds that social environmental factors such as racism, gender, and culture need to be discussed to adapt the treatment for Asian Americans. She also emphasizes the importance of working with clients to help them identify and understand their own personal formulations for the etiology of their BID. By understanding the various influences on the development of one's own body image, clients may be able to challenge previously held notions of beauty and begin to develop their own definitions of what is attractive.

Informative Readings

Cummins, L. H., & Lehman, J. (2007). Eating disorders and body image concerns in Asian American women: Assessment and treatment from a multicultural and feminist perspective. *Eating Disorders, 15,* 217–230.—Reviews literature on the prevalence of eating disorders and negative body image in Asian American women and provides recommendations for culturally sensitive treatment.

Jackson, S. C., Keel, P. K. K., & Lee, Y. H. (2006). Trans-cultural comparison of disordered eating in Korean women. *International Journal of Eating Disorders, 39,* 498–502.—Empirical investigation and theoretical discussion regarding native cultural factors that contribute to the development of eating disorders in Korean and Korean American women.

Jung, J., & Forbes, G. B. (2007). Body dissatisfaction and disordered eating among college women in China, South Korea, and the United States: Contrasting predictions from sociocultural and feminist theories. *Psychology of Women Quarterly, 31,* 381–393.—Empirical investigation and theoretical discussion regarding the impact of Westernization and social change on body dissatisfaction and disordered eating in East Asian women.

Kaw, E. (1993). Medicalization of racial features: Asian American women and cosmetic surgery. *Medical Anthropology Quarterly, 7,* 74–89.—Ethnographic research exploring cultural and institutional factors that influence the decisions by Asian American women to undergo cosmetic surgery.

Lee, C. L., & Zhan, G. (1998). Psychosocial status of children and youths. In L. C. Lee & N. W. S. Zane (Eds.), *Handbook of Asian American psychology* (pp. 137–163). Thousand Oaks, CA: Sage.—Theoretical discussions and reviews of empirical research related to the psychology of Asian Americans.

Mintz, L. B., & Kashubeck, S. (1999). Body image and disordered eating among Asian American and Caucasian American college students. *Psychology of Women Quarterly, 23,* 781–796.—Examines gender differences within race and racial differences within gender on measures of body image attitudes and eating-disordered behaviors.

Phinney, J. S. (1996). Understanding ethnic diversity: The role of ethnic identity. *American Behavioral Scientist, 40,* 143–152.—Description of a model of ethnic identity development along with ways in which the model can be used to help students explore their own ethnicity.

Reddy, S. D., & Crowther, J. H. (2007). Teasing, acculturation, and cultural conflict: Psychosocial correlates of body image and eating attitudes among South Asian women. *Cultural Diversity and Ethnic Minority Psychology, 13,* 45–53.—Empirical research and theoretical discussion regarding sociocultural correlates of body dissatisfaction and eating disorder symptoms in South Asian American women.

Smart, R. (2010). Treating Asian American women with eating disorders: Multicultural competency and empirically supported treatment. *Eating Disorders, 18,* 58–73.—Discussion of clinical and treatment issues to be addressed in treating eating disorders in Asian American women.

Tewari, N., & Alvarez, A. N. (Eds.). (2009). *Asian American psychology: Current perspectives.* New York: Erlbaum.—Comprehensive book on the major issues related to Asian American mental health and includes chapters on Asian American body image by Kawamura and Rice, stereotypes and media images by Aoki and Mio, and parenting and raising families by Hayashino and Chopra.

Yang, C. J., Gray, P., & Pope, H. G. (2005). Male body image in Taiwan versus the West: Yanggang Zhiqi meets the Adonis Complex. *American Journal of Psychiatry, 162,* 263–269.—Empirical research and theoretical discussion regarding body image experiences of Taiwanese versus European American men.

CHAPTER 27

Hispanic/Latino Body Images

DEBORAH SCHOOLER
LYNDA S. LOWRY

Introduction

The dominant North American beauty ideal identifies thinness as the key requirement of feminine beauty and muscularity as the essence of the male physique. Accordingly, men and women are taught not only to want this unattainable body, but to continually strive to reach it through diet, exercise, and a host of commercially available products. These mainstream values, however, may be at odds with the values individuals receive from their own cultures and communities. The present chapter provides a succinct review of existing research on Latino body image. Data on the prevalence of body dissatisfaction and disordered eating among Latinos are discussed, followed by an analysis of the potential antecedents and consequences of body image concerns among Latinos.

Prevalence of Body Image Concerns among Latinos

Initially, body image was considered a concern of White women; subsequent efforts to include women of color in research on body image were first directed primarily at African American women. Although there is now a growing literature examining body image among Latinos, the bulk of this research still relies on comparisons of the prevalence or degree of body image concerns among girls and women of different ethnic groups,

237

with a smaller set of studies comparing boys and men. Findings from such comparison studies have been mixed, with some scholars concluding that Latinos are protected from body image concerns, and others concluding that Latinos experience equal or greater risks than Caucasians.

Latino communities may be more accepting of a wider range of body types than Caucasian communities. Instead of a thin ideal for women, Latino culture, like African American culture, may value a "thick" ideal, comprised of a slender but curvy body, with a thin waist, big breasts and hips, and a round behind. Accordingly, researchers have examined whether Latino adolescents and adults are more satisfied with their own body sizes than Caucasians.

In some studies, Latina girls and women have indeed reported greater body satisfaction compared to Caucasian girls and women. In a sample of midlife African American, Caucasian, and Latina women, for example, it was found that Latina women had the lowest rates of body preoccupation. A second set of studies, however, finds that Latinas experience as many body image concerns as Caucasian girls and women. Latina adolescents frequently describe an ideal body type that is comparable to the White norm and report an interest in weight loss at rates similar to those reported by Caucasian peers. Studies comparing body satisfaction between Latino and Caucasian males have been equally contradictory. Although in some studies, Latino boys and men report more body satisfaction compared to their Caucasian counterparts, the majority of studies find comparable levels of body satisfaction among Latino and Caucasian men.

In addition to research on body satisfaction and ideal body size, ethnic comparisons have also been drawn with regard to eating behavior. Although disordered eating is a complex behavior with multiple causes, disordered eating is often considered to be a behavioral manifestation of body image concerns. Comparison studies indicate that Latinos are at equal or greater risk of developing an eating disorder relative to other ethnic groups. In samples where Latino adolescents report greater body satisfaction compared to Caucasian boys and girls, Latinos still report comparable or higher rates of disordered eating. In a sample of White, Asian, and Latina elementary school girls, Robinson and colleagues found that after controlling for actual body size, Latina girls were significantly more likely than their White and Asian peers to report both wanting to lose weight and actively attempting to lose weight by dieting or fasting. In one study, more than 60% of Latina girls had engaged in unhealthy weight loss behaviors, such as fasting or skipping meals, at some point during the past year. Research suggests that body policing and weight management practices are frequent in Latino families, potentially because of health-related concerns. In the United States, Latinos are at increased risk of being overweight and of developing conditions such as diabetes and coronary disease, and weight loss behaviors may be motivated, in part, by desire to avoid these conditions.

Consequences of Body Image Concerns

As noted above, body dissatisfaction may put Latinos at risk for other mental health concerns, such as disordered eating. Recent evidence suggests that the associations between body dissatisfaction and mental health concerns, however, may be different for Latino youth than for White youth. Specifically, there is growing evidence that body dissatisfaction may be more closely linked to mental health problems among Latinos compared to other ethnic groups. For example, a longitudinal study of nearly 1,400 adolescent girls (including 380 Latina girls) found that preoccupation with thinness predicted onset of an eating disorder more strongly among Latina girls than among Caucasian girls.

A similar pattern emerges when considering self-esteem and depression. Among Latina women, body dissatisfaction is strongly associated with increased levels of depression, and decreased levels of self-esteem and life satisfaction. Latino men with higher body mass indices tend to be less satisfied with their life and report higher levels of depression. Studies using multiethnic samples suggest that disordered eating and depression are more highly correlated among Latinas than among Caucasians or African Americans. These findings suggest that although body dissatisfaction may be marginally less prevalent among some Latino populations, its implications for well-being are no less severe.

Although the mechanisms of these associations are not fully understood, acculturation processes have recently been implicated in the strong associations between body dissatisfaction and mental health concerns reported by Latina girls and women. The acculturation process involves many potential stressors, such as navigating language use, balancing a complex set of cultural norms and scripts, or experiences of discrimination. The difficulties an individual may experience in response to the demands of the acculturation process have been labeled acculturative stress, and research has suggested that high levels of acculturative stress present a mental health risk for U.S. Latinos. Although most studies on the mental health consequences of acculturative stress have focused on depression, there is evidence that acculturative stress might also contribute to the etiology of disordered eating. In one study, Latinas who were dissatisfied with their body were especially likely to report disordered eating if they also reported high levels of acculturative stress. Among Latinas with low levels of acculturative stress, body dissatisfaction and disordered eating were not correlated.

Acculturation, Media Use, and Body Image

In arriving at their own body attitudes, Latinos must negotiate the values provided by the dominant, White culture and those provided by their own families, communities, and cultures. Latinos are often discussed as having a "dual identity," bridging multiple cultures, races, traditions, and communities. Among a sample of adolescents from an ethnically diverse high school, Latino adolescents most frequently selected a bicultural reference group label as opposed to a mainstream or strongly ethnic identification. Consequently, Latinos are presented with two sets of cultural values that may differ greatly in their approach to beauty, body, and appearance. Just as Latinos must negotiate a complex set of cultural values over what is beautiful, they must also navigate among multiple, cultural definitions of what is *saludable* (healthy). Latino research participants indicate that they receive a complex and often contradictory set of messages about the relationships among health, weight, appearance, and diet.

Evidence suggests that Latinas who place greater emphasis on mainstream, Anglo values and norms, as opposed to Latino values and norms, may face greater body image concerns. For example, greater acculturation into mainstream White culture has been associated with higher incidence of disordered eating in both Mexican American and Cuban American women and in diverse samples of Latina adolescents. At the same time, acculturation has also been linked to higher blood pressure, higher cholesterol, and greater incidence of diabetes among Latino adults. Higher rates of adolescent obesity have been found among second- versus first-generation Latinos and scholars argue that higher levels of acculturation and unhealthy diet patterns partially explain the association between generation status and obesity. More acculturated Latino adolescents report eating more fast food and engaging in less physical activity than their less acculturated peers.

Media is one vehicle by which individuals can learn about cultural body ideals, including those of the dominant Anglo culture and those of the Latino culture. Latino youth typically report watching almost 4 hours of television a day, roughly 1 hour more than their Caucasian peers. The media use of Latino youth is generally split between mainstream English-language programming and Spanish-language programming on networks like Telemundo and Univision. Initial studies suggest that mainstream media use may impact the body image of Latino youth. Across several studies, Latino adolescents and young adults who regularly watched more mainstream television and movies and read more mainstream magazines report greater body dissatisfaction than those who consume less of these forms of media. By providing access to mainstream values, media use may be one means of becoming acculturated. At the same time, ethnic identity and acculturation processes may contribute to the ways in which Latinas interact with and are affected by media exposure. Research indicates that Latina adolescents who strongly identify with their ethnic heritage are less influenced by exposure to mainstream media messages about body and appearance.

Less research has examined the effects of Spanish-language media. According to dual-role theory, Spanish language television acts both as an agent of assimilation into the mainstream culture and as a conduit to one's ethnic heritage and community. Content analyses have not yet specifically investigated the portrayals of men's and women's bodies on Spanish-language television or magazines, and opinions from Latino focus groups are mixed. Although some participants have argued that the cultural thick ideal permeates Spanish-language media, presenting a healthier alternative to mainstream media, others have argued that the women depicted in Spanish-language media still conform to mainstream values. Given that Spanish-language media present the potential for presenting an alternate body ideal, future work should specifically investigate the role of Spanish-language media in Latino body image.

Latinos are often discussed as inhabiting the "borderlands," bridging multiple cultures, races, traditions, and communities, and inhabiting both real and metaphorical borderlands. Although most studies have used panethnic samples of "Latino" or "Hispanic" individuals, Latino communities are composed of individuals with diverse ethnic backgrounds, including individuals of Mexican, Caribbean, Central American, and South American descent. Generally, studies either collapse these groups into a panethnic sample or examine a homogeneous sample (e.g., Puerto Rican women), so, as of yet, little is known about how body image might be experienced differently among these populations. In addition to considering individuals identifying themselves as monoethnic (identifying with one ethnicity), or as having a "dual ethnicity" (for example, identifying as Black and Cuban), it is necessary for research to appreciate the role a multiethnic identity (identifying with three or more ethnicities) plays in developing body image values. Similar to findings with monoethnic Latinos, early findings comparing multiethnic youth to youth of other ethnic groups are mixed. Some studies have found higher levels of disordered eating or stronger associations between disordered eating and mental health concerns among multiethnic individuals compared to others. Other studies have not, and future work is needed to understand the complexities of body image among multiethnic youth. Even among Latinos who identify as monoethnic, however, the negotiation of cultural body ideals may not be restricted to mainstream White and Latino values. Recent evidence suggests that Latino adolescents are also engaging with African American cultural values and Black-oriented media in arriving at their own body attitudes. For example, in a study of Latina adolescents, girls who watched more Black-oriented television felt better about their bodies than girls who watched less.

Conclusions

The research findings on Latino body image are varied and, at times, contradictory. Taking acculturation processes into consideration, however, such contradiction seems probable and meaningful. If acculturation stress strengthens the connection between body image concerns and disordered eating, we might expect to find higher incidence of disordered eating among Latinos compared to Whites, despite comparable or healthier levels of body satisfaction. Moreover, if acculturation processes are indeed central to the development of body image and eating behavior among Latinos, we would expect to find different patterns of outcomes in different populations. For example, because of the developmental course of ethnic identity across adolescence, the acculturation processes of an early adolescent might look very different from that of an older adolescent or emerging adult, who may have a clearer sense of identification either with mainstream or Latino culture. Consequently, we might expect to find vastly different patterns of body image outcomes in these two populations. Similarly, acculturation processes might differ between Latinos who live, work, and study within a larger Latino community and those who are immersed in a predominantly White environment. Accordingly, the lack of a single clear conclusion regarding differences in body image outcomes between Latinos and other ethnic groups may reflect the diverse borderlands occupied by Latino adolescents and the lack of a singular "Latino" experience.

Informative Readings

Barry, D. T., & Grilo, C. M. (2002). Eating and body image disturbances in adolescent psychiatric inpatients: Gender and ethnicity patterns. *International Journal of Eating Disorders, 32*, 335–343.—Compares gender and ethnic groups in body image disturbances and eating disorders.

Cachelin, F. M., Phinney, J. S., Schug, R. A., & Striegel-Moore, R. (2006). Acculturation and eating disorders in a Mexican American community sample. *Psychology of Women Quarterly, 30*, 340–347.—Explores the relationship between acculturation processes and disordered eating behaviors among Mexican American women.

Goodman, J. R. (2002). Flabless is fabulous: How Latina and Anglo women read and incorporate the excessively thin body ideal into everyday experience. *Journalism and Mass Communication Quarterly, 79*, 712–727.—A qualitative examination of Latina and Caucasian women's beliefs about cultural ideals of beauty presented in media.

Gordon-Larsen, P., Harris, K. M., Ward, D. S., & Popkin, B. M. (2003). Acculturation and overweight-related behaviors among Hispanic immigrants to the U.S.: The national longitudinal study of adolescent health. *Social Science and Medicine, 57*, 2023–2034.—A longitudinal study of the impact of acculturation on health behaviors such as weight and physical activity.

Jane, D. M., Hunter, G. C., & Lozzi, B. M. (1999). Do Cuban American women suffer from eating disorders? Effects of media exposure and acculturation. *Hispanic Journal of Behavioral Sciences, 21*, 212–218.—Examines the associations between various acculturation processes, including media use, on eating attitudes of Cuban American women.

McKnight Investigators. (2003). Risk factors for the onset of eating disorders in adolescent girls: Results of the McKnight Longitudinal Risk Factor Study. *American Journal of Psychiatry, 160,* 248–254.—Examines the ways in which body preoccupation, culture, and social pressure contribute to onset of eating disorder pathology among ethnically diverse adolescents.

Perez, M., Voelz, Z. R., Pettit, J. W., & Joiner, T. E. (2002). The role of acculturative stress and body dissatisfaction in predicting bulimic symptomatology across ethnic groups. *International Journal of Eating Disorders, 31,* 442–454.—Provides data on the relationship between acculturation and body image disturbances among White, Black, and Hispanic women.

Ricciardelli, L. A., McCabe, M. P., Williams, R. J., & Thompson, J. K. (2007). The role of ethnicity and culture in body image and disordered eating among males. *Clinical Psychology Review, 27,* 582–606.—A review of literature concerning disordered eating behaviors among men from culturally diverse backgrounds.

Rivadeneyra, R., & Ward, L. M. (2005). From Ally McBeal to Sabado Gigante: Contribution of television viewing to the gender role attitudes of Latino adolescents. *Journal of Adolescent Research, 20,* 453–475.—Examines correlates of Latino adolescents viewing of English and Spanish television programming.

Robinson, T. N., Killen, J. D., Litt, I. F., Hammer, L. D., Wilson, D. M., Haydel, F., et al. (1996). Ethnicity and body dissatisfaction: Are Hispanic and Asian girls at increased risk for eating disorders? *Journal of Adolescent Health, 19,* 384–393.—Examines the correlates of disordered eating among an ethnically diverse sample of adolescent girls.

Rubin, L. R., Fitts, M. L., & Becker, A. E. (2003). "Whatever feels good in my soul": Body ethics and aesthetics among African American and Latina women. *Culture, Medicine, and Psychiatry, 27,* 49–75.—Uses qualitative methods to analyze the complex relationship between cultural attitudes and body image among Black and Latina women.

Schooler, D. (2008). Real women have curves: A longitudinal investigation of TV and the body image development of Latina adolescents. *Journal of Adolescent Research, 23,* 132–153.—A longitudinal study examining associations between acculturation and media on Latina girls' body satisfaction.

CHAPTER 28

Body Images in Non-Western Cultures

EILEEN P. ANDERSON-FYE

Introduction

Ideal body images vary cross culturally, yet there is usually shared agreement on local standards. This chapter addresses some of the systematic differences found in body image conceptualization and ideals in non-Western cultures. It then reviews the most pressing contemporary questions in the field regarding the role of globalization in shaping body image cross culturally: Are Western body image ideals being exported to the rest of the world? What are the processes by which local communities adopt or reject Western ideals? What are the implications of the coexistence of competing body image ideals for globalizing and increasingly multicultural communities?

Non-Western Theories of the Body: One Body Per Person?

In order to understand variations of body image ideals cross culturally, it is important to understand that conceptualizations of what a "body" itself is vary among non-Western cultures. Western cultures tend to operate on principles of individualism and think of the body as that which is bounded by one individual's skin; that is, there is one body per person. This conceptualization is consistent with biomedical notions of a universal, individual body as the subject of intervention. In contrast, in more sociocentric societies, a body may be part of collective management practices; that is, there may be two or more people sharing any given body. Most often, families or close others may have substantial influence over another's body through feeding or caring practices. The people involved think of themselves as a group, not as isolated individuals. Accordingly, practices related to health and healing tend to include multiple participants.

A vivid example of this latter, sociocentric point of view is provided by Anne Becker's research in rural Fiji. Becker showed how caring for bodies and specifically maintaining a robust body size was not only a critical task in a subsistence society but also one fundamentally shared by loved ones. If a person lost weight, or was accused of "going thin," in the local vernacular, the problem was understood to be housed in that person's close relationships, not with the individual. The family and other loved ones of that person held the responsibility for the problem—and also the cure—of that person's undesirable loss of weight. By better caring for and feeding the "sick" person, the loved ones participated in healing and maintaining the body that they considered to be part of themselves. In this way, bodies in this community were all shared by a web of close others in a dense social network.

The Fijian case provides an example of how body image is closely tied to local theories of the body. This type of sociocentric conception of the body is particularly common among non-Western, nonindustrialized nations. It stands in sharp contrast to the Western view of the body that holds it to be the property and responsibility of the individual person rather than the social group.

Macrostructural Factors Related to Ideal Body Image

In addition to local conceptions of the body, everyday lived experiences related to structural factors are associated with ideal body shape and size cross culturally. Rarely do we find universals in the cross-cultural record. Rather, the factors of availability of food, health indicators, gender, and industrialization/development are better conceptualized as guiding principles that work along with specific cultural beliefs and practices in the non-Western world to determine ideal body images.

Availability of Food

When food is scarce in a society due to poverty, armed conflict, or a combination of both, ideal body images tend to be more robust. In situations of starvation or limited availability of food, only those with higher social status are able to procure the resources to consume enough or excess food. In these societies, those of lower social status tend to do more physical labor. Those of higher status have lower overall physical activity, thus preserving body mass. In short, bigger is generally perceived to be better. If a nation or region is under the scarcity condition, then it would make sense to expect that distorted body image and related eating disorders involving food refusal might be rare. This argument is a common one to explain the relatively low rates of disordered body image in a number of countries in sub-Saharan Africa, for example.

In contrast, wealthier nations with more abundant food availability tend to have the inverse relationship between status and body size. That is, under the food availability condition, communal body image ideals tend to be slimmer, and food refusal is an indicator of higher status. Further, leisure time for physical exercise is also positively associated with social status. In sum, food scarcity tends to breed larger body ideals, whereas food abundance is related to leaner ideals, though there are exceptions.

Health Indicators

Several global health threats appear to be related to a larger body ideal. Malnutrition, a major contributing factor to many other health problems, has been the most persistent of these. HIV/AIDS, often overlapping with malnutrition, has been identified as another key health threat that can impact body ideals. In areas where a large minority of the population has contracted HIV/AIDS, a robust body size with the locally desired shape can be a marker of relative health. In several studies in sub-Saharan Africa, HIV/AIDS is so highly stigmatized that not only is a thin body potentially marked as diseased, but also a redistribution of fat tissue typical of some of the antiretroviral therapies (which may include increasing fat around the middle and atrophy of extremity and facial fat among other patterns) is marked as undesirable. Therefore, body ideals that privilege body fat distribution toward the hips for females and the extremities for males tend to be preferred. However, younger upwardly mobile subgroups, such as younger career-oriented Black women in urban South Africa, are also turning toward more toned and muscular ideals as alternate non-HIV-positive body images. Epidemic or pandemic disease threat that includes physical emaciation tends to be associated with larger cultural ideal body images in places hit the hardest.

Gender

Body image ideals and the relative importance of body image to other ethnopsychological functioning tend to both vary by gender and be related to culture-specific gender roles. Although body size aspects of ideal body image trend together by gender, body shape aspects of ideal body image tend to vary by gender. In other words, in places such as Samoa where larger body sizes are preferred, the distribution of body mass varies for females and males; females should carry their weight especially around the hips, whereas males should have substantial muscular development. Similarly, when thinner ideals are preferred, women should still be curvaceous and men should be more muscular. Evolutionary anthropologists and psychologists have argued that for females, waist-to-hip ratio is key in ideal body shapes in most parts of the world. An analogous but weaker pattern, waist-to-chest ratio, has been found for men. On the ground for women, the waist-to-hip ratio translates to local ideal body shapes such as the "hourglass figure" that indicate a curvaceous female figure with primary emphasis on the hips. Many non-Western cultures, especially those in Latin America, the Caribbean, sub-Saharan Africa, and the Pacific Islands, are thought to embrace slightly more curvaceous ratios than Western cultures.

Gender role change is thought to be related to body image dissatisfaction (BID) for women. In non-Western cultures, gender role transition for women is likely to involve less support on men and increasing public roles outside of the household such as in Latin America. It may also include a conflict between more traditional private roles and more masculine public roles such as in Japan. Conflicting role expectations are found to be stressful throughout the world. This sort of stress itself, as well as exposure to multiple models of ideal femininity, has been found to impact both how women perceive their own bodies and cultural body ideals. Female bodies can take on heightened personal, familial, and cultural meanings in the midst of gender role transition by indicating traditional versus changing values.

For men, larger body sizes are preferred in most non-Western cultures when compared with women. However, the male trend toward preference for increased muscularity in Western cultures is beginning to be echoed in studies conducted in non-Western cultures around the world. The drive toward muscularity in Western cultures has been linked to disordered body image and dangerous behavior among boys and men and should be taken seriously as patterns emerge in non-Western cultures as well.

Industrialization/Development

Industrialization is often, but not always, a part of economic development in non-Western nations. Both industrialization per se and economic development more generally appear to affect body image ideals in the cross-cultural record. Industrialization is thought to have effects in a number of ways including individualization, regimentation, the increasing influence of biomedicine, and changing gender roles. Economic development tends to not only underscore these factors but also introduces social change and globalization. Especially during engagement with what has been termed the *global economy*, interaction with Western images, ideas, and ideals often increases in the non-Western world.

When a society shifts from an agricultural base to industrialization, understandings of work, time, and individuality tend to shift. While the work of many traditional economies is integrated throughout a full day, week, or longer, industrialization often introduces shift work with precise starting and stopping times. Moreover, the unit doing the work is an individual, not a family or collective, which can help shift sociocentric notions of self and body toward individualistic ones. Work is often monitored carefully from an external hierarchy, and ideally, those who are more efficient are rewarded. This sort of regimentation can also introduce culturally specific notions of work and competition that have been shown to affect body image during processes of economic development.

In places that have undergone industrialization in the last several decades, Western medicine (i.e., biomedicine) often enters. Biomedicine, with its focus on individual bodies and individual preventative behaviors, underscores the notions of body as individualistic and controllable through work and risk reduction. These notions can change body image from something shared and stable to something personal and malleable. Once the body becomes an object of "work," BID becomes more likely. When comparative images are drawn from Western media, those images can become powerful and impact body ideals in the direction of slender sizes and Western-preferred shapes, though this process is not inevitable. Overall, when industrialization and modernization occur around the world, body size and shape ideals tend to shift toward Western ideals, and beliefs about the ability to modify body size and shape shift. Such processes are strongest among upwardly mobile and urban individuals, and substantial intracultural variation regarding body images persists.

Globalization and Body Image

Are Western Body Image Ideals Being Exported to the Rest of the World?

One of the most pressing issues in the consideration of non-Western body images is the role of globalization. Several decades ago, it was hypothesized that globalization would spread BID and related body image and eating disorders in a fairly straightforward fashion around the globe. Early correlative quantitative studies indeed showed that in societies undergoing globalizing cultural and economic change, disordered eating behaviors were beginning to be found among women. Currently, eating disorders are part of the World Health Organization's priority health concerns, particularly among adolescent females. However, ethnographic and multimethod research conducted over the last 25 years has shown that the patterns and processes of globalization impacting non-Western body images are multiple and highly dependent upon local and regional contexts. These more nuanced data are helping in the identification and prevention of disordered body image in non-Western cultures.

What Are the Processes by Which Local Communities Adopt or Reject Western Ideals?

Becker's work in Fiji showed that the influx of global media—even without much of a global economy—can impact conceptions of body image and disordered eating behaviors. In the Fijian case, only 18 months after the introduction of television with Western programming, young women moved from thinking of their bodies as unchangeable and supported by a dense social network to malleable by themselves as individuals. Their desire for thinner, more Western-looking bodies was not due to aesthetic goals but rather a desire for the consumerist and glamorous lifestyles they saw attached to the thin bodies. The slender Western body ideals were a means to an end for them, rather than ends unto themselves. Through careful, multimethod, longitudinal research, Becker has documented a profound change in rates of disordered eating behaviors—related to this shift in body ideals and body image—now on par with rates found in Western nations.

Developed societies such as Hong Kong and Taiwan were among the first non-Western cultures to report eating disorders such as anorexia nervosa (AN). However, Sing Lee and colleagues showed that early on, key body image components of the diagnosis of AN were absent among a significant proportion of those diagnosed. That is, the "fat phobia" that is central to Western understandings of body image and eating disorders was missing, though the disorders held the same dire physiological consequences that they do in the West. Lee and colleagues' work caused scholars and clinicians to question the previously assumed relationship between body image and eating disorders and remains in the conversation of diagnostic retooling currently going on regarding DSM-5.

Currently, Western-style BID (i.e., wanting to be thinner among females and more muscular among males) is found throughout the world, leading many to speculate on the role of "globalization" in creating and spreading pathology. Given the overwhelming findings in this direction, Anderson-Fye fully expected to find a mushrooming of BID and related disordered behaviors in Belize, a rapidly developing nation heavily dependent on the West for its tourism economic base and where female bodies and beauty were already very important culturally. However, instead, in longitudinal ethnographic research, Anderson-Fye found a rejection of Western female body ideals and very low levels of disordered behaviors. Body shape was more important than body size, and bodies could be adorned by clothing if one did not naturally possess a curvaceous "Coca-Cola" figure. Moreover, the drive to restrict food or exercise excessively did not fit with the local psychology and was rejected by most. This research, sometimes considered an "ethnographic veto" of the universality of the spread of disordered body image and eating behaviors due to globalization, showed how local psychological and cultural values could resist powerful Western models.

In contexts of globalizing cultural change, some strata of the population are usually at earlier risk for problems than others. Usually, but not always, intracultural variation risk factors include female gender, adolescence, upward mobility, urban location, and high levels of interaction with global media.

What Are the Implications of the Coexistence of Competing Body Image Ideals?

Understanding non-Western patterns of body image conceptualization, practices, and disorders is not only important for global health concerns, but also for increasingly multicultural Western contexts due to high rates of migration. Current migratory trends bring large numbers of people from non-Western cultures into Western contexts. For example, in the United States, one in five schoolchildren today is from an immigrant family with that number expected to increase to one in three by 2030. Understanding familial and cultural conceptualizations of body image and body ideals can be critical, especially if we consider that with few notable exceptions, migration to Western contexts puts young women and men at risk for body image and eating problems through a number of mechanisms. Prevention and treatment programs that understand local cultural context and variation have been shown to be among the most promising for these youth.

Conclusions

In sum, conceptualizations of body image as well as body image ideals vary enormously throughout the non-Western world. It is critical to remember that Western individualistic notions of body image are not universal, though they do appear to be increasingly common. Local contexts and local uptake of global images of and messages regarding bodies are crucial in understanding body image throughout the non-Western world. Differential acceptance of and resistance to Western body ideals for both females and males throughout the non-Western world are not only important to note but also may be instructive for promotion of protective interventions regarding body image in multicultural contexts, whether due to globalization or immigration.

Informative Readings

Anderson-Fye, E. P. (2004). A coca-cola shape: Cultural change, body image, and eating disorders in San Andrés, Belize. *Culture, Medicine, and Psychiatry, 28*, 561–595.—A longitudinal ethnographic examination of body image and disordered eating among adolescent girls in Belize.

Anderson-Fye, E. P. (2009). Cross-cultural issues in body image and eating problems among children and adolescents. In L. Smolak & J. K. Thompson (Eds.), *Body image, eating disorders, and obesity in youth: Assessment, prevention, and treatment* (2nd ed., pp. 144–174).—Washington, DC: American Psychological Association. Reviews cross-cultural data for body image and eating problems among youth with particular focus on current trends such as extremely high rates of disordered eating in Korea.

Anderson-Fye, E. P., & Becker, A. E. (2003). Sociocultural aspects of eating disorders. In J. K. Thompson (Ed.), *The handbook of eating disorders and obesity* (pp. 565–589). New York: Wiley.—A review of sociocultural trends in body image and eating disorders including summaries of specific world regions.

Anderson-Fye, E. P., & Lin, J. (2009). Belief and behavior aspects of the EAT-26: The case of schoolgirls in Belize. *Culture, Medicine, and Psychiatry, 33*, 623–638.—An empirical article describing use of the EAT-26 for cultural contexts undergoing cultural change by separately assessing beliefs and behaviors.

Becker, A. E. (Ed.). (2004). New global perspectives on eating disorders. *Culture, Medicine, and Psychiatry, 28*, 4.—An edited special issue journal volume that holds major qualitative and ethnographic contributions regarding Curacao, Japan, South Africa, Fiji, and Belize, as well as commentaries by top scholars in the field.

Becker, A. E. (2005). *Body, self, and society: The view from Fiji.* Philadelphia: University of Pennsylvania.—A comprehensive study on conceptions of bodies and body images in a sociocentric cultural context.

Csordas, T. (Ed.). (2001). *Embodiment and experience: The existential ground of culture and self.* Cambridge, UK: Cambridge University.—An edited volume on theories and examples of embodiment and body image in a number of non-Western cultures.

Frederick, D. A., Buchanan, G. M., Sadeghi-Azar, L., Peplau, L. A., Haselton, M. G., Berezovskaya, A., et al. (2007). Desiring the muscular ideal: Men's body satisfaction in the United States, Ukraine, and Ghana. *Psychology of Men and Masculinity, 8*, 103–117.—Illustrates the state-of-the-art methodology for assessing muscularity ideals among men and examines male body dissatisfaction comparatively.

Lee, S., Ho, T. P., & Hsu, L. K. G. (1993). Fat phobic and non-fat phobic anorexia nervosa: A comparative study of 70 Chinese patients in Hong Kong. *Psychological Medicine, 23*, 999–1017.—Classic article establishing non-fat-phobic AN and therefore variable relationships between body image and AN.

Lester, R. J. (2007). Critical therapeutics in two eating disorders treatment centers. *Medical Anthropology Quarterly, 21*, 369–387.—Compares Mexican and U.S. models of body image, disordered eating, and treatment programs.

Lipinski, J. P., & Pope, H. G., Jr. (2002). Body ideals in young Samoan men: A comparison with men in North America and Europe. *International Journal of Men's Health, 1*, 163–171.—Examines drive for male muscularity in cross-cultural contexts.

Nasser, M., Katzman, M. A., & Gordon, R. A. (Eds.). (2001). *Eating disorders and cultures in transition*. New York: Taylor and Francis.—Examines the role of social change in body image and eating disorders in multiple regions of the world.

Puoane, T., Tsolekile, L., & Steyn, N. (2010). Perceptions about body image and sizes among black African girls living in Cape Town. *Ethnicity and Disease, 20*, 29–34.—Examines body image ideals among Black schoolgirls in South Africa and where those ideals originate, with particular focus on social and health status.

Body Image and Congenital Conditions Resulting in Visible Difference

NICHOLA RUMSEY
DIANA HARCOURT

Introduction

Whether present at birth or acquired later in life, a physical appearance that is different from the norm can have considerable ramifications throughout the lifespan. While many adapt positively to the challenges, others experience adverse effects on self-perceptions, including body image and self-esteem, and in relation to social functioning. This chapter summarizes current understanding of the impact of congenital disfigurement and those factors than can promote resilience or exacerbate distress. The implications of this knowledge for the provision of care and a research agenda for the future are outlined. Readers are encouraged to consult Chapter 41 for coverage of body image and adjustment issues associated with disfigurement resulting from burns.

Types of Congenital Conditions Resulting in Disfigurement

Visible differences result from a wide variety of congenital anomalies. The exact incidence is unknown. Some are evident at birth (e.g., a cleft of the lip), whereas others, such as neurofibromatosis, become more visible over time. Malformations of the head and neck are the most common visible birth "defects." A cleft of the lip and/or palate occurs in approximately 1 of 700 births, on one (unilateral) or both (bilateral) sides of the face. Other anomalies include the failure of the cheek and jaw bones to fully develop (e.g., Treacher-Collins syndrome), or the early fusion of the cranial bones (as in Cruzon's syndrome). Some genetic conditions produce an unusual appearance, including Marfan syndrome (elongated face, torso, and limbs) and epidermolysis bullosa, which results in minor or extensive skin blistering. Disfigurement may also result from the delayed maturation of blood vessels (cutaneous haemangiamata), vascular malformations (birthmarks), or the failure of a limb to fully develop. Webbing ("syndactyly") results from the failure of fingers or toes to separate fully, whereas in polydactyly an extra digit is present on the hand or foot.

Defining "Disfigurement"

The boundary around what is and what is not a disfigurement is far from straightforward. For example, at what point do prominent ears constitute an abnormality? A definition adopted by several researchers is of disfigurement as "a difference from a culturally defined norm that is visible to others." The inclusion of "visibility to others" excludes conditions such as body dysmorphic disorder in which the difference is imagined or grossly exaggerated by the affected person (see Chapter 35). The language used to describe differences in appearance has a negative focus (e.g., disfigurement, deformity, and defect). Although debate about the most appropriate terminology is ongoing, researchers and clinicians are encouraged to use descriptors with sensitivity.

Psychosocial Issues and Congenital Disfigurement

The challenge of understanding the impact of disfigurement on body image is complicated by the variety of causes, the range of body sites affected, the anticipated trajectory of the underlying condition and its treatment, the life stage of the affected person, and numerous personal, social, and situational characteristics. Nevertheless, there is a surprising degree of commonality in the issues reported. The growth in the number of qualitative and mixed methods studies has added to the richness of understanding in the field, as have recent efforts to include service users in the research process. However, researchers can only scratch the surface of the lived experience of visible difference, and the contribution to understanding of several moving and very lucid personal accounts published in recent years has been immeasurable.

The impact of disfigurement has been described from a variety of viewpoints. The sociocultural perspective highlights the influence of the prevailing societal context on an individual's interpretation and response to his or her difference. There is no doubt that in our appearance-obsessed, Westernized societies, messages associating good looks with happiness are omnipresent and unremitting, to the detriment of those whose appearance is in some way different. Psychological perspectives have highlighted the impact of disfigurement on emotions, components of the self-system, and behaviors of people with disfigurement, and on the ways in which the visible difference impacts on the cognitions and behaviors of others. Research in the 1980s and 1990s identified a range of negative effects on self-perceptions (including body image) and social functioning, together with a complex interplay of the responses of the affected person and the reactions of others. Social encounters, for example, can be thrown off kilter by real or anticipated negative reactions from others, or by the physical limitations to nonverbal expression caused by the congenital condition. Discomfort on either side may contribute to an unsatisfactory or abbreviated interchange. The avoidant or stilted reactions of others may result in negative spirals of aversive emotional responses, maladaptive thought processes, unfavorable self-perceptions, and longer-term effects on the behavior of the person with the disfigurement, including social avoidance or an overreliance on camouflage makeup.

It is essential to recognize, however, that not all people with visible differences are equally affected. Findings suggest that 30–50% experience significant psychosocial difficulties (depending on the particular aspect of distress measured). Others adjust positively and feel that the disfigurement plays only a small part in their lives. As discussed subsequently, recent research has focused on the identification of factors that differentiate positive from negative adjusters.

The Impact of Visible Difference across the Lifespan

Until recently, researchers have considered people with disfigurements as a population set apart from others with body image concerns, yet many challenges faced during childhood, adolescence, and adulthood are not exclusive to those with a disfigurement. Perhaps the most helpful way to characterize the effects of a visible difference is as an underlying stressor present throughout the lifespan. It may exacerbate the pressures associated with various developmental stages, and it may entail a "weak link" in the psychological armory when under pressure from an accumulation of life events or daily stressors. Many congenital conditions necessitate regular visits to surgeries or hospitals reminding the affected person and his or her family of the "difference." The specter of treatment, such as the next operation, may loom large at particular ages or throughout life.

During childhood, the family environment is a significant influence on the development of body image, and preliminary research suggests that family psychological processes are more influential than surgical interventions in promoting adjustment or exacerbating distress. Parents' feelings about their child's appearance are transmitted and then assimilated by the child from an early age, influencing developing perceptions of body image and self-worth. Families vary considerably in their strategies for dealing with the visible difference of one of their members. Some discuss it openly; others act as if the difference doesn't exist. Children may not raise body image issues for fear of upsetting their parents. Early research suggests that a family environment in which the condition is allowed to have only a minimal impact and in which a positive body image and high self-esteem are not contingent on the disfigurement is likely to be beneficial. Additionally, the child should be encouraged to develop social interaction skills that will prove beneficial in a wider social environment.

Parental influence typically wanes during the school years as children engage increasingly in social comparisons with their peers. During this developmental period there have been reports of more negative self-concepts, less positive social functioning, and higher levels of social withdrawal in children with a cleft compared to their noncleft peers. Reports of teasing by others are commonplace in children with visible differences. While this is an issue for all children, a distinguishing characteristic can make a young person an obvious target for peer harassment. Thus children and young people with visible differences have an increased risk of appearance-related teasing and bullying and for developing negative self-perceptions, including body dissatisfaction, during this time. However, not all young people with a visible difference report teasing, and not all those who are teased find it distressing. Stable friendships are protective, and it is likely that children with positive core self-evaluations interpret negative encounters as less threatening than those who feel their difference is central to their body image. Susceptibility and resilience at this and other developmental stages are complex issues in need of further research.

Physical changes in adolescence can strengthen links between outward appearance and self-perceptions, and a visible difference that sets the affected person apart from the norm can present distinct challenges. Developing independence and autonomy means that adolescents are increasingly likely to have to deal with the responses of others, without the intervention and immediate support of caregivers. Although it could reasonably be expected that this life stage might be particularly challenging, research is equivocal and includes reports that teenagers with a cleft are as satisfied with their appearance and their friendships as their nonaffected peers.

Body image issues may play a significant part in treatment decision making during adolescence. Some interventions are growth dependent and there may be considerable pressure to undergo surgery at a particular developmental stage. Reconstructive procedures can involve damage to one part of the body to reconstruct another, for example, the removal of toes to create fingers for those with congenital hand anomalies. Many young people face multiple interventions in the ongoing quest to "normalize" their appearance and may feel their treatment decisions are driven by the agendas of the surgeon or their parents. The young person may want to look more like and feel more accepted by peers, but may also feel that the difference is part of his or her identity. Some may need support to cope with appearance-altering surgeries; others may need help expressing that they do not want further operations.

A minority of people with congenital disfigurements experience distress in adulthood. Research has associated visible differences with a variety of negative life experiences in the realms of dating, employment, and occupational attainment. The dislike of feeling different, and the desire to achieve "normalcy" by looking unremarkable is strong among those reporting distress. People with visible differences may feel deprived of the ability to manage the assumptions and misconceptions others make on the basis of their appearance. Changing social groups (e.g., starting a new job or moving to a new neighborhood) can be particularly challenging. Considerable effort may be required to leave established support systems for the relative unknown of a new social environment, where a visible difference is likely to be a distinguishing characteristic, a novelty, and a source of curiosity. New strategies must be developed to deal with the reactions of unfamiliar others. A positive body image, high levels of energy, initiative, and good social skills may be required to progress beyond initial meetings to form new friendships and relationships. Some people with congenital disfigurements have reported negative impacts on longer-term relationships, including marrying at a later age, settling for the wrong partner, and experiencing less marital satisfaction than comparison groups. However, there are also reports of people thriving despite some obvious challenges. Positive adjusters become comfortable in their own skin and believe their disfigurement has given them unique and valued characteristics, including communication skills, inner strength, and genuine friendships that do not rely on external appearances.

Research with older adults is currently limited. However, contrary to the notion that older people are less concerned about their appearance, recent findings suggest visible differences can be troubling for many. The focus of concern may shift from the desire to look "attractive" to one of "propriety"—the wish to appear tidy and smart—nevertheless, significant numbers of those with disfigurement experience distress and also feel their concerns are not appreciated by the clinicians who treat them.

Understanding Individual Variation in Adjustment

In recent years, researchers have investigated factors contributing to the considerable variation in adjustment to disfigurement. To date, the majority of this work has focused on adults rather than younger people, largely for pragmatic reasons, including ease of access and the availability of appropriate measures. The headline finding is that the major contributor to adjustment is the cognitive architecture of the person with a disfigurement—the lens through which he or she views the world. The psychological characteristics differentiating those experiencing higher levels of distress from those who are positively adjusted include levels of optimism, the extent to which their view of themselves is dominated by thoughts about appearance, concern about negative evaluations by others, and feelings of social acceptance.

The intuitive belief that the severity of a disfigurement predicts the extent of distress is still widespread among the public and health care providers; however, there is little support for this in the literature. Previously, the consensus among researchers was that disfigurements that are readily visible to others, most notably on the face, were the most likely to result in distress. However, fearing negative evaluation in social situations, some go to great lengths to conceal their disfigurement with clothing or camouflage, even from their partners. Although this reduces their distress in public, intimate relationships may be affected by fears of exposure. More research is needed to understand the relationship between disfigurement and intimacy. Subjective perceptions of the visibility of a disfigurement to others are a more powerful predictor than objective measures. Thus, experts in the field recommend the routine inclusion of subjective measures in any assessment of distress.

Other long-held beliefs are also being challenged by research. While higher mean levels of distress are reported by women and younger people, many men and older people are also distressed by disfigurement. In summary, assumptions about adjustment based on the etiology, location, and severity of the condition are misplaced, as are those relating to age, gender, and treatment history of the affected person. The implication is that routine assessment and support should be available for all.

Clinical Implications and Health Care Provision

In their regular contacts with people with disfiguring conditions, health care professionals have a vital role to play in promoting positive body image and psychological adjustment in people with disfigurements. Currently, prospective patients are offered a variety of appearance-enhancing surgical or medical solutions in response to psychological and social difficulties. Provided in isolation, they may reinforce the notion that quality of life necessarily improves when physical appearance is enhanced. This offers a simplistic view of adjustment and increases the pressure on prospective patients to undergo treatment that might "improve" their looks. Although some shifts in the ethos of care have been made (e.g., each U.K. cleft team now includes a psychologist as a core member), more effort is required to shift from an exclusive emphasis on fixing the problem of disfigurement through surgical intervention to promoting positive psychosocial adjustment through a variety of techniques. Chapter 46 provides further discussion of treatment considerations for persons with disfiguring conditions.

Future Research Questions

Although the psychological characteristics that promote adjustment in people with disfigurements have come into clearer focus, the detail remains blurred. Research efforts in this area must continue, particularly in relation to the emergence and development of factors contributing to resilience in children and young people. This raises a particular set of challenges, including the need for longitudinal research, the ongoing need to develop measures with an appropriate focus on appearance concerns, and methods of engaging younger participants. To this end a range of innovative methods designed to encourage participation are being developed, including online focus groups and the compilation of collections of photographs and scrapbooks by participants. To complement the emphasis on individual factors in adjustment, efforts to further understand the influence of race, culture, and social class should be redoubled.

It is tempting to dichotomize those affected as predominantly "positive" or "negative" adjusters; however, a dynamic interplay of experiences characterizes the daily lives of many. Fluctuations between states of relative adjustment and distress remain to be fully understood. In the interest of reducing perceived and real gaps between people with and without disfigurement, the current focus on commonalities in body image is to be encouraged. Researchers should also bear in mind that despite their enthusiasm for understanding the impact of disfigurement, participants may also have other body image concerns, and the latter may be more distressing.

Conclusions

Far from living in a society that promotes valuing diversity in appearance, we are in the grip of a culture ever more obsessed with physical attractiveness. Levels of body image concern and overall adjustment in people with congenital anomalies vary considerably and are predicted much more strongly by psychological factors than the physical characteristics of any difference. While many are well adjusted, this population has an increased risk for a range of poorer psychosocial outcomes. Disfigurement and its treatment can represent underlying stressors across the lifespan, making repeated calls on energy reserves and coping resources.

Informative Readings

Eiserman, W. (2001). Unique outcomes and positive contributions associated with facial difference: Expanding research and practice. *Cleft Palate Craniofacial Journal, 3*, 236–244.—A "call to arms" for researchers and clinicians to focus on the positives associated with disfigurement as well as the challenges.

Feragen, K. B., & Borge, A. I. (2010). Peer harassment and satisfaction with appearance in children with and without a facial difference. *Body Image: An International Journal of Research, 7*, 97–105.—A discussion of the complex interplay of social experiences and satisfaction–dissatisfaction with appearance, including a consideration of risk and protective factors.

Lansdown, R., Rumsey, N., Bradbury, E., Carr, A., & Partridge, J. (Eds.). (1997). *Visibly different: Coping with disfigurement*. Oxford, UK: Butterworth-Heinemann.—A discussion of the definitions and causes of visible differences, a summary of approaches to intervention, and a series of personal accounts.

Moss, T. P. (2005). The relationship between objective and subjective ratings of disfigurement severity and psychological adjustment. *Body Image: An International Journal of Research, 2*, 151–159.—An exploration of the relative contribution of patient and clinician ratings of the severity of a condition and distress in 400 outpatients.

Mouradian, W. E. (2001). Deficits versus strengths: Ethics and implications for clinical practice and research. *Cleft Palate Craniofacial Journal, 38*, 255–259.—A consideration of the ethical ramifications of focusing on the problems and difficulties associated with disfigurement.

Murrey, L., Arteche, A., Bingley, C., Hentges, F., Bishop, D., Dalton, L., et al. (2010). The effect of cleft lip on socio-emotional functioning in school aged children. *Journal of Child Psychology and Psychiatry, 51*, 94–103.—A rare longitudinal study of the social adjustment of 93 children with a cleft and 77 controls, highlighting the additional contribution of communication difficulties.

Ong, J. L., Clarke, A., Johnson, M., White, P., Withey, S., & Butler, P. (2007). Does severity predict distress? The relationship between subjective and objective measures of severity in patients treated for facial lipoatrophy. *Body Image: An International Journal of Research, 4*, 239–248.—A quantitative study with repeated measures over a 2-year period, demonstrating the importance of subjective assessments of appearance.

Partridge, J. (1990). *Changing faces*. London: Penguin Books.—An eloquent personal account of the journey from injury to adjustment by the chief executive of the charity Changing Faces.

Rumsey, N., & Harcourt, D. (2005). *The psychology of appearance*. Maidenhead, UK: Open University Press.—A comprehensive summary and critical evaluation of research and understanding and a review of methodological challenges inherent in research relating to appearance and disfigurement.

Strauss, R. R., & Fenson, C. (2005). Experiencing the "good life": Literary views of craniofacial conditions and quality of life. *Cleft Palate Craniofacial Journal, 42*, 14–18.—A qualitative approach to understanding how people with craniofacial conditions view positive aspects of life using literary selections from fiction.

PART V

BODY IMAGE DYSFUNCTIONS AND DISORDERS

CHAPTER 30

Body Image
and Social Functioning

STACEY TANTLEFF-DUNN
DANIELLE M. LINDNER

Introduction

Decades of research consistently show that an individual's physical appearance is related to various aspects of his or her social functioning. Physical attractiveness is associated with greater popularity, lower levels of loneliness, and greater feelings of overall social connectedness. Even small children demonstrate preferences for peers who are more attractive in studies examining play behavior. A smaller but increasingly compelling literature suggests that, in addition to the impact of *actual* attractiveness, the way an individual feels about his or her body also relates to social functioning. Generally, people who feel more positively about their bodies report greater comfort and confidence in their interpersonal interactions, whereas those who feel more negatively about their bodies report greater discomfort in and avoidance of social situations. The focus of this chapter is to provide theoretical perspectives from which we can better conceptualize the relationship between body image and social functioning, summarize the relevant literature, and discuss the implications for treatment and future research.

Social Cognition: A Conceptual Framework for Understanding Body Image and Social Functioning

Over 50 years ago, Fritz Heider described social cognition as our perceptions of others' attitudes, intentions, emotions, behaviors, and manner of

263

relating to us. As we try to understand our social world we rely heavily on the schemas we have developed about others and about ourselves, including schemas about body image (see Chapter 5). How we feel about ourselves and our bodies can impact both our own behavior in social interactions, as well as our perceptions of the behavior of others. For example, if a young woman who is experiencing a significant amount of body dissatisfaction goes to a party and a male friend asks her to dance, how might she respond? Given her existing set of beliefs, she may assume he extended the offer only because he feels sorry for her, not because he enjoys her company. She may in turn grow anxious and respond to him in a less socially engaging manner or she may decline his offer altogether. Alternatively, she may feel so anxious or self-conscious at the party due to her dissatisfaction with her body that she appears aloof and unapproachable. If not asked to dance, she may interpret it as confirmation that she is unattractive. This scenario points to the reciprocal nature of the relationship between body image and social functioning.

One way our body image schemas develop is through social interactions. Social interactions have been described as a "looking glass" through which our experiences with others reflect back important messages about ourselves and, more specifically, about our appearance. While the opinions of others certainly shape our views of ourselves, the opposite is also true. Self-perceptions can color our perceptions of others' reactions to us, or, in some circumstances, can impact the type of reactions we receive. This is demonstrated in Kleck and Strenta's classic study on the role of "negatively valued characteristics" in perceptions of interpersonal interactions. In their experiment they used makeup to create the appearance of a scar on the faces of a group of research participants. The researchers then removed the scars without participants' knowledge before they engaged in conversation with a confederate. Participants who believed they had a facial scar reported that it negatively impacted the quality of their social interaction relative to comparison groups of participants who were instructed to tell the confederate that they suffered from allergies or epilepsy. The latter participants also reported that their condition had a negative impact on the social interaction, but they reported that their condition impacted the level of nervousness and tenseness displayed by the confederate, whereas participants in the scar condition reported changes in the confederate's gazing behavior. This early work highlighted the impact that an imagined (i.e., self-perceived) physical defect may have on social interactions.

A study conducted by Nezlek explored the relationship between overall body satisfaction and social interaction. Male and female college students were asked to record information about the frequency and quality of their social interactions in a daily diary. Participants with greater body satisfaction reported that their day-to-day interpersonal interactions felt more intimate. Body-satisfied women also reported increased social confidence and perceived that they had greater influence in their social interactions than women with less body satisfaction. This study and that of Kleck and Strenta indicate that body image can act as a filter through which we evaluate the nature and quality of our interactions and possibly even our relationships.

Body Image and Social Functioning in Clinical Samples

Research involving clinical populations for whom body image may be a particular area of concern, such as individuals diagnosed with eating disorders or body dysmorphic disorder (BDD), clearly demonstrates the link between body image and social functioning. Women with eating disorders, who characteristically are dissatisfied with their bodies, report greater social anxiety and public self-consciousness. Women who report body shame, which often accompanies body dissatisfaction, also tend to report greater social withdrawal. McClintock and Evans's investigation of the characteristics underlying social phobia and eating disorders revealed that low body esteem is associated with symptoms of social phobia, including fear of negative evaluation by others and low self-acceptance.

Similarly, in patients with BDD (see Chapter 35), which is characterized by significant concerns about appearance, social phobia is the second-most common comorbid diagnosis. Even when an additional diagnosis of social phobia is not warranted, BDD includes significant impairment in social and occupational functioning. Social impairment may take the form of avoiding social situations that may highlight an individual's perceived flaw, engaging in compensatory behaviors, or perceiving seemingly ambiguous comments made by others as threatening or as negative feedback related to appearance. Anecdotally, work with patients with BDD suggests a cycle in which concerns about appearance lead to dysfunctional social behavior that then results in social interactions that serve to validate perceptions of rejection. Feeling rejected then fuels concerns about physical appearance and leads to continued behavioral avoidance.

Findings regarding social functioning in other clinical and medical populations in which body image dissatisfaction (BID) may be present are somewhat limited. Corry and colleagues described that many burn survivors report increased self-consciousness and avoidance of social situations secondary to real or perceived stigmatization (see also Chapter 41). In a study by Huang and colleagues, men who were HIV-positive experiencing lipodystrophy reported poorer body image, quality of life, and greater situational body image dysphoria relative to men who were HIV-positive without lipodystrophy. Additionally, Hartl and colleagues identified body image as one of several predictors of long-term social functioning in patients with breast cancer.

Overweight or obese individuals, who are more likely to be dissatisfied with their bodies than are nonobese people, also report social difficulties related to their weight and body image (see Chapters 20 and 21). A study by Annis and colleagues compared body image and psychosocial functioning among currently overweight, previously overweight, and never overweight women. Currently overweight women reported the most body dissatisfaction as well as less social self-esteem and life satisfaction. Moreover, among currently and formerly overweight women, poorer social functioning was related to a history of greater weight-related stigmatization. Controlling for body image evaluations attenuated these associations. Other studies have found that overweight or obese individuals are more avoidant of social situations, perceive greater social rejection, and in some cases, report decreased quality of relationships. In general, overweight and obese individuals report more difficulties with social functioning than their average-weight peers. Given the increasing incidence of obesity, these relationships are increasingly important to understand. Of particular interest is the extent to which body image mediates, or at the very least moderates, the relationship between obesity and negative social consequences.

Body Image and Social Functioning in Nonclinical Samples

Several potential social consequences of poor body image have been identified in nonclinical samples. Negative body image evaluation and a high level of investment in appearance are associated with public self-consciousness, introversion, social anxiety, poor general and social self-esteem, and low confidence in interpersonal interactions. Body dissatisfaction and dysfunctional investment in appearance are also related to dysphoria in or avoidance of situations in which appearance is salient as well as an overall decrease in one's quality of life.

It is worth noting that the aforementioned relationships are correlational in nature and that most of the available information about the relationship between body image and social functioning comes from scale-development research that includes social functioning as a part of the construct validation process. In the few studies that focused on social functioning, results are largely consistent with findings from the scale-development papers. For example, Davison and McCabe found that among adolescent girls, positive body image was predictive of more positive same- and other-sex relationships. For adolescent boys, positive body image only predicted more positive relationships with members of the other sex. Appearance-related social comparison was not a significant predictor of social functioning for either gender. In another study comparing social functioning between adolescent females with high and low body dissatisfaction, Schutz and Paxton found that girls with high body dissatisfaction reported higher levels of social anxiety and insecurity in addition to negative friend characteristics including friend alienation and the perception that thinness was important in interpersonal relationships.

Despite the importance of moving beyond correlational studies, few researchers have done so. One exception is Carron and colleagues' examination of college-age women's anxiety in various social situations, including wearing a bathing suit at the beach alone or with friends. Relative to being alone, participants reported that being in a group of female friends or being in a group of mixed company would yield a reduction in anxiety, whereas there was no reduction in anxiety when participants imagined wearing a bathing suit on the beach with male friends. Participants believed that if they were with others, any appearance-related evaluation would be spread across the members of the group, a phenomenon labeled "diffusion of evaluation." The results of this study indicate that group situations might be slightly less intimidating for women, but the attractiveness of the group members may affect the amount of diffusion of evaluation.

An Attachment Theory Perspective on Body Image and Social Functioning

In his writings about attachment theory, Bowlby argued that early attachment sets the stage for later social functioning and also plays a role in the development of psychopathology. Bartholomew and Horowitz expanded upon Bowlby's seminal work to examine attachment styles in adult relationships. They conceptualized adult attachment as consisting of two orthogonal dimensions, the first being one's view of the self as either positive and worthwhile or negative and unworthy. The second dimension is one's view of others, which can also be either positive (i.e., others will accept me) or negative (i.e., others will reject me). These two dimensions combine to produce four attachment styles that range from secure attachment in which individuals view themselves positively and view others as positive and accepting, to three types of insecure attachment in which views of the self and/or others are negative and nonaccepting.

In general, secure attachment is associated with more positive body image and insecure attachment is associated with more negative body image. Cash, Theriault, and Annis found that, for both men and women, a secure attachment style is associated with greater body satisfaction, less dysfunctional investment in appearance, and less body image dysphoria. In contrast, men and women with a preoccupied attachment style (they viewed themselves negatively but viewed others positively and sought acceptance from them) reported less body satisfaction, more dysfunctional investment in appearance, and greater body image dysphoria. McKinley and Randa extended this work by priming female participants to think about their experiences in specific relationships prior to completing measures of attachment and body image. They found that attachment anxiety and avoidance were good predictors of body image when participants thought about close friendships, but not romantic relationships.

Although conclusions about causality cannot be drawn from correlational data, based on the very nature of attachment theory it seems unlikely that body dissatisfaction causes difficulties in attachment; rather, individuals with body dissatisfaction may have had early attachment difficulties that persist and impact adult interpersonal relationships and self-image. Consistent with this assertion, Troisi and colleagues found that women diagnosed with an eating disorder were more likely to retrospectively report insecure attachment and separation anxiety symptoms. It is important to understand how the attachment styles reported by individuals with varying degrees of BID may manifest themselves in interpersonal relationships. Body-satisfied individuals with a secure attachment style may have an internalized sense of self-worth that is not contingent upon the acceptance of others. They are likely to have an easier time developing close, trusting relationships relative to individuals with greater body dissatisfaction and a preoccupied attachment style who may lack an internalized sense of self-worth but still desire close relationships. When their interpersonal needs are not met, they are likely to feel worse about themselves in general and about their bodies in particular.

Conclusions and Future Directions

Regardless of their actual appearance or attractiveness, people who are dissatisfied with their bodies or who place significant emphasis on the role of appearance in overall self-concept generally report poorer social functioning than those who are satisfied with their bodies or for whom appearance is less important. Poorer social functioning often takes the form of anxiety in certain social situations or avoidance of anxiety-provoking situations altogether. Research on social anxiety indicates that those who are especially anxious in social situations often report difficulty maintaining friendships, poorer performance during conversations, decreased perceptions of social support, and for women, less disclosure in social situations. They are also more likely to make negative appraisals of social situations, which may serve to create additional anxiety and make social interactions more aversive. For women, increases in body dissatisfaction often occur during adolescence when peer relationships become increasingly complex (e.g., navigating romantic vs. platonic relationships). The anxiety experienced in social interactions as a result of body dissatisfaction may further complicate the process.

Our review of the literature reveals that although researchers have a basic understanding of the relationship between poor body image and difficulties in social functioning, there are several avenues for additional research. The small number of studies examining aspects of social functioning as a primary variable of interest in relation to body dissatisfaction is surprising. Although there are several measures designed to assess various aspects of psychosocial functioning in relation to body image (see Chapters 15 and 18), the measures are often used in such a way that the implications of results for social functioning are addressed in a very limited manner. In addition, few studies address potential mediators of the relationship between body image and social functioning. For example, research indicates that social comparison is related to body dissatisfaction. It is important to consider how frequent social comparisons may impact interpersonal relationships. Feelings of jealousy, guilt, or resentment, for example, may result from social comparison and undermine the development of close, trusting relationships with comparison targets who may be same-sex friends.

There are two primary methodological limitations of the research related to body image and social functioning, the first being that the majority of existing data still come from samples of predominantly White female college students. Despite expansion to additional populations (e.g., clinical groups), the growth is limited. Research on how body image impacts social functioning in both sexes of different ages and ethnicities is still needed. Secondly, the literature consists mainly of correlational studies. Further prospective and experimental research is needed to shed light on the nature of the reciprocal relationship between body image and social functioning. Such research will inform efforts to minimize negative social consequences for individuals with normative levels of body dissatisfaction and to treat those with severe BID. In addition to the frequently used cognitive-behavioral strategies to address BID (see Chapter 47), interpersonal psychotherapy may be particularly helpful for addressing the many ways relationships impact body image and how poor body image adversely affects the nature and quality of social interactions. Similarly, it is worth exploring the effectiveness of social skills training to facilitate positive social relationships that may contribute toward preventing BID.

Informative Readings

Annis, N. M., Cash, T. F., & Hrabosky, J. I. (2004). Body image and psychosocial differences among stable average weight, currently overweight, and formerly overweight women: The role of stigmatizing experiences. *Body Image: An International Journal of Research, 1*, 155–167.—Provides information about differences in body image and social functioning among women with differing weight histories.

Carron, A. V., Estabrooks, P. A., Horton, H., Prapavessis, H., & Hausenblas, H. A. (1999). Reductions in social anxiety of women associated with group membership: Distraction, anonymity, security, or diffusion of evaluation? *Group Dynamics, Theory, Research, and Practice*, *3*, 152–160.—Compares and discusses body image in various interpersonal contexts (e.g., alone, single-sex groups, mixed groups).

Cash, T. F., Theriault, J., & Annis, N. M. (2004). Body image in an interpersonal context: Adult attachment, fear of intimacy, and social anxiety. *Journal of Social and Clinical Psychology*, *23*, 89–103.—Provides information about the relationships among body image, adult attachment style, and social anxiety.

Davison, T. E., & McCabe, M. P. (2005). Relationships between men's and women's body image and their psychological, social, and sexual functioning. *Sex Roles*, *52*, 463–475.—Uses regression models to explore the role of body image in social functioning.

Davison, T. E., & McCabe, M. P. (2006). Adolescent body image and social functioning. *Journal of Social Psychology*, *146*, 15–30.—Describes the relationship between body image and same- and other-sex relations in adolescent boys and girls.

Kleck, R. E., & Strenta, A. (1980). Perceptions of the impact of negatively valued physical characteristics on social interaction. *Journal of Personality and Social Psychology*, *39*, 861–873.—Presents a series of experiments highlighting the impact of an imagined physical defect on social perceptions.

McClintock, J. M., & Evans, I. M. (2001). The underlying psychopathology of eating disorders and social phobia: A structural equation analysis. *Eating Behaviors*, *2*, 247–261.—Highlights the shared difficulties experienced by those having symptoms of eating disorders and social phobia, including fear of negative evaluation.

McKinley, N. M., & Randa, L. A. (2005). Adult attachment and body satisfaction: An exploration of general and specific relationships. *Body Image: An International Journal of Research*, *2*, 209–218.—Examines the relationship between different types of attachment and body image.

Nezlek, J. B. (1999). Body image and day-to-day social interaction. *Journal of Personality*, *67*, 793–817.—Uses a daily diary methodology to examine body image and its impact on aspects of social functioning, including feelings of confidence and influence in interpersonal interactions.

Schutz, H. K., & Paxton, S. J. (2007). Friendship quality, body dissatisfaction, dieting, and disordered eating in adolescent girls. *British Journal of Clinical Psychology*, *46*, 67–83.—Examines the quality of same-sex friendships in relation to body image and eating behavior.

Troisi, A., Di Lorenzo, G., Stefano, A., Nanni, R. C., Di Pasquale C., & Siracusano, A. (2006). Body dissatisfaction in women with eating disorders: Relationship to early separation anxiety and insecure attachment. *Psychosomatic Medicine*, *68*, 449–453.—Discusses the etiological role of separation anxiety and insecure attachment in the development of eating and body image difficulties.

CHAPTER 31

Body Image and Sexual Functioning

MICHAEL W. WIEDERMAN

Introduction

How could body image *not* be intimately tied to sexual functioning? After all, it is through our bodies that we both experience sexual sensation and provide sexual stimulation to partners. It becomes more complex, however, when we consider what might be included in the concepts of "body image" and "sexual functioning."

First, in considering any links between sexual functioning and body image, there may be an important distinction between *body image* as a term for the global assessment of one's own physical attractiveness, or desirability as a sexual partner, versus how one feels about one's own genitals or erogenous zones (those body parts that are typically sexualized and considered particularly important for sexual arousal). Feeling unattractive generally may be relevant to sexual functioning, yet feelings about specific body parts such as genitals and breasts (for women) may also be relevant to sexual functioning in their own ways.

Just as "body image" might mean different things, so may "sexual functioning." The term *sexual functioning* might include how one's body physically responds to sexual stimulation, or the degree of sexual pleasure or satisfaction one experiences, or even the amount and types of sexual experience one has had. Conceivably, sexual functioning in the present may be influenced by the amount and types of sexual experiences one has had in the past. In understanding connections between body image and sexual functioning, it may be important to start with consideration of basic sexual experience.

271

Initial research on potential relationships between body image and sexuality was focused on global physical attractiveness as correlated with sexual experience, such as age at first sexual activity with a partner, total number of sexual partners, and current sexual relationship status. Early researchers generally found small correlations between people's physical attractiveness and sexual experience; attractive people tended to report greater sexual experience involving partners. This relationship made sense because sexual activity with partners requires being attractive to potential partners. However, those initial studies relied on not only self-reports of sexual experience but also self-reports of attractiveness. This could be a problem because other research had demonstrated only very weak relationships (if at all) between self-rated attractiveness and how peers rated those same individuals.

To investigate the relative importance of self-rated attractiveness, which might be considered global body image, compared to attractiveness as judged by others, Hurst and I conducted a study involving nearly 200 female college students. While the women were completing self-report surveys, they were unknowingly being rated on their physical attractiveness by a male and a female peer. The women were also weighed and their height measured before leaving so that we knew their actual body size. In general, we found that the women's body size and peer-rated attractiveness were much better predictors of sexual experience with partners than was the women's body image.

We interpreted our research findings as indicating that, when it came to basic sexual experiences with a partner, attractiveness to potential partners seemed to be more important than how young adult women evaluated and felt about their own body. However, it was possible that less attractive women held different sexual values or goals, thereby resulting in less sexual experience. Fortunately, we included measures of sexual attitudes, which turned out to be unrelated to the size or rated attractiveness of the women.

To date there has not been analogous research in which males' body images, body sizes, and observer-rated attractiveness have been considered simultaneously. Such research may be more complicated for male respondents than for females. Whereas females who are dissatisfied with their overall body appearance almost invariably wish to be thinner, forms of male body image dissatisfaction presumably are more variable. Some men may indeed wish to be thinner (as high levels of fat may be considered unattractive for both women and men), whereas others may wish to be larger in the sense of increased muscularity or a larger body frame (as ideals of masculinity include muscularity and height). Indeed, Cash, Maikkula, and Yamamiya studied college men's and women's body image concerns during sexual activity and found that, whereas the men were equally self-conscious about their weight and muscle tone, the women were substantially more self-conscious about their weight than their muscle tone.

In summary, several studies have revealed small relationships between physical attractiveness and extent of sexual experience. There are some indications that perceptions of attractiveness by peers are more important than self-perceptions of attractiveness, but the research on this topic has been limited primarily to college students, and particularly females. What about body image and sexual functioning within a particular sexual experience?

Body Image and Immediate Sexual Functioning

Once involved with a sexual partner, a person's sexual functioning includes the ability to get physically aroused, experience orgasm, and find the experience pleasurable and satisfying. How would body image be thought to relate to these experiences? First, body image concerns may prompt an individual to avoid particular sexual activities or settings, thereby resulting in less experience with positive sexual functioning. Second, body image concerns may be distracting during sexual interactions, a phenomenon sex therapists refer to as *spectatoring*.

Spectatoring was first considered as a problem that might inhibit a male's ability to obtain an erection. For a man who had experienced difficulty obtaining or maintaining erections in the past, a sexual interaction with a partner may trigger concerns about his erection in this instance. Such concerns might prompt the man to monitor the quality of his erection, thereby distracting his attention from his partner and his own experience of pleasure. Of course this distraction could be expected to further impair his erection.

Because the perceived "success" of a male–female sexual interaction usually depends on an erect penis, spectatoring for men may revolve around monitoring erection quality. For women, however, being a desirable sexual partner may have less to do with performance or degree of physical arousal, and more to do with being an attractive ("sexy") visual stimulus. Spectatoring for a woman may often involve monitoring how her body might appear to her sexual partner (see Chapter 6 on "self-objectification"). Indeed, Meana and Nunnink examined the self-reported frequency of performance-based versus appearance-based spectatoring among a large sample of college students. Compared to men, women reported higher levels of both types of distraction during sexual activity. The men indicated greater likelihood of performance-based than appearance-based spectatoring.

When it comes to assessing the extent to which one feels self-conscious about physical appearance during sexual intimacy with a partner (see Chapter 15), at least three different self-report measures have been published. Higher scores on each indicate what might be termed *body image self-consciousness*, or focusing one's attention on how one's body appears to one's partner. Such spectatoring is expected to reduce focus on the person's own sexual arousal and pleasure.

Since 2000, the results of several studies have been published, each looking at body image concerns as related to sexual functioning with partners. Despite different samples and different measures, the results have been consistent: Women and men who report greater body image self-consciousness during physical intimacy with a partner also report more problems with sexual functioning and less pleasure and enjoyment of sexual activity. The forms of self-reported sexual problems investigated in these studies have included decreased arousal, less frequent orgasms, greater aversion to sex, less desire for sex, and increased anxiety during sex.

One way to approach examination of possible links between body image and sexual functioning is to study changes in sexual functioning after relatively sudden changes in body image. Stofman and colleagues took such an approach by surveying women who had undergone cosmetic surgery to improve the appearance of either their breasts, midsection (torso and upper legs), or their face. The three samples were relatively small (19–26 women each), but even though virtually all respondents indicated an improvement in their overall body images as a result of their surgery (see Chapter 45), there were some substantial differences among the three groups when it came to sexual functioning. Compared to the women who underwent facial surgery, substantially more women who had undergone procedures to improve the appearance of their breasts or midsections reported increases in the frequency of sexual activity, sexual satisfaction, frequency of orgasm, and willingness to engage in new sexual practices with a partner. Unfortunately, the data were based on self-reported perceptions of changes from before surgery to the present time, so it is unknown how well they correspond to actual changes in sexual functioning from pre- to postsurgery.

Several different studies all point to relationships between body image self-consciousness during physical intimacy with a romantic partner and sexual dissatisfaction and problems in sexual functioning, but there's more. In a few studies, sexual assertiveness or sexual self-efficacy was also examined. Women who indicated greater body image self-consciousness also reported feeling less able to communicate assertively with sexual partners, or to be an active agent within sexual encounters with partners. Indeed, in one large sample of women seeking services at community family planning clinics, those who indicated more general focus on how their body looked to others also reported less consistent condom use and greater likelihood of having engaged in sexual activity after drinking alcohol or taking other drugs.

In summary, based on several lines of research, there have been some consistent findings regarding body image self-consciousness and sexual functioning. First, compared to men, this form of spectatoring appears to be more common among women. Second, among women, greater body image self-consciousness during sexual activity is related to greater likelihood of sexual problems and sexual dissatisfaction, as well as decreased assertiveness during sexual activities with partners. Lastly, this specific body image self-consciousness during sexual activity appears to mediate relationships between more general body image and sexual functioning. In other words, because global body image is correlated with body image self-consciousness during sexual activity, and body image self-consciousness during sexual activity is correlated with sexual functioning, measures of global body image tend to be correlated with sexual functioning. However, when researchers have statistically accounted for body image self-consciousness during sexual activity, correlations between global body image and sexual functioning have decreased substantially or disappeared altogether.

Genital and Breast Body Image

Less research has focused on body image related specifically to genitals and to women's breasts than on general body image or body image self-consciousness during physical intimacy with a partner. Still, because of the obvious relevance of genitals and women's breasts for sexual activities with partners, it is important to consider potential links to sexual functioning.

To date, only a few studies have queried respondents about perceptions of their own genitals. One Internet survey of more than 52,000 respondents indicated that 55% of men were satisfied with their penis size, with the remaining men desiring a larger penis. Men who perceived their penises as relatively larger were most likely to be satisfied with their penis size. Interestingly, 85% of female respondents indicated being satisfied with the size of their male partners' penises. Only 30% of the women were satisfied with their own breasts, whereas 56% of men were satisfied with their female partners' breasts. Younger and thinner women were most likely to desire larger breasts than they had, whereas older and heavier women were most likely to indicate dissatisfaction with the droopiness of their breasts. Not surprisingly, women with greater breast dissatisfaction were least likely to undress in front of their romantic partners and most likely to try to conceal their breasts during sexual activity with partners.

Two studies on genital body image have involved college student respondents, and both revealed that men indicated more positive self-evaluations of their genitals than did women (although genital body image was generally positive for both men and women). In both studies, respondents with more extensive sexual experience tended to indicate more positive genital body image. In one study, among college student women, the only aspects of genital body image with which at least 20% of respondents indicated dissatisfaction was "amount of pubic hair" and "odor of genitals," whereas for men only "length of nonerect penis" and "appearance of nonerect penis" demonstrated a similar frequency of dissatisfaction.

Unanswered Questions

In the past decade there has been considerably more research on body image as related to sexual functioning than there was during the previous decade. Still, many questions remain unanswered. For example, the bulk of research has been based on college student respondents, most of whom were female and White. The extent to which apparent relationships between body image and sexual functioning also apply to noncollege student women and men, of various ages, sexual orientations, and ethnicities, remains less certain. Research on general body image satisfaction among women of different ethnicities has indicated particular patterns of ethnic differences (see Chapters 25–28), so hypothesizing such ethnic differences in the relevance of body image in women's sexual functioning seems logical.

It is important to remember that the types of body image concerns that interfere with sexual functioning vary by gender. For women, the most common body image concerns in sexual situations seem to revolve around being too large or fat, breasts that are too small or too droopy, and genitals that do not match cultural ideals of femininity (e.g., too much pubic hair, vaginal odor, and labia that are too large). In contrast, men's most common body image concerns in sexual situations seem to revolve around having too much fat, too little muscularity, and too small a penis. Because such conclusions are based on young adult (college student) samples, the extent to which they apply to older men and women is unclear, and further research is needed. Similarly, what about potential effects of exercise, as well as whether individuals have always had such concerns or whether they result from relatively recent bodily changes?

Another important question is how feedback and interactions with romantic and sexual partners influence body image as it relates to sexual functioning. For example, research by Pole, Crowther, and Schell examined perceptions of married women concerning comments from the family members and spouses of those women pertaining to the women's appearance. Even after statistically controlling for the women's body size, perceptions of spousal criticism were predictive of negative body image for these women. However, the actual views of the husbands toward their wive's appearance were not measured. Also, the focus of the research was *not* on appearance and potential criticism during sexual intimacy, although such questions beg asking. Similarly, what about effects of feedback from men's sexual partners on the men's body image? These are just a few of the most obvious issues in need of further research.

Clinical Implications

The existing research on body image and sexual functioning has important clinical implications. First, clinicians should be aware that body image concerns during physical intimacy with romantic or sexual partners may be a substantial problem for a sizeable minority of women and some men. This may be especially true among people presenting for sex therapy, couples counseling, or treatment for anxiety disorders or eating disorders. Individuals experiencing such concerns may not express them explicitly, perhaps because they believe the "real problem" to be that their body is sexually unappealing to partners, and so there would be no point in raising such concerns to a professional who could not "fix" their appearance (e.g., help them lose weight or develop muscle definition).

Just as mental health professionals should be aware of body image concerns as related to sexual functioning, clinicians should not assume that people with heavier bodies necessarily experience body image concerns that interfere with sexual functioning, or that thinner people do not. The potential effects of particular settings, sexual activities, and partners on physical self-consciousness need to be assessed individually. Assessing and addressing such issues within the context of the sexually intimate couple seems most promising, especially to the extent that one or both partners hold inaccurate assumptions about the other partner's perceptions and feelings.

In addition to clarifying perceptions and improving communication about body image in the bedroom, clinicians addressing body image concerns in sex therapy may consider gradually increased exposure, systematic desensitization, cognitive restructuring, or mindfulness and acceptance interventions (see Chapter 47). To the extent that particular sexual settings or activities produce anxiety in the client, thereby prompting cognitive distraction and resulting decreases in arousal and satisfaction, proven techniques of anxiety reduction are warranted.

Informative Readings

Cash, T. F., Maikkula, C. L., & Yamamiya, Y. (2004). "Baring the body in the bedroom": Body image, sexual self-schemas, and sexual functioning among college women and men. *Electronic Journal of Human Sexuality*, 7. (2004, June 29).—Presents a new measure and supporting data pertaining to self-consciousness over body exposure during sexual activities with partners.

Dove, N., & Wiederman, M. W. (2000). Cognitive distraction and women's sexual functioning. *Journal of Sex and Marital Therapy*, 26, 67–78.—A study of college women's appearance-based and performance-based cognitive distraction during sexual activity.

Filiault, S. M. (2007). Measuring up in the bedroom: Muscle, thinness, and men's sexual lives. *International Journal of Men's Health*, 6, 127–142.—A rare example of research focused on men's body image as related to sexual functioning.

Frederick, D. A., Peplau, A., & Lever, J. (2008). The Barbie mystique: Satisfaction with breast size and shape across the lifespan. *International Journal of Sexual Health, 20,* 200–211.—Presents the results of an Internet survey of over 52,000 respondents.

Koch, P. B., Mansfield, P. K., Thurau, D., & Carey, M. (2005). "Feeling frumpy": The relationships between body image and sexual response changes in midlife women. *The Journal of Sex Research, 42,* 215–223.—Research focusing on midlife women's perceptions of change in both body image and sexual functioning.

Lever, J., Frederick, D. A., & Peplau, L. A. (2006). Does size matter? Men's and women's views on penis size across the lifespan. *Psychology of Men and Masculinity, 7,* 129–143.—Presents the results of an Internet survey of more than 52,000 respondents.

Meana, M., & Nunnink, S. E. (2006). Gender differences in the content of cognitive distractions during sex. *The Journal of Sex Research, 43,* 59–67.—A revealing comparison of men and women as to distracting concerns during sexual activity.

Morrison, T. G., Bearden, A., Ellis, S. R., & Harriman, R. (2005). Correlates of genital perceptions among Canadian post-secondary students. *Electronic Journal of Human Sexuality, 8.* (2005, May 24).—One of the few studies focused on respondents' perceptions of their own genitals.

Pole, M., Crowther, J. H., & Schell, J. (2004). Body dissatisfaction in married women: The role of spousal influence and marital communication patterns. *Body Image: An International Journal of Research, 1,* 267–278.—Although limited in scope, an important attempt to gauge how husbands may influence women's body image satisfaction.

Stofman, G. M., Neavin, T. S., Ramineni, P. M., & Alford, A. (2006). Better sex from the knife? An intimate look at the effects of cosmetic surgery on sexual practices. *Aesthetic Surgery Journal, 26,* 12–17.—Despite some methodological limitations, a rare follow-up on patient perceptions of sexual changes after cosmetic surgery.

Stuart, R. B., & Jacobson, B. (1994). *Weight, sex, and marriage: A delicate balance.* New York: Guilford Press.—Written by a husband–wife team of clinicians, an insightful examination of how women's body weight might serve multiple functions in regulating the sexual lives of couples.

Wiederman, M. W. (2000). Women's body image self-consciousness during physical intimacy with a partner. *The Journal of Sex Research, 37,* 60–68.—Presents a new measure and supporting data pertaining to young women's self-consciousness over being nude in front of sexual partners.

Wiederman, M. W., & Hurst, S. R. (1998). Body size, physical attractiveness, and body image among young adult women: Relationships to sexual experience and sexual esteem. *The Journal of Sex Research, 35,* 272–281.—Includes consideration of measured body size and judges' ratings of physical attractiveness.

Yamamiya, Y., Cash, T. F., & Thompson, J. K. (2006). Sexual experiences among college women: The differential effects of general versus contextual body images on sexuality. *Sex Roles, 55,* 421–427.—Examines body image and sexual functioning, with a unique focus on women's first-time sexual experience with a particular partner.

CHAPTER 32

Body Image
and Anorexia Nervosa

SHERRIE SELWYN DELINSKY

Introduction

Eating disorders are associated with serious medical and psychosocial morbidity and tremendous health care costs. Medical complications of eating disorders may be life threatening and among mental disorders, eating disorders are associated with the highest risk of premature death, both due to medical complications and elevated rates of suicide in this population. In addition to the physical toll, eating disorders are associated with elevated depression and anxiety, social and occupational impairment, and reduced quality of life.

Body image disturbance (BID) is a core diagnostic feature of eating disorders such as anorexia nervosa (AN) and bulimia nervosa (BN), and it is also a risk factor for the development of these eating disorders. Persistence of BID is associated with relapse in AN and BN, and yet BID is less likely to resolve with treatment than other behavioral symptoms of these disorders. Thus, there is a consensus in the field that more effective treatments targeting BID are needed in order to improve overall treatment outcome and especially to prevent relapse.

Body Image Criteria for Diagnosis of AN

AN is an eating disorder characterized by refusal to maintain a minimally normal weight for age and height, as well as amenorrhea in postmenarcheal females. The two additional criteria required for a diagnosis of AN pertain to body image: (1) "intense fear of gaining weight or becoming fat, even though underweight," and (2) "disturbance in the way in which one's body weight or shape is experienced, undue influence of body weight or shape on self-evaluation, or denial of the seriousness of the current low body weight," according to the *Diagnostic and Statistical Manual of Mental Disorders* (DSM-IV-TR) (p. 589).

The variety of concepts described in these criteria reflects the multidimensional nature of body image. That is, BID can manifest as a disturbance of perception, cognition, affect, behavior, or a combination of these dimensions.

Perception is the mental image of one's body or body parts, as well as the sensations associated with inhabiting one's body. Perceptual aspects of body image include a sense of taking up space, body composition (e.g., sensations of muscularity or flabbiness), shape of body parts (e.g., "roundness" or protrusion), as well as connectedness (e.g., whether body parts are perceived as individual components or interconnected).

Cognitions include beliefs about the appearance of one's body (e.g., that parts of the body are excessively unattractive) as well as the meaning of this appearance (e.g., being excessively round means being unacceptable and worthless). In individuals with eating disorders, these beliefs tend to be overvalued ideas about the importance of weight and/or shape as they relate to self-evaluation, and tend to be associated with excessive preoccupation. Overvalued ideas can be rigidly held and difficult to modify. An individual with AN who overvalues the importance of weight and shape is likely to base his or her self-worth on achieving, and then maintaining, a very low body weight. Achievement of such a weight may become the defining accomplishment in life, and the loss of that accomplishment through dreaded weight gain represents failure and loss of essential aspects of identity and worth.

Denial of the seriousness of low weight is a cognitive manifestation of BID that is unique to AN. Low weight is often interpreted as being benign or desirable, and many patients with AN report no difference between perceived and desired size, indicating that they do not want their bodies to be much different from how they see them. Such individuals tend to discount the negative consequences of AN and report that others, including loved ones and medical professionals, are making "much ado about nothing." Similarly, such individuals discount social, occupational, or educational impairment or impact of low weight on quality of life.

Affect includes feeling fat, disgusted, ashamed, and self-conscious, especially in situations that trigger thoughts about weight/shape (e.g., seeing one's reflection, being seen by others) or after eating certain foods. Behaviors include various methods of checking one's weight or appearance, or alternatively, avoiding or preventing exposure to one's weight/appearance.

Do Individuals with AN Overestimate Body Size?

One aspect of body image perception, body size overestimation, has been a controversial topic, especially given the theoretical and treatment implications of this phenomenon (see Chapter 17). Only half of studies included in an empirical review by Farrell, Lee, and Shafran reported that individuals with AN overestimate their size, compared with healthy controls, whereas the other half of studies found no overestimation or in some cases, underestimation of size relative to healthy controls. Discrepant findings have been attributed to heterogeneity of assessment methods, including whether whole body or body parts are assessed, as well as problems with ecological validity of assessment methods, but other influential factors have been identified. For example, Smeets has argued that most research has assessed *memory* for body size, rather than *perception* of body size, as these are related yet separate constructs. Recent neuroimaging research corroborates that a stored distorted prototypical image may be associated with functional abnormalities in the brains of patients with AN.

Is Fear of Weight Gain (Fat Phobia) a Necessary Criterion for AN?

Not all individuals with AN-like illness present with fear of weight gain as their rationale for food refusal or low weight. In fact, significant cultural variation in symptom presentation has been observed, particularly the absence of "fat phobia," especially in non-Western cultures like China. Much of this research has been authored or coauthored by Dr. Sing Lee, who is credited for extensive descriptions of this phenomenological variant of AN, which is typically referred to as "non-fat-phobic AN." Rationales for food refusal that do not pertain to body image are diverse, and include somatic complaints (e.g., nausea, bloating), religious beliefs, desire for control, and desire to influence family dynamics. The absence of fat phobia has also been linked to its lack of cultural prominence as an expression of distress, poor insight, or intentional nondisclosure of symptoms. Observations of non-fat-phobic AN have led many theorists, especially Lee and colleagues, to view AN, as currently defined by DSM-IV-TR, as a culture-bound syndrome, and have endorsed flexibility regarding diagnostic criterion for AN.

A recent review of the literature evaluating whether data support modification of diagnostic criteria for AN by Becker and colleagues found that non-fat-phobic AN is actually widely geographically distributed. Furthermore, there appears to be a consistent profile of eating disorder psychopathology among non-fat-phobic AN that is present across cultures and is associated with low weight comparable to conventional AN. Finally, a large meta-analysis by Thomas and colleagues concluded that individuals with non-fat-phobic AN appear to exhibit less severe eating pathology than individuals meeting all criteria for AN, a finding consistent with cross-sectional research suggesting that individuals who meet all criteria for AN except fat phobia have a better naturalistic course of illness than individuals with full-syndrome AN. Self-reported fear of weight gain typically is absent in children as well, according to the review of the literature by the Workgroup for Classification of Eating Disorders in Children and Adolescents, and it has been suggested that harmful weight loss behaviors likely provide more reliable diagnostic information than self-reported insights of psychological motivations in children and adolescents. Based on this cumulative data, the American Psychiatric Association DSM-5 Eating Disorders Work Group has proposed that the next iteration of the classification system (DSM-5) include persistent behavior intended to avoid weight gain as an alternative to self-reported fear of weight gain.

Is BID in AN Comparable to BID in Other Eating Disorders?

Studies directly comparing body image across eating disorder diagnostic groups have yielded mixed results (see also Chapters 33 and 34). In contrast to a meta-analysis by Cash and Deagle, which reported greater overall body dissatisfaction among patients with BN compared to those with AN (but no difference in perceptual size estimation), a recent study by Hrabosky and colleagues found that individuals with AN and BN reported comparable levels of BID, distress, preoccupation, investment, disturbance, and quality of life. The only significant difference between the AN and BN groups was that individuals with BN were more likely than those with AN to cope with body image-related stress by eating or overeating.

What Are Effective Treatments for BID in AN?

The extant, albeit limited, literature suggests that cognitive-behavioral therapy (CBT) is more effective than no treatment or nonspecific treatments for BID (see Farrell, Shafran, and Lee for a review). Traditional CBT packages for BID include psychoeducation, cognitive restructuring, imagery, exposure, and behavioral experiments (see Chapter 47). Research on stand-alone body image treatments for individuals with AN is virtually nonexistent. This is due mostly to the fact that treatment of AN is typically comprehensive and multidisciplinary, comprised of nutritional rehabilitation, medical management, and psychological treatment elements. Few randomized controlled trials of these comprehensive treatments have been conducted in general, due to the numerous challenges of studying this population, the most problematic being study recruitment and retention. Treatment outcomes are generally considered inadequate, especially relative to other eating disorders such as BN and binge-eating disorder (BED). Consequently, randomized controlled trials or dismantling studies as part of larger treatment outcome studies of AN are urgently needed to elucidate which specific body image interventions are most efficacious with this population.

A handful of studies, however, have evaluated change in BID in naturalistic settings of individuals receiving inpatient or residential treatment for AN. The results have been mixed. Two inpatient studies showed no improvement in body image among patients with AN, whereas another residential study reported improvements in weight and shape concerns. In all of these studies, patients gained significant weight during treatment, and it is possible that lack of deterioration of body satisfaction reflects at least tolerance of weight gain. Thus, it is likely that the context of actual physical change during weight gain presents unique challenges to body image that are not observed in patients with BN. (*Note.* Patients with BN tend to show more unequivocal body image improvement during intensive treatment.) These findings touch upon an intriguing question: Can improvements in body image occur during the weight gain phase of treatment for AN or are attitudinal shifts only achieved after patients enter their healthy weight range? Overall, more research on change in body image is needed among patients receiving intensive treatment for AN, across levels of care, in order to identify the relation and timing of weight gain to body image improvement.

What Are Mechanisms That Maintain BID in AN?

The development and implementation of more effective treatments for BID among individuals with eating disorders, especially AN, is considered a priority. Two trends in the research on body image treatments have emerged: (1) development of treatment protocols based on theoretical or empirical mechanisms of how BID is maintained (see Shafran and colleagues), and (2) evaluation of treatment protocols with mixed eating disorder diagnosis samples or with nonclinical samples exhibiting extreme weight and shape concerns.

The first proposed mechanism than maintains BID is selective attention. Selective attention to disliked body parts exacerbates preoccupation with those body parts and breeds negative cognitions and affect during confrontation with those body parts. Research indicates that individuals with eating disorder symptoms are more likely to focus on disliked body parts when looking in the mirror than individuals without eating disorder symptoms. Additional research indicates that individuals with eating disorders have attentional biases for weight and eating-related information, but these biases are amenable to treatment. In a recent study by Shafran and colleagues, CBT addressing selective attention to disliked body parts and sensations reduced attentional bias, although, interestingly, no specific attentional training intervention was needed to achieve the improvement, and the improvement was largely independent of eating symptom change.

In addition to selectively focusing on appearance and disliked body parts, individuals with eating disorders report greater negative emotions and cognitions than non-eating-disordered controls when viewing their bodies in the mirror. This is the second hypothesized mechanism. Research on cerebral blood flow following exposure to one's own body indicates hyperactivation in patients with AN in brain areas associated with response to aversive events, suggesting that exposure activates the attention network and somatosensory system. Negative emotions associated with exposure, however, can be reduced over the course of exposure. Key and colleagues reported a pilot study of "mirror confrontation" within an inpatient treatment of AN in which weight-restored patients received standard body image treatment with or without the use of the mirror-confrontation exercise. The mirror-confrontation group showed significant improvement at the 6-month follow-up, compared to the standard treatment group, which did not exhibit significant change in body image. Delinsky and Wilson also reported the effectiveness of a mirror-exposure therapy using a mindfulness-based approach to mirror exposure with women with extreme weight and shape concerns. Similarly, a cognitive-behavioral body image group therapy incorporating body exposure (using mirror and video feedback) resulted in significant declines in negative body-related cognitions and emotions among women with eating disorders.

The negative emotions and cognitions experienced while confronting one's appearance reinforce the belief that the body is unacceptable and should be avoided or more carefully monitored, often leading to the third hypothesized mechanism that reinforces negative body image—excessive avoidance or checking. Avoidance may take the form of wearing baggy or unattractive clothing, not looking at one's own body or reflection clothed or unclothed, or avoiding situations in which others might see one's body, such as in changing rooms, while swimming, or with sexual partners. Avoidance reinforces negative body image because opportunities to evaluate or modify negative beliefs or affect are circumvented. Therefore, individuals do not receive feedback that could facilitate a modification of their negative opinions. Checking may take the form of mirror scrutiny, weighing, measuring one's own body parts, pinching, or jiggling. Given the tendency to selectively attend to disliked aspects of appearance and to experience negative cognitions and emotions, checking behaviors are part of the cycle of distress and preoccupation. Individuals with AN demonstrate high levels of avoidance and checking behaviors. Behavioral interventions that directly target checking and avoidance effectively reduce these specific behaviors, as well as improve overall shape and weight concerns and distress.

A fourth proposed mechanism that maintains BID is body size overestimation, which is thought to arise from body checking and is reinforced through the other mechanisms described above. Shafran and colleagues' recent trial of a brief cognitive-behavioral intervention designed to target these mechanisms indicates initial promise: the group of individuals with high shape concerns who received CBT showed improvement compared with a control group, and these improvements were maintained over 3 months. The treatment components included attentional retraining to view one's body more holistically in front of a mirror, mindfulness techniques to distance from negative cognitions and affect during mirror exposure, psychoeducation about the mechanisms that reinforce negative body image, and behavioral assignments to reduce body checking and avoidance. Video feedback was also provided to give patients novel and realistic feedback about their bodies, especially relative to their predictions. Replication of this study, especially with patients with AN and in the context of a larger clinical trial or dismantling study, is clearly warranted.

Conclusions

In sum, BID is a risk factor for the development and persistence of AN, as well as a core diagnostic feature of the illness. Given the multidimensional nature of body image, disturbance manifests differently across individuals. For example, although currently a diagnostic criterion, fear of weight gain is not present in all cases, and typically is not present in children. This phenomenological variant, known as "non-fat-phobic" AN, has led to reconsideration of the eating disorder classification system, as well as proposals to include a behavioral alternative to this criterion. The extant research also indicates that body size overestimation is not universal, although denial of the seriousness of underweight and overvaluation of the importance of low weight are common presentations. No stand-alone body image treatments for AN have been evaluated. CBT has the most empirical support as a treatment for BID in nonclinical and mixed eating disorder diagnosis samples. The most promising innovations in treating BID focus on mechanisms hypothesized to maintain disturbance: selective attention, negative cognitions and affect in the face of exposure, body checking and avoidance, and body size overestimation.

Informative Readings

American Psychiatric Association. (2000). *Diagnostic and statistical manual of mental disorders* (4th ed., text rev.). Washington, DC: Author.—The widely accepted manual delineating diagnostic criteria for mental disorders, including AN.
American Psychiatric Association DSM-5 Work Group. (2010). *Proposed draft revi-*

sion. Retrieved March 5, 2010, from *www.dsm5.org/ProposedRevisions/Pages/ EatingDisorders.aspx.*—Proposed draft revisions of DSM-5 criteria by the Eating Disorders Work Group.

Becker, A. E., Thomas, J. J., & Pike, K. M. (2009). Should non-fat-phobic anorexia nervosa be included in DSM-5? *International Journal of Eating Disorders, 42,* 620–635.—A comprehensive literature review and meta-analysis of the data regarding fear of weight gain as a diagnostic criterion for AN.

Cash, T. F., & Deagle, E. A., III. (1997). The nature and extent of body-image disturbance in anorexia nervosa and bulimia nervosa: A meta-analysis. *International Journal of Eating Disorders, 22,* 107–125.—A meta-analysis of the data comparing individuals with AN to those with BN on measures of body image.

Delinsky, S. S., & Wilson, G. T. (2006). Mirror exposure for the treatment of body image disturbance. *International Journal of Eating Disorders, 39,* 108–116.—An experimental study of the effects of a mindfulness-based mirror-exposure treatment compared with a nondirective control for individuals with extreme weight and shape concerns.

Farrell, C., Lee, M., & Shafran, R. (2005). Assessment of body size estimation: A review. *European Eating Disorders Review, 13,* 75–88.—A comprehensive and critical appraisal of the literature on body size estimation in eating disorders.

Farrell, C., Shafran, R., & Lee, M. (2006). Empirically evaluated treatments for body image disturbance: A review. *European Eating Disorders Review, 14,* 289–300.—A comprehensive literature review of empirically tested treatments for individuals with levels of BID.

Hrabosky, J. I., Cash, T. F., Veale, D., Neziroglu, F., Soll, E. A., Garner, D. M., et al. (2009). Multidimensional body image comparisons among patients with eating disorders, body dysmorphic disorder, and clinical controls: A multisite study. *Body Image: An International Journal of Research, 6,* 155–163.—An empirical study comparing the multidimensional nature of body image functioning among individuals with AN, BN, or body dysmorphic disorder (BDD), relative to psychiatric controls recruited from 10 treatment centers in the United States and England.

Hsu, L. K., & Lee, S. (1993). Is weight phobia always necessary for a diagnosis of anorexia nervosa? *American Journal of Psychiatry, 150,* 1466–1471.—A narrative review of the history of core features of AN and evaluation of the literature of the weight phobia criterion as it relates to the psychopathology of the illness across cultures.

Key, A., George, C. L., Beattie, D., Stammers, K., Lacey, H., & Waller, G. (2002). Body image treatment within an inpatient program for anorexia nervosa: The role of mirror exposure in the desensitization process. *International Journal of Eating Disorders, 31,* 185–190.—An experimental study of the effects of a mirror-confrontation treatment compared with a control treatment among weight-restored patients during inpatient hospitalization.

Shafran, R., Farrell, C., Lee, M., & Fairburn, C. G. (2009). Brief cognitive behavioural therapy for extreme shape concern: An evaluation. *British Journal of*

Clinical Psychology, 48, 79–92.—Evaluation of a brief CBT compared with applied relaxation for individuals with extreme shape concerns.

Shafran, R., Lee, M., Cooper, Z., Palmer, R. L., & Fairburn, C. G. (2008). Effect of psychological treatment on attentional bias in eating disorders. *International Journal of Eating Disorders, 41,* 348–354.—Empirical studies of attentional bias and CBT to treat attentional bias among individuals with eating disorders compared with controls.

Smeets, M. A. M. (1997). The rise and fall of body size estimation research in anorexia nervosa: A review and reconceptualization. *European Eating Disorders Review, 5,* 75–95.—A narrative literature review on body size estimation in AN.

Thomas, J. J., Vartanian, L. R., & Brownell, K. D. (2009). The relationship between eating disorder not otherwise specified (EDNOS) and officially recognized eating disorders: Meta-analysis and implications for DSM. *Psychological Bulletin, 135,* 407–433.—A meta-analysis of 125 studies conducted from 1987 to 2007 evaluating the psychopathology of EDNOS with that of other officially recognized eating disorders (AN, BN, and BED).

Workgroup for Classification of Eating Disorders in Children and Adolescents (WCEDCA). (2007). Classification of child and adolescent eating disturbances. *International Journal of Eating Disorders, 40,* S117–S122.—Reviews current classification schemes for eating disturbances and disorders in children and adolescents and related literature in child development.

CHAPTER 33

Body Image and Bulimia Nervosa

JANIS H. CROWTHER
NICOLE M. WILLIAMS

Introduction

According to the most recent edition of the *Diagnostic and Statistical Manual of Mental Disorders* (DSM-IV), bulimia nervosa (BN) is characterized by repeated episodes of binge eating and the regular use of inappropriate compensatory techniques to counteract the effects of food consumption, particularly weight gain. Binge eating, a cardinal symptom of BN, involves the uncontrolled consumption of an excessively large amount of food in a given period of time. It may be precipitated by restrained eating and negative emotions, and occurs, on average, twice a week in this disorder. An additional diagnostic criterion is the emphasis placed upon body weight and shape in the individual's negative evaluation of self. DSM-IV specifies two subtypes of BN: the purging type, which involves the regular use of self-induced vomiting or the misuse of laxatives, diuretics, or enemas; and the nonpurging type, which involves the regular use of fasting or excessive exercise. Currently, there are two proposed revisions to the diagnostic criteria for BN in the fifth edition of the DSM: the first reduces the required minimum frequency of binge episodes from twice weekly to once weekly over the previous 3 months, and the second eliminates the specification of subtypes.

Eating disorders, including BN as well as anorexia nervosa (AN) and eating disorder not otherwise specified (EDNOS), are one of the most common disorders among females in Western society. BN affects between

1 and 3% of adolescent and young adult women, and its subclinical forms, characterized by frequencies of bingeing and compensatory strategies that fall below threshold, affect even larger percentages of females. Approximately 90% of the cases of BN are female.

Within their cognitive-behavioral theory (CBT) of BN, Christopher Fairburn and associates have focused on the overvaluation of body shape, weight, and eating, viewing it as the "core psychopathology" of BN and a fairly stable construct. They point out that individuals who do not have eating disorders use multiple life domains (e.g., relationships with family and friends, educational and work performance, physical appearance, hobbies, and other interests) to evaluate their self-worth. In contrast, individuals with eating disorders rely excessively on their body shape, weight, and eating habits and their ability to control them as the singular domain upon which they base their self-evaluation. As a result, the lives of individuals with BN become consumed with the relentless pursuit of extremely high standards for shape, weight, and eating, dysfunctional thoughts regarding these domains, and strict dietary and weight control. A recent study by Grilo and colleagues confirms the significant role of overvaluation of shape and weight in BN, as 95% of the participants with BN and 86% of the participants with subthreshold BN exceeded the overvaluation thresholds used in this research.

Body Image Disturbance in BN

In contrast to the overvaluation of weight and shape, which has been conceptualized not only as a symptom but also as an important maintenance factor for BN, women with BN also experience body image disturbance (BID), including disturbances in the perceptual, cognitive-affective, and behavioral realms. First, women with BN often overestimate their body size, reporting that their current figure or specific body parts, such as the waist, stomach, hips, and thighs, are larger than is objectively true. Interestingly, although perceptual body size distortion historically has been considered a core feature of AN and the diagnostic criteria for AN include disturbance in one's experience of body weight or shape (see Chapter 32), a meta-analysis of 66 studies by Cash and Deagle found that participants with BN and AN exhibited significantly greater body image distortion than control samples, with the average patient with an eating disorder distorting (i.e., overestimating) her size to a greater extent than approximately 73% of the controls. The two eating disorder groups did not differ significantly from one another in their relative body image distortion. In addition, because participants with eating disorders did not differ from controls in their estimation of the size of neutral objects, it would appear that the body image distortion is not due to a generalized sensory-perceptual deficit. Instead, it may be due to cognitive-attitudinal factors, whereby the internalization of the thin ideal with its preference for extreme thinness leads one to selectively and inaccurately interpret one's body or body parts as larger than is true.

Second, women with BN also experience body dissatisfaction, operationally defined here as the negative and dysfunctional feelings and beliefs about one's shape and weight. Generally, research has found that although substantial proportions of females across the lifespan report body dissatisfaction, women with BN report body dissatisfaction at significantly higher levels than women without eating disorders. In their meta-analysis, Cash and Deagle found that the average individual with BN evaluated her body more negatively than 90% of controls, a level of body dissatisfaction that exceeded that reported by women with AN. Women with BN report "feeling fat," an experience that may fluctuate within and across days, and express significant distress and concerns about their shape and weight.

Consistent with CBT, women with BN also report many negative automatic thoughts and dysfunctional assumptions about their weight and shape (e.g., "I am too fat," or "If I stop purging, I'll gain weight, and people will think negatively about me"), and they report negative body-related cognitions at much higher frequencies than women without eating disorders. Although Hilbert and Tuschen-Caffier found that generally women with BN reported body-related cognitions more frequently than a non-eating-disordered control group, they also found that after mirror exposure to their physical appearance, women with BN reported a greater increase in negatively valenced body-related cognitions that persisted at follow-up.

Third, women with BN exhibit both body image avoidance and body checking. In the last decade, there has been increased attention to the behavioral dimensions of body image. Body avoidance involves behaviors that allow an individual to avoid seeing her shape and/or weight, including wearing baggy clothes, refusing to weigh herself or to look at herself in the mirror or other reflective surfaces, and avoiding physical intimacy. In contrast, body checking involves repeated attention to one's body size, shape, and weight, with such attention being excessive and critical, and includes such behaviors as examining oneself in the mirror, feeling for bones, pinching one's arms or stomach, or monitoring the spread of one's thighs when sitting. Although less widely investigated than body image distortion and body dissatisfaction, research has found that women with eating disorders, including BN, engage in body image avoidance and body checking at higher frequencies than women without eating disorders.

Shafran, Fairburn, Robinson, and Lask interviewed women with eating disorders about body checking and body avoidance and found that 92% of the patients reported checking their bodies to evaluate their shape or look for signs of weight gain, whereas 62% reported actively avoiding shape and weight checking, most often at times when they had gained weight. It seems paradoxical that women with eating disorders would engage in both body checking and body avoidance; yet, in their study, women with eating disorders report alternating between body checking and body avoidance.

According to Fairburn, Shafran, and colleagues, body checking and body avoidance may be "direct expressions" of the overvaluation of shape and weight. These behavioral dimensions contribute to the maintenance of BN through two mechanisms. First, as a result of body checking, individuals pay selective attention to the parts of their body that they dislike, which increases their body dissatisfaction. Second, as a result of body avoidance, individuals do not pay attention to information that might challenge or disconfirm their body image concerns. A recent experimental study conducted by Jansen and her associates provides some initial support for the role of selective attention. Using a remote eye-tracking device, the researchers recorded the amount of time that women who were eating symptomatic and women who served as controls spent viewing their most beautiful and most ugly body parts. They found that although the controls spent comparable amounts of time viewing their self-identified ugliest and most beautiful body parts, the eating-symptomatic group spent significantly more time looking at their self-identified ugliest body part (including upper legs, hips, belly, and knees) than at their self-identified most beautiful body part.

Theoretical Models of BID and BN

There are several empirically supported models that incorporate BID in the etiology or maintenance of BN. According to Stice's dual-pathway model, body dissatisfaction results from increased pressure to be thin from family, peers, and the media, and from the internalization of the thin ideal. These factors contribute to body dissatisfaction because the messages encouraging thinness from family, peers, and the media increase one's dissatisfaction with one's body and because most women cannot attain the thin beauty ideal espoused for women in Western society.

Body dissatisfaction then leads to bulimic pathology via one of two pathways. First, because of body dissatisfaction, an individual begins to diet because she holds the belief that dieting is an effective way to lose weight. Dieting may lead *directly* to binge eating either because of the feelings of caloric deprivation associated with severe restriction in the amount of food consumed or because the violation of strict dietary guidelines may result in disinhibited eating. Dieting may also lead *indirectly* to binge eating through the negative affect associated with caloric deprivation or its association with the threats to self-esteem associated with chronic dieting failures. Second, body dissatisfaction is often associated with negative affect, largely due to the significance of physical appearance to an individual's self-evaluation in our society. Negative affect may lead directly to overeating and binge eating because eating functions to self-soothe and nurture or to distract or avoid negative emotions.

Vohs, Bardone-Cone, Joiner, and colleagues also incorporate body dissatisfaction in their interactive model of bulimic symptom development. This model conceptualizes perfectionism as a "dispositional tendency" that is activated when one has an unmet body standard. The model predicts that perfectionism, body dissatisfaction, and self-esteem interact in the development of bulimic symptomatology. Thus, perfectionism would result in bulimic symptoms only if individuals experience body dissatisfaction. However, those perfectionists with high self-esteem would view their weight and shape as changeable, implementing effective techniques to address their goals. Conversely, perfectionists with low self-esteem would lack confidence that they can reach their goal and their feelings of inadequacy and associated negative affect could contribute to binge eating.

Finally, Fairburn and his colleagues primarily focus on the factors that maintain BN. In their theory, overvaluation and control of shape, weight, and eating leads to severely restrictive dieting, in which individuals limit both the quantities and types ("safe" vs. "forbidden" goods) of foods they consume, and the use of other forms of compensatory weight control strategies, including purging via self-induced vomiting, laxative and diuretic misuse, and excessive exercising. Like the dual-pathway model, binge eating results from the pattern of severe dietary restriction and the need to adhere to rigid and inflexible dietary rules. When individuals experience dietary lapses, such lapses are viewed as a failure of their ability to control their intake, and may trigger binge episodes (e.g., "Well, I've already ruined my diet today, so I might as well eat what I want"). The consequences of a binge include the use of compensatory weight control strategies to counteract the potential weight gain associated with the binge as well as an exacerbation of concerns about shape, weight, and eating and a return to severe dietary restriction.

There is considerable empirical support for the role of BID in increasing risk for bulimic pathology and maintaining the disorder. In a meta-analysis that utilized experimental and prospective studies, Stice concluded that body dissatisfaction is an important risk and maintenance factor for eating pathology. Although the effect sizes were generally small, the results of this meta-analysis supported the body dissatisfaction–bulimic pathology path of the dual-pathway model as body dissatisfaction predicted increases in dieting and negative affect and the onset and increase in bulimic symptomatology. In addition, consistent with the interactive model of bulimic symptomatology, perfectionism emerged as a risk and maintenance factor.

Conclusions and Future Directions

Given the current state of this literature, there are several implications for assessment, treatment, and research. First, given that BID is a multidimensional construct, it is important that clinicians working with women with BN conduct a comprehensive body image assessment, including overvaluation of weight and shape, body image distortion, body dissatisfaction, and body checking and avoidance. Second, given the importance of BID in the maintenance of BN, clinicians working with women with BN must familiarize themselves with techniques to address this "core psychopathology." Fairburn and colleagues have argued for a reformulation and greater emphasis on addressing the overvaluation of weight and shape and its manifestations, particularly body checking and body avoidance. Thus, clinicians utilizing cognitive-behavioral therapy for BN should not only focus on identifying and challenging automatic thoughts and dysfunctional assumptions about shape, weight, and eating but also consider the use of additional techniques, including exploring the meaning and consequences of overvaluation of shape and weight, addressing shape and weight checking, and considering the frequency and role of appearance-focused social comparisons.

Finally, research should continue to focus on increasing our understanding of BID in BN. One potentially fruitful avenue involves the use of experimental methodologies to investigate the proposed mechanisms through which various aspects of BID contribute to the development and maintenance of BN. Future research might build on recent theoretical and empirical work by examining further the associations among body checking, body avoidance, selective attention, and body dissatisfaction. For example, Shafran and her colleagues conducted an experimental analysis of body checking and found that body checking led to increased body dissatisfaction among a nonclinical sample. A second avenue involves the use of ecological momentary assessment, a methodology that involves sampling phenomena and experiences when they occur in the naturalistic environment, not only to investigate the manifestation of various aspects of BID among women with BN but also to explore the prospective relationships among BID, negative affect, disordered eating, and the use of compensatory weight control strategies. For example, a series of studies conducted in our laboratory using ecological momentary assessment have found that body checking is normative among a nonclinical sample of young women, with women endorsing body-checking behaviors at high rates and often in response to social comparisons; that appearance-focused social comparisons occur frequently among young women experiencing body dissatisfaction; and that upward appearance-focused social comparisons are associated with body dissatisfaction, thoughts of dieting, and thoughts of exercise. Future research might examine these topics among women with eating disorders.

Informative Readings

American Psychiatric Association. (2000). *Diagnostic and statistical manual of mental disorders* (4th ed., text rev.). Washington, DC: Author.—Provides information about the diagnostic and associated features and course of BN.

Cash, T. F., & Deagle, E. A., III. (1997). The nature and extent of body-image disturbances in anorexia nervosa and bulimia nervosa: A meta-analysis. *International Journal of Eating Disorders, 22,* 107–125.—Presents a meta-analytic review of 66 studies of perceptual and attitudinal aspects of BID among anorexic and bulimic samples.

Eating Disorders Work Group. (2010). DSM-5 proposed diagnostic criteria for bulimia nervosa. Retrieved June 1, 2010, from *www.dsm5.org/ProposedRevisions/ Pages/proposedrevision.aspx?rid=25.*—Describes proposed revisions to the diagnostic criteria and the rationale for the changes.

Fairburn, C. G. (2008). *Cognitive behavior therapy and eating disorders.* New York: Guilford Press.—Presents a treatment protocol for enhanced cognitive-behavioral therapy, including detailed recommendations for addressing the core psychopathology of overvaluation of weight and shape.

Fairburn, C. G., Cooper, Z., & Shafran, R. (2003). Cognitive behaviour therapy for eating disorders: A "transdiagnostic" theory and treatment. *Behaviour Research and Therapy, 41,* 509–528.—Describes the core psychopathology of eating disorders and presents a transdiagnostic theory that has relevance not only to our understanding and treatment of BN but to other eating disorders as well.

Grilo, C. M., Crosby, R. D., Masheb, R. M., White, M. A., Peterson, C. B., Wonderlich, S. A., et al. (2009). Overvaluation of shape and weight in binge eating disorder, bulimia nervosa, and sub-threshold BN. *Behaviour Research and Therapy, 47,* 692–696.—Findings relevant for the clinical significance of overvaluation of shape and weight for BN.

Hilbert, A., & Tuschen-Caffier, B. (2005). Body-related cognitions in binge-eating disorder and bulimia nervosa. *Journal of Social and Clinical Psychology, 24,* 561–579.—Describes an investigation of the cognitive aspects of BID in women with BN, women with binge-eating disorder, and women without an eating disorder.

Hrabosky, J. I., Cash, T. F., Veale, D., Neziroglu, F., Soll, E. A., Garner, D. M., et al. (2009). Multidimensional body image comparisons among patients with eating disorders, body dysmorphic disorder, and clinical controls: A multisite study. *Body Image: An International Journal of Research, 6,* 155–163.—A multisite study examining body image functioning among individuals with AN, BN, body dysmorphic disorder, and psychiatric controls.

Jansen, A., Nederkoorn, C., & Mulkens, S. (2005). Selective visual attention for ugly and beautiful body parts in eating disorders. *Behaviour Research and Therapy, 43,* 183–186.—Describes a study using eye movement registration to examine body shape-related processing biases in normal weight females with and without eating problems.

Shafran, R., Fairburn, C. G., Robinson, P., & Lask, B. (2004). Body checking and its avoidance in eating disorders. *International Journal of Eating Disorders, 35,* 93–101.—Reports the results of two studies on body checking and avoidance among women with eating disorders.

Shafran, R., Lee, M., Payne, E., & Fairburn, C. G. (2007). An experimental analysis of body checking. *Behaviour Research and Therapy, 45,* 113–121.—Describes an experimental investigation of the effects of a high and low body-checking condition on body size estimation and body dissatisfaction.

Stewart, T. M., & Williamson, D. A. (2004). Assessment of body image disturbances. In J. K. Thompson (Ed.), *Handbook of eating disorders and obesity* (pp. 495–514). Hoboken, NJ: Wiley.—Reviews assessment measures for various aspects of BID.

Stice, E. (2001). A prospective test of the dual-pathway model of bulimic pathology: Mediating effects of dieting and negative affect. *Journal of Abnormal Psychology, 110,* 124–135.—Describes the dual-pathway model and provides prospective findings in support of the model.

Stice, E. (2002). Risk and maintenance factors for eating pathology: A meta-analytic review. *Psychological Bulletin, 128,* 825–848.—Presents a meta-analytic review of risk and maintenance factors for eating disorders, including body dissatisfaction.

Vohs, K. D., Bardone-Cone, A. M., Joiner, T. E., Jr., Abramson, L. Y., & Heatherton, T. F. (1999). Perfectionism, perceived weight status, and self-esteem interact to predict bulimic symptoms: A model of bulimic symptom development. *Journal of Abnormal Psychology, 108,* 695–700.—Describes a longitudinal study investigating an interactive model of bulimic symptom development.

CHAPTER 34

Body Image and
Binge-Eating Disorder

JOSHUA I. HRABOSKY

Introduction

Binge-eating disorder (BED), a research category in the fourth edition of the *Diagnostic and Statistical Manual of Mental Disorders* (DSM-IV), is defined by recurrent binge eating without the presence of maladaptive compensatory weight control behaviors characteristic of bulimia nervosa (BN). Binge eating is defined as eating an unusually large amount of food given the circumstances while experiencing a subjective sense of loss of control during the eating episode. Binge-eating episodes are further characterized by eating more rapidly than normal; eating beyond a sense of fullness; eating despite the absence of hunger; hiding the extent to which one is eating; and/or experiencing disgust, depression, or guilt associated with one's eating. In its current state, the DSM-IV requires binge eating must occur, on average, at least 2 days per week for no less than 6 months; however, the recently proposed revisions for the DSM-5 require binge episodes must occur, on average, at least once per week for no less than 3 months.

BED has received support as a prevalent and chronic psychiatric disorder, especially in comparison to BN and anorexia nervosa (AN). Binge eating is associated with numerous additional clinical problems, including depressive symptomatology, low self-esteem, and poor quality of life. Research has further found high rates of psychiatric comorbidity in individuals with BED compared to individuals without BED. BED is predominantly associated with overweight and obesity, and is, consequently, associated with greater risk of medical morbidities and mortality. (See

Chapter 21 for a discussion of adulthood obesity and body image.) In fact, obese patients with BED suffer from greater health dissatisfaction, poorer health-related quality of life, and higher rates of major medical disorders (e.g., hypertension, diabetes, cardiac problems) than obese patients without BED. Further, BED is associated with increased health care utilization, making it a major target for treatment and prevention within the larger subset of obese individuals.

Shape and Weight Overvaluation

Research on the presence and mediating role of body image in BED has historically focused on the degree of *concern* with one's body weight and/or shape. This has been most commonly defined by the Eating Disorder Examination's (EDE) shape and weight concern subscales, which comprise items purportedly assessing a range of constructs, including fear of weight gain, preoccupation with shape or weight, dissatisfaction with shape and weight, and discomfort seeing one's body. The EDE, both in its interview and self-report (EDE-Q) forms, has been the most often-used instrument for measuring the psychopathology of BED. Thus, its shape and weight concern subscales have historically been the primary source of knowledge about body image in BED. Individuals with BED have been found to report significantly greater degrees of shape and weight concern than both overweight and normal-weight individuals without BED, while similar in degree to individuals with AN and BN.

Within the past decade and, to a greater degree the past couple of years, the focus of research on understanding body image in BED has shifted to the excessive influence of shape or weight on one's self-evaluation, or *overvaluation*. Shape/weight overvaluation has been defined as the importance one places on her or his physical appearance (specifically, one's body shape and weight) in defining her- or himself. Overvaluation, or *investment*, is associated with, yet distinct from, the degree of satisfaction or dissatisfaction with one's appearance. In fact, although many may endorse dissatisfaction with their body shape or weight, only a portion will report that the appearance of their shape or weight significantly impacts their self-worth. Moreover, as Masheb and Grilo found in a longitudinal study of body image in BED, shape/weight overvaluation appears to be more stable and more closely associated with self-esteem than body dissatisfaction.

Shape/weight overvaluation has been found to be of critical importance in characterizing and maintaining AN and BN, as well as the more prevalent eating disorder not otherwise specified (EDNOS). Consequently, this construct (i.e., "undue influence of body weight or shape on self-evaluation") is currently included in the DSM-IV (p. 545) as a diagnostic criterion for both AN and BN. Yet, debate continues regarding the specific diagnostic criteria for the BED diagnosis, including whether, like AN and BN, it too should be characterized by overvaluation of shape and weight.

Recent research has supported shape/weight overvaluation as a distinguishing clinical feature within patients with BED. Hrabosky, Masheb, and colleagues found 58% of a sample of 399 treatment-seeking patients with BED endorsed clinical overvaluation. This subset of patients reported greater eating-related and general psychopathology than those experiencing subclinical overvaluation. Several recent studies including clinical and community-based samples have replicated, as well as extended, the findings of Hrabosky and colleagues, comparing these two BED subgroups with overweight individuals without BED, individuals with BN or subthreshold BN, and psychiatric controls. These studies found individuals with BED, regardless of degree of overvaluation, suffer from greater eating pathology than overweight individuals and psychiatric controls. Further, patients with BED endorsing clinical overvaluation differed little from patients with BN on measures of eating pathology and general psychological disturbance. High levels of shape/weight overvaluation in BED is associated with greater body dissatisfaction, eating pathology, depressive symptomatology, social dysfunction, and rates of lifetime psychiatric comorbidity; poorer self-esteem and quality of life; and increased health care utilization. Many of these associations persist after controlling for depression/negative affect. Interestingly, although patients with BED experiencing clinical overvaluation endorsed greater distress associated with binge eating, several studies have found no differences between patients with clinical overevaluation and those with subclinical overvaluation in the frequency of binge eating. Nor do these groups differ significantly in body mass index.

These findings have resulted in a call for the addition of a diagnostic *specifier* for BED in DSM-5, identifying a distinct subgroup of individuals who suffer from a key cognitive feature commonly associated with clinically relevant psychological and behavioral disturbances. Whereas some have suggested that shape/weight overvaluation should be included as a diagnostic *criterion*, doing so would exclude a substantial proportion of individuals who engage in recurrent binge eating and suffer from clinically significant behavioral and psychosocial problems. Nonetheless, the existing data support the clinical significance of shape/weight overvaluation in BED.

Body Image Coping Strategies in BED

Although shape/weight overvaluation is considered core to the psychopathology of disordered eating, body image coping strategies are hypothesized to be its behavioral expression. Individuals suffering from body image distress engage in a range of mental or behavioral strategies to cope with various threatening situations. Such maladaptive coping practices include body checking, body avoidance, appearance correcting, and camouflaging, and serve multiple purposes. Mountford and colleagues found female patients with an eating disorder, including a subset of patients with BED, engage in body checking in an effort to decrease anxiety through reassurance, avoid negative consequences that may occur without body checking, and control dietary intake and weight. Body checking, like other self-regulating strategies, allow the individual to escape or reduce, albeit momentarily, the psychological or emotional distress associated with the individual's physical appearance, consequently maintaining negative body image attitudes through negative reinforcement.

Reas and colleagues found self-report items assessing body checking and body avoidance in a sample of treatment-seeking patients with BED were significantly but differentially associated with disordered eating behaviors. Checking behavior was positively associated with dietary restraint, whereas body avoidance was positively associated with binge eating. Reas and colleagues hypothesized that patients' fluctuating feelings of loss of control are associated with the appearance-managing strategy they exercise. Mountford and colleagues similarly found a significant correlation between dietary restraint and appearance checking. They further discovered that restraint was positively associated with the degree to which individuals believe body checking helps control their dietary intake and weight. Despite temporarily reducing anxiety through reassurance, body checking purportedly magnifies perceived imperfections, motivating the individual to engage in further dietary restriction. On the other hand, efforts in avoiding appearance-related triggers, thoughts, or emotions may include binge eating. Disinhibited eating has been posited as a means of experiential avoidance (e.g., attempts to ignore body image-related thoughts or triggering situations).

Patients with BED particularly engage in maladaptive coping strategies for managing body image distress. Reas and colleagues found a substantial subset (57%) of patients with BED endorsed pinching areas of their body to check for fatness, whereas an even larger subset (89%) reported often avoiding wearing clothes that make them aware of the shape of their body. Comparing the body image experiences of treatment-seeking obese patients with and without BED, Hrabosky, Cash, and colleagues found patients with BED were significantly more likely than their non-BED counterparts to cope with body image threats by engaging in body avoidance, experiential avoidance, appearance-fixing behaviors, and self-regulation through eating.

Stability of Body Image Over Time

BED has been supported as a stable disorder, comparable in duration and chronicity to other eating disorders (i.e., AN, BN, and EDNOS). Although research has focused primarily on the duration and resolution of eating disorder features characteristic of BED and central to its diagnosis, body image problems also appear to persist. Striegel-Moore and colleagues examined the course of body image before, at the time of, and prior to the time of diagnosis of an eating disorder in adolescent females. The authors found that, similar to young women diagnosed with BN, women with BED endorsed significantly greater weight dissatisfaction than healthy comparisons at all time points ranging from 2 years prior to diagnosis of BED to 2 years after diagnosis. Moreover, the data suggested these group differences increased over time, reflecting worsening body image in BED.

To gain insight into the long-term course of BED and BN, Fichter and colleagues compared these groups of female patients, along with healthy controls, at presentation for treatment and at 12-year follow-up. Although patients with both BED and BN displayed significant reductions over time in self-report measures of body dissatisfaction and drive for thinness, patients with BED suffered from poorer body image than their BN counterparts at both time points. In addition, higher body dissatisfaction was predictive of general severity of BED at 12 months follow-up. Most interesting, however, was the authors' finding that, despite the resolution of eating disorder symptoms, a subset of patients with a previous diagnosis of BED continued to endorse a thinner body shape ideal than healthy comparisons. Cognitive processes, such as body image may, therefore, be more chronic and persisting than the problematic behaviors with which they are correlated.

Body Image and Treatment of BED

Body Image and Treatment Outcome

Specialized treatments, such as cognitive-behavioral therapy (CBT) and interpersonal psychotherapy (IPT) have received empirical support as efficacious interventions for producing statistically and clinically significant reductions in, or full remission of, binge eating. Yet, a sizeable proportion of patients do not fully respond to treatment. Efforts have begun toward identifying patient predictors of treatment outcome and the mechanisms by which treatments result in behavioral change.

Both shape/weight concern and shape/weight overvaluation have received support as predictors of treatment outcome of BED. Dingemans and colleagues found that full remission of binge eating following group CBT was fully mediated by changes in weight concerns from pre- to post-treatment and marginally by changes in shape concerns. Weight and shape concerns did not, however, predict binge-eating status 1 year post-treatment. Hilbert and colleagues examined putative pre- and midtreatment predictors of post- and follow-up response to CBT and IPT. The authors found that, among those individuals with low (compared to high) interpersonal problems, greater shape/weight concern at both pre- and midtreatment was predictive of posttreatment nonresponse. Similar to the previous study, Hilbert and colleagues found shape/weight concern was not predictive of binge-eating status 1 year following treatment's end.

In addition to being a significant correlate of concurrent psychopathology and dysfunction, shape/weight overvaluation has received support as a predictor of treatment outcome. Masheb and Grilo categorized patients receiving guided self-help CBT or behavioral weight loss (BWL) into clinical and subclinical overvaluation groups based on baseline reports, and found patients endorsing pretreatment shape/weight overvaluation suffered from greater eating pathology at the end of treatment. These analyses were repeated with a sample of patients who received CBT and BWL group therapy and, regardless of treatment condition, baseline overvaluation status was predictive of posttreatment binge-eating frequency.

Treatment of Body Image in BED

Within CBT for BED, the primary aim of treatment for body image disturbances involve identifying and correcting maladaptive assumptions associated with body shape and weight (see Chapter 47 on body image CBT). However, as noted above, cognitive-behavioral formulations of body image in BED have identified behavioral aspects (e.g., body checking and avoidance) in the maintenance of body image disturbance and binge eating. Body exposure techniques have been increasingly implemented within the context of CBT of eating disorders with the aim of addressing both cognitive and behavioral aspects of body image disturbance. Central to body exposure is the in vivo provision of visual feedback, often via a mirror, of one's physical appearance. While the initial goals of body exposure are to correct distorted perception and reduce avoidance, Hilbert and colleagues contend additional purposes include inducing changes in negative body-related schema as well as habituation of negative body-related feelings. In an initial study of the impact of body exposure on mood, appearance-based self-esteem, and negative thinking, Hilbert and colleagues delivered the intervention over two sessions to patients with BED and healthy controls. Results indicated that, while within sessions, patients with BED suffered from increased negative mood and decreased appearance self-esteem, mood significantly improved after follow-up in patients with BED and, regardless of group, appearance self-esteem increased. Further, negative mood and frequencies of negative cognitions reduced and appearance self-esteem increased by the time of the second exposure session. The authors concluded, despite decreases in the frequencies of negative cognitions, changes in cognitive content may require further body exposure and/or cognitive restructuring.

Hilbert and Tuschen-Caffier extended the results of this study, randomly assigning women with BED to receive CBT with body exposure or CBT with cognitive restructuring. The two treatment conditions resulted in statistically similar and substantial improvements in shape/weight concerns and body dissatisfaction at posttreatment and were maintained at 4-months posttreatment. Similarly, negative body image thoughts decreased in frequency by follow-up. Although the study was limited by small sample sizes (12 patients per group), the authors contend the results suggest that the previously established CBT protocol will not be necessarily enhanced through the alternative use of body exposure rather than cognitive restructuring.

Conclusions and Future Directions

Despite the absence of a body image-related criterion for BED in the DSM-IV, a burgeoning body of research has been directed toward understanding the role of body image in this particular eating disorder. Nonetheless, there are limitations in the existing literature and numerous empirical questions remain. Previous research has relied heavily on psychometrically flawed measures of body image. The proposed subscale structure of the EDE has failed to be replicated, whereas another commonly used measure, the Body Shape Questionnaire, has been criticized for its length and the inclusion of unnecessary items unrelated to its proposed unidimensional construct (i.e., body image preoccupation). Alternatively, more psychometrically sound measures of the multifaceted body image construct should be considered. Using previously validated measures of related, yet discrete, body image dimensions, Hrabosky and colleagues found that obese patients with BED endorsed more severe global and body area-specific body dissatisfaction, greater body-related situational distress and appearance investment (i.e., overvaluation), and poorer body image-related quality of life than their non-BED counterparts.

Further research is necessary to understand the clinical significance of shape/weight overvaluation in BED. While both binge eating and body image disturbance have been supported as correlates of general psychological distress and impaired psychosocial functioning, little is known about the degree to which these two variables uniquely influence distress and dysfunction within BED. Mond and colleagues found shape/weight concern to be a stronger mediator of the influence of obesity on psychosocial functioning than binge eating. Treatments for BED are evaluated in their effectiveness in inducing reduction or remission of binge eating; yet early outcome research with BN suggests that despite remission of behavioral symptoms by the conclusion of treatment, the continued presence of shape/weight overvaluation results in increased risk of relapse in behavioral symptoms. Future research should consider examining outcome of shape/weight overvaluation following treatments for BED, as well as whether the continued presence of overvaluation posttreatment predicts relapse.

Despite increased empirical efforts to understand the mechanisms of binge episodes in natural settings (i.e., through the use of ecological momentary assessment [EMA] rather than relying on retrospective self-report measures), no known research has examined reactivity to body image-triggering situations as a precipitant to maladaptive eating in BED. Future research should explore the situational reactivity of patients with BED through EMA, examining the schema-driven cognitive processes in both patients who endorse and deny clinically significant shape/weight overvaluation, as well as the degree to which body image-related thoughts and emotions precipitate binge episodes.

Informative Readings

Dingemans, A. E., Spinhoven, P., & van Furth, E. F. (2007). Predictors and mediators of treatment outcome in patients with binge eating disorder. *Behaviour Research and Therapy, 45*, 2551–2562.—An initial examination of the putative mediators and predictors of outcome of CBT for BED.

Fichter, M. M., Quadflieg, N., & Hedlund, S. (2008). Long-term course of binge eating disorder and bulimia nervosa: Relevance for nosology and diagnostic criteria. *International Journal of Eating Disorders, 41*, 577–586.—A comprehensive 12-year longitudinal study comparing the course of BED and BN in an inpatient sample.

Hilbert, A., Saelens, B. E., Stein, R. I., Mockus, D. S., Welch, R. R., Matt, G. E., et al. (2007). Pretreatment and process predictors of outcome in interpersonal and cognitive behavioral psychotherapy for binge eating disorder. *Journal of Consulting and Clinical Psychology, 75*, 645–651.—A study of pre- and midtreatment patient characteristics as predictors of treatment outcome.

Hilbert, A., & Tuschen-Caffier, B. (2004). Body image interventions in cognitive-behavioural therapy of binge-eating disorder: A component analysis. *Behaviour Research and Therapy, 42*, 1325–1339.—The only known study examining the unique effectiveness of body image exposure and cognitive restructuring as components of CBT for BED.

Hilbert, A., Tuschen-Caffier, B., & Vögele, C. (2002). Effects of prolonged and repeated body image exposure in binge-eating disorder. *Journal of Psychosomatic Research, 52*, 137–144.—The first study of its kind examining the psychological mechanisms and effectiveness of body image exposure in BED.

Hrabosky, J. I., Cash, T. F., Sarwer, D. B., Clauss, L. J., Gibbons, L. M., & Infield, A. L. (2007, November). *Multidimensional assessment of body image in binge eating disorder and obesity*. Poster presented at the 41st Annual Convention of the Association for Behavioral and Cognitive Therapies, Philadelphia, PA (available from the author at *jhrabosky@lifespan.org*).—A study of the presence, specificity, and severity of multiple body image dimensions in BED and non-BED obesity.

Hrabosky, J. I., Masheb, R. M., White, M. A., & Grilo, C. M. (2007). Overvaluation of shape and weight in binge eating disorder. *Journal of Consulting and Clinical Psychology, 75,* 175–180.—An initial study supporting the clinical significance of shape/weight overvaluation in BED, and the first to support the inclusion of shape/weight overvaluation as a diagnostic specifier in the DSM-5.

Masheb, R. M., & Grilo, C. M. (2003). The nature of body image disturbance in patients with binge eating disorder. *International Journal of Eating Disorders, 33,* 333–341.—One of the first studies to examine the clinical significance of shape/weight overvaluation in BED.

Masheb, R. M., & Grilo, C. M. (2008). Prognostic significance of two sub-categorization methods for the treatment of binge eating disorder: Negative affect and overvaluation predict, but do not moderate, specific outcomes. *Behaviour Research and Therapy, 46,* 428–437.—The first study demonstrating shape/weight overvaluation as a predictor of outcome for treatment of BED.

Mond, J. M., Rodgers, B., Hay, P. J., Darby, A., Owen, C., Baune, B. T., et al. (2007). Obesity and impairment in psychosocial functioning in women: The mediating role of eating disorder features. *Obesity, 15,* 2769–2779.—Discovered that shape/weight concerns, but not binge eating, mediate the relationship between obesity and psychosocial functioning.

Mountford, V., Haase, A., & Waller, G. (2006). Body checking in the eating disorders: Associations between cognitions and behaviors. *International Journal of Eating Disorders, 39,* 708–715.—Developed and validated a measure of automatic thoughts that purportedly motivate and maintain body checking.

Reas, D. L., Grilo, C. M., Masheb, R. M., & Wilson, G. T. (2005). Body checking and avoidance in overweight patients with binge eating disorder. *International Journal of Eating Disorders, 37,* 342–346.—An initial study of the frequency and correlates of body checking and avoidance in BED.

Striegel-Moore, R. H., Franko, D. L., Thompson, D., Barton, B., Schreiber, G. B., & Daniels, S. R. (2004). Changes in weight and body image over time in women with eating disorders. *International Journal of Eating Disorders, 36,* 315–327.—A longitudinal study of the parallel changes in weight and body image in patients with AN, BN, BED, and no eating disorder.

CHAPTER 35

Body Image and Body Dysmorphic Disorder

KATHARINE A. PHILLIPS

Introduction

Body dysmorphic disorder (BDD), also known as dysmorphophobia, is a body image disorder that has been described around the world for more than a century. DSM-IV defines BDD as preoccupation with an imagined defect in appearance; if a slight physical anomaly is present, the person's concern is markedly excessive. The preoccupation must cause clinically significant distress or impairment in social, occupational, or other important areas of functioning, and cannot be better accounted for by another mental disorder, such as anorexia nervosa (AN). BDD's delusional variant is classified as a psychotic disorder—a type of delusional disorder, somatic type. Patients with delusional BDD receive diagnoses of both BDD and delusional disorder.

The major proposed changes for BDD's diagnostic criteria in DSM-5, slated for publication in 2013, are the following: (1) addition of a criterion that describes repetitive behaviors, (2) addition of an insight specifier that indicates that BDD may encompass a range of insight (including delusional BDD beliefs), and (3) addition of a specifier for muscle dysmorphia (MD). These proposals are subject to change, as the development of DSM-5 is still underway.

Prevalence

BDD appears to be relatively common. In six epidemiological studies, BDD's prevalence was 0.7–2.4%. Smaller studies in nonclinical student samples have found a higher prevalence of 2–13%. In one study, 2.2% of 566 high school students currently had BDD. BDD also appears relatively common among inpatients on general psychiatry units (13–16%) and among outpatients with atypical major depressive disorder, social phobia, and obsessive compulsive disorder (OCD). However, as discussed below, BDD often goes unrecognized and undiagnosed.

BDD also appears to be relatively common in medical settings. A prevalence of 9–12% has been reported in dermatology settings, 9.5% in a cosmetic dental setting, and 7.5% in an orthodontia setting. In cosmetic surgery settings in the United States, 7–8% of patients have been found to have BDD, and in international cosmetic populations, the reported prevalence is 3–53%.

Case Example[1]

Ms. A., a 26-year-old single White female, presented with a chief complaint of "I look ugly and deformed." She was obsessed with her "crooked" nose, "ugly" eyes, "pimply" skin, "bushy" facial hair, and "fat" thighs. She estimated that she thought about her perceived appearance flaws for 10 hours a day and checked them in mirrors for 5 hours a day. She repeatedly sought reassurance from family members about how she looked but could not accept reassurance that she looked normal. She compulsively compared herself with other people, applied makeup for hours a day, picked her skin with pins to try to make it look better, covered her face with her hand, and spent an hour a day tweezing facial hair. As a result of her appearance concerns, she had dropped out of high school. After getting her general equivalency diploma (GED) she enrolled in college classes but could not take a full course load because her obsessions distracted her from studying and because she felt too self-conscious and ugly to go to class. Ms. A. avoided friends, dating, and most other social interactions. She was chronically suicidal and had attempted suicide because, as she said, "I'm ugly, and I look like a freak."

Clinical Features

Appearance Preoccupations

Individuals with BDD are preoccupied with thoughts that some aspect(s) of their appearance is unattractive, deformed, or ugly, when in reality the perceived flaws are minimal or nonexistent. Preoccupations most com-

---

[1]The material in the case description has been disguised and is a fictional/composite case.

monly involve aspects of the face or head, most often the skin, hair, or nose (e.g., acne, scarring, thinning hair, or a large or crooked nose). However, any body part can be the focus of concern, and most patients are preoccupied with multiple areas.

BDD preoccupations are distressing, time consuming, and typically difficult to resist or control. The preoccupations are usually associated with low self-esteem, shame, embarrassment, and fear of rejection. BDD beliefs span a spectrum of insight, from good insight through absent insight (i.e., delusional beliefs). Most patients have poor insight or are delusional, not recognizing that the flaws they perceive are actually minimal or nonexistent. Individuals with delusional BDD beliefs (i.e., complete conviction that their view of their appearance is accurate) are largely similar to those with nondelusional BDD beliefs across a broad range of clinical features. A majority of patients have ideas or delusions of reference, thinking that other people take special notice of the supposed defects—for example, stare at them or mock them.

Repetitive Behaviors

Virtually all individuals with BDD perform repetitive and time-consuming behaviors that aim to check, hide, obtain reassurance about, or fix the perceived defect. Common behaviors are excessive checking of the perceived flaw in mirrors, other reflecting surfaces, or directly; excessive grooming; reassurance seeking; comparing with others; and skin picking. Nearly all patients attempt to camouflage the perceived deformity (e.g., with a hat, hair, makeup, body position, or clothing); this behavior can be conceptualized as an avoidance behavior but may also be repetitive (e.g., frequent makeup reapplication). Although the goal of such behaviors is to diminish anxiety provoked by the appearance concerns, these behaviors may increase anxiety.

Psychosocial Functioning and Quality of Life

Functioning and quality of life in BDD vary but are typically markedly poor. In a study of 76 individuals with BDD, most of whom had a primary diagnosis of BDD, 36% had not worked in the past month because of psychopathology, and 32% wanted to attend school but were unable to attend because of psychopathology. On the Social Adjustment Scale—Self-Report, mean social adjustment scores are more than two standard deviations below community norms. In two studies, 27–31% of individuals with BDD had been completely housebound for at least 1 week because of BDD symptoms, and 48% of adults and 44% of adolescents with BDD had been psychiatrically hospitalized. Individuals with BDD have poorer mental health-related quality of life than norms for patients with type II diabetes, a recent myocardial infarction, or clinical depression (major depressive disorder and/or dysthymia).

Suicidality

Although data on suicidality are limited, in clinical cross-sectional samples lifetime rates of suicidal ideation (78–81%) and suicide attempts (24–28%) are very high. In the only prospective study of individuals ascertained for BDD, the annual rate of completed suicide was markedly elevated (0.3%) and higher than that for other psychiatric disorders. In a retrospective study in two dermatology practices over 20 years, most patients who suicided had acne or BDD.

Demographic Features, Course of Illness, and Comorbidity

The two largest epidemiological studies of BDD (N = 2,510 and N = 2,552) found a point prevalence of 2.0% in women versus 1.5% in men, and 1.9% in women versus 1.4% in men, respectively. Studies in clinical samples of convenience in adults have had widely varying proportions of males and females, with some studies containing more females and others more males. In the two largest series, 55% of 293 subjects and 64% of 200 subjects were female. In clinical samples, a majority of patients is single.

BDD usually begins during adolescence and can occur in childhood. In the only observational prospective study of BDD's course, the probability of full remission from BDD over 1 year of follow-up was only .09, and the probability of partial remission was .21. However, BDD's course is more favorable when patients receive appropriate treatment (see below).

Most patients have co-occurring mental disorders, most commonly major depressive disorder, a substance use disorder, social phobia, or OCD. A majority of patients have a personality disorder, most often avoidant personality disorder.

Muscle Dysmorphia

Chapter 22 provides a review of body image in relation to muscularity. MD is a form of BDD that occurs nearly exclusively in males. It consists of preoccupation with the idea that one's body is insufficiently muscular or lean, or is "too small," despite being normal looking or even very muscular. One study found that men with MD were significantly more likely than men with BDD but not MD to lift weights excessively (71 vs. 12%), diet (71 vs. 27%), and exercise excessively (64 vs. 10%). Those with MD had significantly poorer quality of life and notably higher lifetime rates of suicide attempts (50 vs. 16%) and substance use disorders (86 vs. 51%), including anabolic steroid abuse/dependence (21 vs. 0%). Thus, this form of BDD appears to be associated with severe psychopathology.

Body Image Disturbance in BDD

Little is known about body image disturbance (BID) in BDD, even though it is a central feature of the disorder. In a study that used the Multidimensional Body-Self Relations Questionnaire and compared individuals with BDD to published norms, subjects with BDD were significantly less satisfied with their appearance, and men with BDD were significantly more invested in their appearance. Compared to norms, males and females with BDD felt less physically healthy; females were less alert to being ill and were less invested in a healthy lifestyle.

In a study that compared BDD and eating disorders, individuals with BDD, AN, or bulimia nervosa (BN) had significantly elevated disturbance in most body image dimensions compared to gender-matched clinical controls. Both the BDD and eating disorder groups had severe BID, including similar degrees of body dissatisfaction and distress. However, participants with BDD reported more body image impairment than those with eating disorders, including greater investment in appearance for self-worth and a more deleterious effect of body image on quality of life.

Preliminary findings suggest that individuals with BDD may experience abnormalities in visual processing and executive functioning, which may possibly contribute to their BID. In a study that used the Rey–Osterrieth Complex Figure Task, subjects with BDD tended to focus on details rather than the overall organization of visual stimuli. Similarly, a functional magnetic resonance imaging (fMRI) study of facial processing found a bias for detail encoding and analysis rather than holistic visual processing strategies in subjects with BDD versus healthy controls. These findings raise the possibility that appearance-related beliefs in BDD may arise, at least in part, from hyperattentiveness to minor details of physical appearance.

Assessing BDD

Although BDD appears to be relatively common, it usually goes undiagnosed. Several studies examined the issue of whether BDD is recognized in clinical settings. These studies interviewed a series of patients to determine whether they had BDD and then ascertained whether those with BDD had the diagnosis recorded in his or her clinical record. In all of the studies, no patient who was identified by the investigators as having BDD had the diagnosis recorded in his or her clinical record. The most common reasons patients do not disclose BDD symptoms to their clinician are embarrassment, fear of being negatively judged, feeling the clinician will not understand their appearance concerns, and not knowing that treatment for body image concerns is available. Thus, clinicians need to systematically screen patients for BDD.

The following questions can be used to assess whether a patient has DSM-IV BDD:

1. Ask: "Are you very worried about your appearance in any way?" OR: "Are you unhappy with how you look?" Invite the patient to describe the concern and ask whether there are other body areas he or she dislikes.
2. Ascertain that the patient is preoccupied with the perceived flaws by asking "How much time would you estimate you spend each day thinking about your appearance?" OR: "Do these concerns preoccupy you?" (A useful guide is to require about an hour or more a day as a criterion for the diagnosis.)
3. Ask: "How much distress do these concerns cause you?" Ask specifically about resulting anxiety, social anxiety, depression, feelings of panic, and suicidal thinking.
4. Ask about effects of the appearance preoccupations on the patient's life—for example: "Do these concerns interfere with your life or cause problems for you in any way?" Ask specifically about effects on work, school, other aspects of role functioning, relationships, intimacy, family and social activities, and household tasks.

The appearance concerns should not be better accounted for by AN or BN. However, BDD and eating disorders may co-occur, in which case both disorders should be diagnosed. While not required for the diagnosis, clues to BDD's presence include the repetitive behaviors described above, ideas or delusions of reference, being housebound, depressed mood, anxiety, panic attacks, social anxiety, and self-consciousness in social situations.

Several screening measures for BDD are available. If they suggest that a patient has BDD, the diagnosis should be confirmed via clinical interview. These measures are (1) Phillips's self-report Body Dysmorphic Disorder Questionnaire (BDDQ), (2) Cash's self-report Body Image Disturbance Questionnaire (BIDQ), and (3) the interviewer-administered screening questions from the Structured Clinical Interview for DSM-IV (SCID) by First and colleagues.

Diagnostic measures, which are semistructured and clinician administered, include (1) the aforementioned SCID, (2) Phillips's BDD Diagnostic Module, (3) Rosen and Reiter's Body Dysmorphic Disorder Examination (BDDE), and (4) the first three items of Phillips's Yale–Brown Obsessive Compulsive Scale Modified for Body Dysmorphic Disorder

(BDD-YBOCS). Sheehan's MINI Plus likely underdiagnoses BDD, because it requires symptoms that are not required by DSM-IV criteria and are not necessarily characteristic of BDD.

Treatment of BDD

Pharmacotherapy

Two controlled studies indicate that serotonin-reuptake inhibitors (SRIs, SSRIs) are often efficacious for BDD; these medications are currently considered the medication of choice for BDD. In a 12-week, double-blind, parallel-group study ($n = 67$ randomized subjects), fluoxetine was significantly more efficacious than placebo for BDD symptoms. In a double-blind, crossover trial ($n = 29$ randomized subjects), the SRI clomipramine was more efficacious than the non-SRI antidepressant desipramine. Four systematic open-label SRI studies have been published ($n = 15–30$), two with fluvoxamine, one with citalopram, and one with escitalopram. Across the above studies, in intention-to-treat analyses BDD response rates ranged from 53 to 77%, with statistically significant improvement in BDD severity in all studies. Significant improvement also occurred in insight, depressive symptoms, suicidal ideation, anxiety, anger–hostility, psychosocial functioning, and mental health-related quality of life in all or most studies that examined these variables. Of note, SRI monotherapy also appears efficacious for delusional BDD.

Cognitive-Behavioral Therapy

Cognitive-behavioral therapy (CBT) appears efficacious for BDD and is currently considered the psychotherapy of choice for BDD (see Chapter 47). Most published studies have included cognitive restructuring as well as exposure (e.g., to avoided social situations) and response prevention (e.g., not seeking reassurance), with these approaches tailored specifically to BDD symptoms. In a study that randomized 54 patients to eight weekly 2-hour group sessions of CBT or a wait-list condition, CBT was more efficacious than no treatment. A study that randomized 19 patients to individual CBT or a wait-list condition found that CBT produced greater improvement than no treatment. Case series and case reports similarly suggest that CBT is efficacious for BDD. The number and frequency of sessions vary greatly across studies, from 12 weekly hour-long sessions to 12 weeks of daily 90-minute sessions.

More recently developed treatment strategies (which are used in addition to the above approaches) include perceptual retraining with mirrors, habit reversal for BDD-related skin picking or hair plucking, cognitive approaches that target core beliefs, and incorporation of behavioral experiments into exposure exercises. However, treatment components of CBT need more study, and studies that compare the efficacy of CBT to that of other therapies are also needed.

Other Treatments

The efficacy of other types of therapy or medications for BDD has not been well studied. A majority of patients with BDD seek and receive cosmetic treatment for their BDD concerns, most commonly dermatologic treatment and cosmetic surgery. As discussed in Chapter 45, available data suggest that these treatments are usually ineffective and may even worsen BDD symptoms.

Conclusions and Future Directions

Although research on BDD is rapidly increasing, it is still limited and at an early stage. Investigation of virtually all aspects of this disorder is greatly needed. Needed studies include additional placebo-controlled pharmacotherapy studies, studies of other medications, studies that compare CBT to other types of therapy, and studies of the combination of psychotherapy and pharmacotherapy. There is a particularly pressing need for research in children and adolescents, including treatment studies.

Because BID is likely central to BDD's pathophysiology and maintenance, this is a key area for future inquiry. Neuroimaging studies are needed, as are other investigations of mechanisms in BDD—neurobiological, psychological, and sociocultural—as knowledge of this disorder's pathogenesis may ultimately guide much-needed treatment and prevention strategies.

Informative Readings

Feusner, J. D., Townsend, J., Bystritsky, A., & Bookheimer, S. (2007). Visual information processing of faces in body dysmorphic disorder. *Archives of General Psychiatry*, *64*, 1417–1425. A controlled study of visual information processing of faces in BDD.

Hollander, E., Allen, A., Kwon, J., Aronowitz, B., Schmeidler, J., Wong, C., et al. (1999). Clomipramine vs. desipramine crossover trial in body dysmorphic disorder: Selective efficacy of a serotonin reuptake inhibitor in imagined ugliness. *Archives of General Psychiatry*, *56*, 1033–1039.—The first controlled pharmacotherapy study of BDD.

Hrabosky, J. I., Cash, T. F., Veale, D., Neziroglu, F., Soll, E. A., Garner, D. M., et al. (2009). Multidimensional body image comparisons among patients with eating disorders, body dysmorphic disorder, and clinical controls: A multisite study. *Body Image: An International Journal of Research, 6*, 155–163.—One of two studies to directly compare clinical features in patients with BDD and those with an eating disorder, with a consideration of multiple dimensions of body image.

National Collaborating Centre for Mental Health. (2006). *Core interventions in the treatment of obsessive compulsive disorder and body dysmorphic disorder.* Available at *www.nice.org.uk/page.aspx?o=289817.*—A national (United Kingdom) clinical practice guideline from the National Institute for Health and Clinical Excellence, National Health Service.

Neziroglu, F., & Cash, T. F. (Eds.). (2008). Body dysmorphic disorder: Causes, characteristics, and clinical treatments [Special section]. *Body Image: An International Journal of Research, 5*, 1–58.—Five articles reviewing research on key topics related to BDD.

Phillips, K. A. (2009). *Understanding body dysmorphic disorder: An essential guide.* New York: Oxford University Press.—A comprehensive guide to BDD for both professionals and lay readers.

Phillips, K. A., Albertini, R. S., & Rasmussen, S. A. (2002). A randomized placebo-controlled trial of fluoxetine in body dysmorphic disorder. *Archives of General Psychiatry, 59*, 381–388.—One of two controlled pharmacotherapy studies, and the only placebo-controlled treatment study, of BDD.

Phillips, K. A., McElroy, S. L., Keck, P. E., Jr., Pope, H. G., Jr., & Hudson, J. I. (1993). Body dysmorphic disorder: 30 cases of imagined ugliness. *American Journal of Psychiatry, 150*, 302–308.—The first descriptive series of BDD using modern assessment methods.

Phillips, K. A., & Menard, W. (2006). Suicidality in body dysmorphic disorder: A prospective study. *American Journal of Psychiatry, 163*, 1280–1282.—A report on suicidal ideation, suicide attempts, and completed suicide in the only prospective observational study of the course of BDD.

Phillips, K. A., Menard, W., Fay C., & Weisberg, R. (2005). Demographic characteristics, phenomenology, comorbidity, and family history in 200 individuals with body dysmorphic disorder. *Psychosomatics, 46*, 317–332.—A report on a broad array of clinical features in 200 individuals with BDD.

Pope, H. G., Phillips, K. A., & Olivardia, R. (2000). *The Adonis complex: The secret crisis of male body obsession.* New York: Free Press.—An overview of BDD, MD, and eating disorders in men for professionals and lay readers.

Rief, W., Buhlmann, U., Wilhelm, S., Borkenhagen, A., & Brähler, E. (2006). The prevalence of body dysmorphic disorder: A population-based survey. *Psychological Medicine, 36*, 877–885.—A large survey of the prevalence and clinical correlates of BDD.

Rosen, J. C., Reiter, J., & Orosan, P. (1995). Cognitive-behavioral body image therapy for body dysmorphic disorder. *Journal of Consulting and Clinical Psychology, 63*, 263–269.—One of two published controlled psychotherapy studies of BDD.

Veale, D., Gournay, K., Dryden, W., Boocock, A., Shah, F., Willson, R., et al. (1996). Body dysmorphic disorder: A cognitive behavioural model and pilot randomized controlled trial. *Behaviour Research and Therapy, 34*, 717–729.—One of two published controlled psychotherapy studies of BDD.

CHAPTER 36

Body Image and Appearance- and Performance-Enhancing Drug Use

TOM HILDEBRANDT

JUSTINE LAI

Introduction

Appearance- and performance-enhancing drugs (APEDs) include a wide range of substances used to alter one's outward appearance or improve one's ability to achieve or succeed in domains where performance is based on physical appearance and strength, such as athletics or enforcement professions (e.g., police officer, fireman, or bouncer). These substances can vary substantially in their legality, potency, risks, and mechanisms of action. They are typically described in the context of anabolic–androgenic steroid (AAS) use, but the term *APED* describes a wider range of substances that include categories such as over-the-counter weight loss or fat-burning substances (e.g., mau huang), illegal fat-burning substances (e.g., thyroid hormones), nonsteroidal anabolics (e.g., insulin or human growth hormone), and more general muscle-building nutritional supplements (e.g., protein powder), along with AASs (e.g., testosterone, Nandrolone). Although the use of these substances is often associated with professional sports scandals, they are primarily used to change appearance by individuals who are not paid to compete in athletics.

The use of APEDs has evolved tremendously over the past 25 years with the burgeoning nutritional supplement market capitalizing on increased knowledge of the specific biological mechanisms involved in muscle growth and body fat reduction. Furthermore, the delegation of AASs in 1990 as a Schedule III controlled substance has made their use for the pursuit of an idealized body a federal offense in the United States. This has generated mainstream awareness of how these substances function to alter appearance. Under these regulations, the pursuit of an ideal body can actually be considered a crime and may be one of the few circumstances where the sociopolitical environment has heavily influenced the public view of this pursuit. For example, men and women who suffer from an eating disorder are considered to have a mental illness, while cosmetic practices such as plastic surgery or enhancement are widely accepted in certain sectors of society. APED use is unique in its designation as a criminal behavior. Although these labels are associated with their respective degrees of stigma, there is significant variation in the potential societal consequences for each subgroup.

The role of body image in APED use is complex. Disturbances in body image are theorized to be a specific risk factor for onset and chronic maintenance of APED use. Data are just beginning to emerge in support of these theories, but not without challenges. New APEDs are being developed regularly in an effort to meet the demands of the marketplace (legal and illegal), to help professionals needing to evade detection on doping tests, and to reduce the side effects associated with the more potent substances. In addition, the wide variation in APED user's body ideals highlights the basic problem of population heterogeneity. For example, bodybuilders may use APEDs to achieve extreme levels of muscularity and low body fat, whereas another user may simply desire to lose weight and reduce overall body fat, and a third type may want to be bigger and stronger with little concern for his or her level of body fat. Even less is known about women who use these substances and their intentions; whether they are pursuing a similar diversity in bodily ideals as men or instead subscribe to the thin ideal. Finally, APED use is typically part of a larger lifestyle dedicated to overall health, higher quality of life, and improved appearance. Adherence to this lifestyle includes regular exercise and strict dietary control, two behaviors traditionally associated health and well-being. The legitimate health benefits of this type of lifestyle make it more difficult to identify problematic APED use and determine when APED use will lead to significant health risks.

Body Image and Initiation of APED Use

Cross-sectional evidence implicates body dissatisfaction in the initiation of both adolescent and adult AAS use. Less is known about the role of body dissatisfaction in other forms of APED use, particularly legal APEDs, although it is assumed to play a prominent role. One of the more pressing questions about initiation of APED use is how one transitions from the widely available and legal APEDs (e.g., nutritional supplements) to illegal forms of APED use (e.g., AASs). Legal APED users with high body dissatisfaction may be more motivated to seek out and initiate illegal APED use than body-satisfied legal APED users. The combination of body dissatisfaction and body investment might further increase the likelihood for illegal APED use or provide an independent risk for APED use. However, investment in appearance or achievement might be the crucial factor, motivating illegal APED use even among those who are satisfied with their body.

Age is likely to be an important moderator of the relationship between body image and initiation of AAS use. Adolescents are at higher risk for acute negative consequences from illegal APED use (e.g., personality changes, aggression, suicide), although the exact reason is unclear. The role of sex hormones in puberty and the development of the adolescent brain are potential biological explanations for this risk. A poor body image among adolescents might provide a specific vulnerability for APEDs, but social relationships are also likely to play a role in bringing about AAS use. For instance, peer groups are a common source of education and validation for the efficacy and safety of APEDs, and therefore may influence initiation among vulnerable individuals. Adolescents are more likely to participate in organized sports, and there is some epidemiological data to suggest that those participating in specific sports are at higher risk for illicit APED use. The transition from legal into illegal APED use for adults is less understood. Men and women who begin using in their later stages of life may be motivated by an attempt to maintain youth or prevent aging. The desired body types may be more realistic and less extreme at this stage, so the influence of body image may be more in the form of the functional role of the body (e.g., strength, vitality, sex drive) over extreme dissatisfaction with outward appearance. Peer circles may also influence illegal APED initiation at these ages through specific gym or fitness communities, or perhaps even membership within certain social groups, such as among male gay or bisexual populations, where high value is placed on certain body ideals. These influences have only recently begun to be recognized and studied.

Body Image and Maintenance of APED Use

Chronic APED use is likely the cause of most negative psychological and physical outcomes. Because no longitudinal data exist for these chronic users, the current understanding of this phenomenon is mostly theoretical. Animal data on AASs suggest that these substances are mildly reinforcing, that they increase the likelihood of natural reinforcers such as exercise, sex, or aggression, and may increase the reinforcing value of other illicit substances such as stimulants or cocaine. Physically, chronic AAS use can impair cardiac or liver function depending upon the type of drug or route of administration (i.e., oral vs. injection). Some of these effects, particularly those associated with the cardiovascular system, are mediated by simultaneous engagement in intense exercise, the use of stimulants to reduce body fat, and the use of AASs. Because side effects are common with illicit APED use, many initiate ancillary drug use to protect the body from the wear and tear of heavy training and APED use. These may be borrowed from a wide range of medical or alternative medicine sources and become part of the APED use pattern despite little direct relation to appearance or performance. One example is the use of prescription pain killers that may be used to treat the injuries incurred from heavy weight training. This expansive use of pharmacotherapy is where APED use clearly becomes part of the individual's lifestyle.

As with initiation, body dissatisfaction, satisfaction, and appearance investment are likely to play a role in chronic APED use. Negative reinforcement is perhaps the most parsimonious conceptualization for how these body image dimensions influence drug use. As an individual approaches his or her physical ideal, he or she attributes much of this success to the use of these drugs. This success is followed by a common experience of distress upon APED discontinuation, due to loss of physical gains made during acute APED use. To avoid this discomfort, the individual continues to use APEDs. This psychological dependence is believed to be part of the initial stages of AAS addiction, although the construct continues to be the subject of further research and debate. The intensity of dissatisfaction when APEDs are discontinued or the intensity of satisfaction when taking APEDs will vary based on the APED user's investment in his or her body. This investment can originate from the APED user's identity (e.g., bodybuilder, professional athlete, fitness model), which lends credibility to the distress or satisfaction experienced by the user; loss of APED effects can reduce success and the effectiveness of APED use can improve success at achieving the standards of the APED user's identity. For example, loss of muscle mass might reduce job opportunities for a fitness model or lead to a drop in performance for an athlete.

An alternative theoretical approach is to consider illegal APED use a chemical form of plastic surgery. There are a number of parallels between these phenomena, including the semipermanence of the physical changes, reports of satisfaction by the majority of users, the potential for serious side effects, and the origins in traditional medicine. Under this conceptualization, illegal APED use can be justified as a reasonable and safe practice when monitored appropriately, but potentially dangerous for those with pathological levels of body image disturbance (BID). Based on the emerging muscle dysmorphia (MD) literature, a subtype of body dysmorphic disorder, it does seem that MD is associated with particularly high rates of APED use. Whether these individuals are more likely to develop chronic patterns of APED use remains to be studied, but if so, these types of data might support a direct link between BID and problematic use.

However, when considering parallels with plastic surgery, it is important to note the lack of medical oversight for APED use. Although there is a wealth of information available to illicit APED users through the Internet and various print materials, such as "steroid bibles," no medical specialties are equipped to manage existing forms of illicit APED use. Some professionals regularly prescribe AASs. For example, doctors providing care for individuals who are HIV-positive prescribe certain low-dose AASs to their patients for weight-maintenance and general vitality, and other doctors prescribe low doses of testosterone as hormone replacement therapy among older or hypogonadal males. However, the low dosages and restrictions on the range of drugs prescribed make it difficult to generalize the experience of these patients to the general APED-using population.

Conclusions and Future Directions

APEDs include a diverse range of substances with different characteristics and APED users are perhaps an equally diverse population. This heterogeneity manifests in their patterns of drug use and the types of BID experienced by users. There are at least four unique subtypes of APED user: (1) recreational user with low BID, (2) primarily concerned with body fat and more anxious about his or her body, (3) primarily concerned with muscle mass and more invested in his or her body, and (4) concerned with both leanness and muscularity and having the most anxiety and highest investment in his or her body. The types of APEDs, overall amount of APED use, and specific risks associated with APED use map onto these subgroups. Some of the more pressing questions in this field deal with developing an appropriate model for determining pathological forms of APED use. Although AAS dependence is one approach to this problem, this diversity challenges the traditional addiction model and suggests a primary role of BID. This psychological feature makes APED use unique among drugs of abuse.

The results of this subtyping research generally suggest that there is significant heterogeneity among male APED users in their motivations, types of APEDs used, and BID. The vast majority of this research has been conducted on adult weightlifting men. Women who use APEDs may do so for very different reasons and body image may also play a motivational or maintaining role. Because APEDs are linked to AASs, which are synthetic male sex hormones, very little clinical or observational research has been done with women who use APEDs. There has been some debate about whether rates of AAS use are increasing among female high school students and this remains unresolved. Higher reported rates may simply reflect the fact that teenagers overendorse AAS-related survey questions due to the availability of legal supplements that mimic the effects of AASs.

In addition to the limits posed by the diversity of APED-using populations, the biggest obstacle to improving our understanding of APED use is the stigma associated with use. Most users are extremely cautious about revealing their use, often denying use of APEDs to maintain the perception that their body results from natural and legally obtained gains. This secrecy is in stark contrast to traditional drugs of abuse that are typically initiated in social and party atmospheres. Not only does this secrecy inhibit research recruitment and participation, it also presents a significant obstacle to treatment-seeking or prevention efforts. The use of APEDs, particularly in the context of severe BID, may be associated with significant mental and physical health consequences. If APED users are reluctant to seek treatment or even engage their existing network of social support for help, then they are likely to experience even more impairment as a consequence of their use. A number of these barriers exist as a function of the sociopolitical environment aimed at identifying and punishing cheating athletes. A second, and more pervasive, obstacle may include the association between this form of drug use and identification with masculine norms that devalue help-seeking behavior. It is likely that any effective clinical interventions or prevention efforts developed for this population will need to address this stigma.

Another issue to address is that the lifestyle associated with APED use can actually lead to improved quality of life, and may provide a structure and discipline for those who might otherwise be engaged in more externally harmful behavior. The rapidly rising rates of obesity in modern society highlight the lack of regular exercise and healthy eating habits among most sectors of the population, whereas almost all APED users adhere to a strict and consistent exercise regimen, along with management of their diet in order to create a caloric and micronutrient balance necessary to approximate their ideal body. The key question is how to identify those who are likely to cross this threshold into an unhealthy extreme. Identifying the exact role of body image in APED use is critical for future understandings of who is likely to transition from legal to illegal forms of APEDs, identifying the specific risk profiles among those who do initiate this behavior, explaining the role of exercise and diet in maintaining or enhancing drug effects, and developing targeted interventions for prevention and treatment of problematic APED use.

Informative Readings

Cafri, G., Thompson, J. K., Ricciardelli, L., McCabe, M., Smolak, L., & Yesalis, C. (2009). Pursuit of the muscular ideal: Physical and psychological consequences and putative risk factors. *Clinical Psychology Review*, 25, 215–239.—Reviews the muscular-ideal construct and some of the potential consequences of pursuing this ideal such as anabolic steroid use.

Hildebrandt, T., Alfano, L., & Langenbucher, J. (2010). Body image disturbance among 1000 appearance and performance enhancing drug users. *Journal of Psychiatric Research, 44*, 841–846.—A subtyping study that identifies four unique profiles of BID among current APED users.

Hildebrandt, T., Langenbucher, J. W., Carr, S. J., & Sanjuan, P. (2007). Modeling population heterogeneity in appearance- and performance-enhancing drug (APED) use: Applications of mixture modeling in 400 regular APED users. *Journal of Abnormal Psychology, 110*, 717–733.—A subtyping study that identifies four unique profiles of APED use among current and experienced APED users.

Hildebrandt, T., Schlundt, D., Langenbucher, J., & Chung, T. (2006). Presence of muscle dysmorphia symptomology among male weightlifters. *Comprehensive Psychiatry, 47*, 127–135.—A subtyping study that identifies five subtypes of male weightlifters with the most pathological group having symptoms consistent with MD.

Hildebrandt, T., Walker, D. C., Alfano, L., Delinsky, S., & Bannon, K. (2010). Development and validation of a male specific body checking questionnaire. *International Journal of Eating Disorders, 43*, 77–87.—A measure development study describing the validation of a male-specific measure of BID.

Kanayama, G., Barry, S., Hudson, J. R., & Pope, H. G., Jr. (2006). Body image and attitudes toward male roles in anabolic–androgenic steroid users. *American Journal of Psychiatry, 163*, 697–703.—A study identifying the relationship between masculine identity and body image among steroid users.

Kanayama, G., Brower, K. J., Wood, R. I., Hudson, J. R., Jr., & Pope, H. G., Jr. (2009). Anabolic–androgenic steroid dependence: An emerging disorder. *Addiction, 104*, 1966–1978.—A suggested modification of the DSM-IV drug dependence criteria for anabolic steroids to include BID, exercise, and dietary control.

McCreary, D. R., Hildebrandt, T. B., Heinberg, L. J., Boroughs, M., & Thompson, J. K. (2007). A review of body image influences on men's fitness goals and supplement use. *American Journal of Men's Health, 1*, 307–316.—A review paper summarizing the heterogeneity in male body image ideals and the role of drug use in the pursuit of these ideals.

Peters, R., Copeland, J., & Dillon, P. (1999). Anabolic–androgenic steroids: User characteristics, motivations, and deterrents. *Psychology of Addictive Behaviors, 13*, 232–242.—A field study of 100 anabolic steroid users that describes the basic motivations for using anabolic steroids.

Walker, D. C., Anderson, D. A., & Hildebrandt, T. (2009). Body checking behaviors in men. *Body Image: An International Journal of Research, 6*, 164–170.—A study that shows a relationship between body checking and the use of APEDs in college students.

PART VI

BODY IMAGE ISSUES IN MEDICAL CONTEXTS

CHAPTER 37

Body Image Issues in Dermatology

ANDREW R. THOMPSON

Introduction

The term *skin condition* rather than *skin disease* is used here, so as to be inclusive of the full range of conditions typically seen in dermatology, which includes both conditions where there is a clear organic cause, and conditions where the cause is primarily psychological in nature. The term *skin conditions* is also used here to include conditions affecting hair. Skin conditions are common, affecting about a third of people at any one time. The role played by psychological factors in dermatological conditions is complex and the field of psychodermatology has been described as being concerned with three groups of overlapping conditions: (1) those that are primarily psychological in nature such as trichotillomania (hair pulling) and delusional disorders such as parasitosis; (2) those that have a psychophysiological element, where stress may play an exacerbating or even initiating role, such as in certain alopecias (hair loss) and uticaria (hives); and (3) those where psychological issues are secondary, associated with the effect of living with the condition, such as in vitiligo (loss of skin pigment) and psoriasis (a condition where the skin is sore and broken in patches).

Body image distress is most likely to be associated with the first and last of these groups, although the focus of this chapter is on the latter group, as conditions that are primarily psychological in nature are dealt with elsewhere (see, for example, Chapter 35). It is important to realize that the physical appearance of the skin and hair are almost always visible

323

to others and are used as markers of various roles and status positions, and not just health but age, gender group membership, and so on. Cash, for example, has written about the symbolism conveyed by hair ("from monks to skinheads, prisoners of war to warriors...," 2001, p. 161) in his discussion of the influence of hair loss on body image.

Clearly then, an obvious impact of living with a skin or hair condition can be its visible or disfiguring effect on appearance; it is this aspect of body image that is the focus of this chapter. One of the centrally important issues discussed below is that both the perceptions of the person living with a dermatological condition and the perceptions of others play a role in the adaptation process.

How Is Body Image Affected by Skin Conditions?

Physical Effects

The physical effects of dermatological conditions are wide ranging both within and between conditions; thus, detailed descriptions of these conditions are beyond the scope of this chapter. Some conditions such as psoriasis and vitiligo are typically chronic diseases that tend to wax and wane in their course. In some conditions, such as psoriasis and eczema, there can be periods when the skin is extremely sore and broken; these episodes are typically associated with functional impairment. In other conditions like acne vulgaris there can be highly noticeable blemishes.

Some dermatological conditions are congenital, such as port-wine stains, and are fixed in their presentation and not usually associated with serious physical complications but are nonetheless very socially noticeable. Disorders of the hair and scalp also fall under the remit of the dermatologist; both hirsutism (excess hair production) and alopecia (hair loss) tend to be highly visible to others. Hair is often culturally associated with gender and both hirsutism and alopecia may pose threats particularly to femininity.

Untoward Treatment Effects

Treatment can involve engaging in unpleasant and time-consuming procedures such as the use of messy and malodorous creams, which may be visible and alter the texture and feel of the skin, acting as another variable influencing body image. For example, in evidence that was submitted to the U.K. All Party Parliamentary Group on Skin, one respondent reported: "Smearing on the evil-smelling, sticky, staining stuff could take up to two or more hours a day, soaking in it another hour or so" (2003, p. 5).

Other treatments such as PUVA, which involves taking psoralens (photosensitizing agents) followed by controlled exposure to UVA light, are time consuming, involve frequent clinic attendance, and can have immediate unpleasant side effects such as itching and possible long-term risks of increased cancer. Indeed, many dermatological drugs are known to have unpleasant side effects and although these can be managed with other treatments, they nonetheless present an additional short-term burden to the patient. Isotretinoin, a drug used to treat acne, has been associated with a number of side effects, including dry lips and eye soreness; use of this drug requires ongoing monitoring because of possible effects on mood.

Social Effects

In one of the earliest studies of the psychosocial impact of living with psoriasis, Jobling revealed that interpersonal difficulties were commonly reported. Several experimental and observational studies have subsequently shown that people often react negatively toward someone with a visible skin condition. In 2005, Grandfield, Thompson, and Turpin demonstrated that people typically exhibit immediate negative associations with skin conditions. Using photographs of clear skin and skin conditions, explicit and implicit attitudes were measured. The Implicit Association Test was used to examine implicit attitudes, an experimental technique allowing the relative strengths of associations between concepts to be measured, thus revealing biases usually moderated by social desirability. The findings suggest that there are negative implicit attitudes or at least automatic negative stereotypes activated when people encounter skin conditions. This suggests that there are either evolutionary or deep cultural predispositions behind the typical social reactions people living with skin conditions encounter.

The reactions exhibited can go well beyond initial stares and actually become abusive and discriminatory, and sadly it is not unusual for children living with skin conditions to report being teased or bullied. Numerous qualitative studies bear testimony to the fact that both adults and children living with skin conditions experience rude name-calling. Whether the result of misunderstanding or malice, people with skin conditions have also reported experiencing discrimination in the workplace. Recently the U.K. Trade Union Unite, along with the Psoriasis Association, lobbied to have the employment rights of people with psoriasis protected. Given the reality that for people living with skin conditions there is a real chance of receiving intrusive negative reactions from others, it is perhaps not surprising that visibility to others is one of the few objective factors identified in the literature as being associated with psychological distress.

Cultural Influences

Beliefs about illness are linked to psychosocial adjustment, and there is evidence that such beliefs vary in connection with cultural and ethnic factors (see Part IV, Chapters 25–28). Unfortunately, there is a dearth of studies in this area although in some qualitative studies conducted, subtle cultural differences in illness perceptions have been reported. For example, Porter and Beuf (1991) reported that for Black Americans living with vitiligo, although there were few objective differences in the patterns of distress in comparison with other groups, there existed lay belief that vitiligo resulted from engaging in sexual activity with Whites. Recently, Thompson and his colleagues studied how British Asian women adapt to living with vitiligo and determined that values related to appearance, status, and myths linked to the cause of the condition were subtly related to cultural beliefs and practices. For example, participants described pressures relating directly to the practice of arranged marriage in terms of the meaning of having an appearance-altering condition.

Psychological Effects

Higher levels of psychological distress have been reported by some people living with skin conditions. In 2000, Picardi and his colleagues reported the results of a large-sample study of persons with a wide variety of skin conditions. About a quarter of patients had clinically significant levels of psychological distress. The psychological difficulties commonly reported in the literature include anxiety (particularly, social anxiety), depression, lowered self-esteem, and feelings of shame, as well as stated body image concerns. Suicidal ideation is unfortunately not uncommon. For example, Rapp and colleagues reported that one in four of their participants with psoriasis had indicated being suicidal at some point.

Although there is a risk of psychological distress associated with skin conditions, there is considerable individual variation and the majority of people cope well. Nonetheless, living with a skin condition is stressful and likely to involve some degree of psychological impact. Some studies suggest that even when people are coping well, there is likely to be a demand on psychological resources, for example, in the need to manage the reactions of others or flare-ups of the condition itself. Indeed, there is considerable evidence from across a range of long-term health conditions that living with uncertainty is itself very stressful.

Individual Variation in Body Image Distress

As with other long-term disfiguring conditions, there does not appear to be a straightforward association between medical and demographic factors, such as condition type and severity, age, and gender, with body image distress. Numerous studies have found only a weak association between clinician-rated disease severity and psychological functioning but a strong relationship between patient-rated severity and psychological distress. Thus, an objectively minor blemish may be seen as "hideous" by one patient, whereas an objectively severe condition may be seen by another patient as "not so bad."

Identification of the variables that are important in adjustment can lead to the development of useful assessment tools and effective interventions. Figure 37.1 shows a simple heuristic model developed by the present author to delineate the factors that are likely to be involved in accounting for individual adjustment in skin conditions.

This figure depicts the role of early experiences and cultural stereotypes. Children may internalize negative reactions toward their skin and values expressed about appearance to develop unhelpful beliefs about their appearance and the role of appearance. In situations where the child has experienced early and repeated social rejection or appearance-related teasing, there may be risk of developing body-specific shame proneness that clinical experience suggests may become generalized to long-term appearance sensitivity.

The literature is full of contradictions in relation to the role played by demographic factors with some studies finding effects for gender and age and others not. However, some skin conditions predominately occur in adolescence, a developmental period with considerable focus on appear-

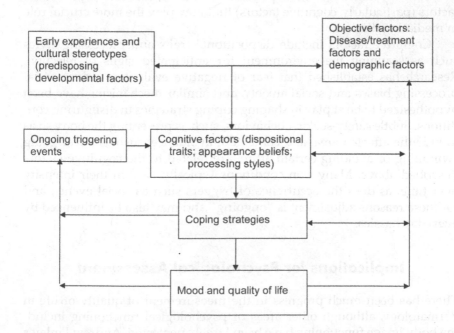

FIGURE 37.1. Model of the interacting factors implicated in the origin and maintenance of skin-specific affect/distress. Adapted from Thompson (2009) with permission from *Dermatological Nursing*.

ance and social acceptance, and there is no doubt that there is certainly an increased risk of experiencing psychological distress in at least the short term for teenagers as they "pass through this stage." Interestingly, several studies now suggest that developing acne vulgaris later in life or having the condition continue into early adulthood may be associated with higher levels of distress than found during adolescence. For example, Hassan and colleagues found higher levels of appearance-specific distress in their participants ages 20 years and over. For those who acquire a skin condition in later life, distress may be related to the activation of existing underlying negative beliefs, or discrepancies arising from beliefs about the difference in value between current perceived appearance status and desired status. It may also be related to cultural stereotypes of acne being an adolescent condition rather than to a simple relationship between duration and distress.

In relation to gender, several studies indicate that women may be more vulnerable to experiencing distress than men, perhaps because of cultural expectations; however, there are an equal number of studies that indicate men are at risk. Cash, in his review of androgenetic alopecia, summarizes the literature that indicates that both men and women can experience considerable psychological distress in response to loss of hair. Importantly, the literature in the area of alopecia also indicates that it is psychosocial factors (particularly, cognitive factors) that may play the more crucial role in mediating distress.

Cognitive factors include dispositional traits and processing styles such as scanning the environment for anticipated signs of rejection. Research has established that fear of negative evaluation drives social processing biases and social anxiety, and similar mechanisms have been hypothesized to be at play in shaping coping strategies in disfiguring conditions. Subtle safety-seeking behaviors, such as presenting the body so as to hide the affected area, and contextual avoidance, such as never going swimming or avoiding certain attire, are related to the cognitive factors described above. Many skin conditions typically vary in their intensity over time, as does the occurrence of triggers such as social events, and for these reasons adjustment is "ongoing" and may also be influenced by everyday hassles.

Implications for Psychological Assessment

There has been much progress in the measurement of quality of life in dermatology, although other areas of psychological functioning including body image functioning have been largely neglected. Andrew Finlay's group at The University of Cardiff developed the Dermatology Life Quality Index (DLQI), an instrument used in a large number of studies and standardized in several countries. The DLQI has 10 items, one of which directly asks about embarrassment and self-consciousness and other questions cover avoidance, so it is possible to use the DLQI to identify where there might be body image concerns.

Health-related quality of life measures like the DLQI are undoubtedly useful to researchers. However, the predominant effects of skin conditions may be emotional, and such measures may underestimate distress and are no substitute for interview-based clinical assessment. In addition, routine assessment gives permission to patients to discuss psychosocial issues and provides an opportunity for emotional disclosure. An empathetic and sensitive clinical assessment can also serve to normalize reactions reducing the stigma associated with the idea of "not coping."

As there is evidence that clinical severity is not a good guide of psychological functioning, it is much better to ask the patient about perceived severity rather than to rely on objective measures. Doing so may give a quick and useful guide to the degree of body image distress. When conducting an assessment, it is important to be aware of all aspects of the model shown in Figure 37.1 and to use a biopsychosocial perspective. Behavioral factors, including the degree to which avoidance is present, should be explored along with cognitive factors, such as the patients' thoughts about themselves and their appearance. Emotional factors, such as the presence of anger, low mood, and shame also require exploration. Lastly, factors such as the presence of actual or perceived social maltreatment and the degree of support require assessment. Where there are high levels of body image distress, it is also important to assess for self-injury and suicidal intent and risk. The ability to conduct an assessment of suicide risk is now a required competency within specialist registrar training for dermatologists in the United Kingdom.

In addition, concerns about skin and hair are often a preoccupation for persons with body dysmorphic disorder (BDD). These individuals often seek help from dermatologists and cosmetic surgeons to remedy their perceived "flaws." As discussed in Chapters 35 and 45, screening for BDD is essential in these practices, as these very distressed individuals seldom benefit from medical or surgical treatments.

Implications for Intervention

Figure 37.1 emphasizes how coping strategies and the ongoing stress of managing reactions of others play an important role in adaptation to the appearance-altering condition. Specialist dermatology nurses with additional training can help patients develop coping strategies both to manage the reactions of others and to manage stress. Relaxation and stress management techniques such as progressive muscle relaxation, biofeedback, mindfulness meditation, and visual imagery have all been used to assist dermatology patients. In addition, relatively simple behavioral techniques such as habit reversal can be useful in reducing itching and unhelpful scratching and picking, and have been shown to have efficacy in assisting children and adults with eczema.

Where there are long-standing dispositional factors, or feelings of rejection, or complex cognitive processing factors in operation, psychotherapy interventions such as cognitive behavioral therapy (see Chapter 47) or interpersonal therapy may be required, and this usually necessitates a referral to a suitably qualified psychotherapist or clinical psychologist. Ideally this professional should have some formal connection to the extended dermatology team, so as to minimize stigmatization that may arise from being referred to a "mental health specialist." Numerous studies have investigated the effectiveness or efficacy of psychological interventions on skin conditions, although the majority of these have been case studies or uncontrolled studies. Only a small number of randomized control trials of psychotherapies have been reported with dermatology patients and those that have been conducted have used a variety of techniques, approaches, and measures, thus making it difficult to draw conclusions.

Conclusions

Clearly, body image distress can be associated with skin and hair conditions. Consideration of psychological issues needs to be a routine part of training and practice in dermatology. Models of service delivery need to be established that provide patients with an opportunity to receive low-intensity psychosocial intervention in the clinic and have access to linked specialist psychological intervention if required. Further research is needed in order to develop and evaluate interventions at all levels of patient care.

Informative Readings

All Party Parliamentary Group on Skin. (2003). *Report on the enquiry into the impact of skin diseases on people's lives*. London: HMSO.—Governmental report seeking to raise awareness of skin disease issues and providing a broad account of the psychosocial impact of skin conditions.

Cash, T. F. (2001). The psychology of hair loss and its implications for patient care. *Clinics in Dermatology, 19*, 161–166.—Practical narrative review of hair loss and its relationship with body image, including recommendations for psychological assessment and treatment.

Chida, Y., Steptoe, A., Hirakawa, N., Sudo, N., & Kubo, C. (2007). The effects of psychological intervention on atopic dermatitis: A systematic review and meta-analysis. *International Archives of Allergy and Immunology, 144,* 1–9.—Reviews eight types of intervention in eight articles and suggests psychological intervention is promising.

Ersser, S. J., Latter, S., Sibley, A., Satherley, P. A., & Welbourne, S. (2007). Psychological and educational interventions for atopic eczema in children. *Cochrane Database of Systematic Reviews, 3,* 1–39.—Review indicating the utility of psychological techniques such as relaxation in reducing the distress associated with childhood eczema.

Grandfield, T., Thompson, A. R., & Turpin, G. (2005). An attitudinal study of responses to a range of dermatological conditions using the Implicit Attitudes Association Test. *Journal of Health Psychology, 10,* 821–829.—An experimental study demonstrating the automatic reactions exhibited toward skin conditions.

Hassan, J., Grogan, S., Clark-Carter, D., Richards, H., & Yates, V. M. (2009). The individual health burden of acne appearance-related distress in male and female adolescents and adults with back, chest and facial acne. *Journal of Health Psychology, 14,* 1105–1118.—Study demonstrating that acne can have a significant impact on adolescents and young adults and that nonvisible acne of the back can be particularly distressing.

Hongbo, Y., Thomas, C. L., Harrison, M. A., Salek, M. S., & Finlay, A. Y. (2005). Translating the science of quality of life into practice: What do DLQI scores mean? *Journal of Investigative Dermatology, 125,* 659–664.—Study showing how the DQLI research tool can be used by clinicians to inform treatment needs.

Jobling, R. G. (1976). Psoriasis: A preliminary questionnaire study of sufferers' subjective experience. *Clinical and Experimental Dermatology, 1,* 233–236.—Early study providing testimony to the psychological impact of living with a chronic skin condition.

Kent, G. (2002). Testing a model of disfigurement: Effects of a skin camouflage service on well-being and appearance anxiety. *Psychology and Health, 17,* 377–386.—Shows camouflage reduces distress but may not address underlying fear of negative evaluation.

Picardi, A., Abeni, D., Melchi, C. F., Puddu, P., & Pasquini, P. (2000). Psychiatric morbidity in dermatological outpatients: An issue to be recognized. *British Journal of Dermatology, 143,* 983–991.—Study showing 25% psychological morbidity as measured by the General Health Questionnaire (GHQ-12) in a large sample of dermatology patients.

Porter, J., & Beuf, A. (1991). Racial variation in reaction to physical stigma: A study of degree of disturbance by vitiligo among Black and White patients. *Journal of Health and Social Behavior, 32,* 192–204.—Study exploring not only racial variation (of which there was little) but also demonstrating the role played by psychological factors beyond demographic and disease-specific factors.

Rapp, S. R., Exum, M. L., Reboussin, D. M., Feldman, S. R., Fleischer, A., & Clark, A. (1997). The physical, psychological and social impact of psoriasis. *Journal of Health Psychology, 2,* 525–537.—Explores the impact of living with a chronic skin condition.

Thompson, A. R. (2009). Managing the psychosocial impact of skin conditions: Theory and the nursing role. *Dermatological Nursing, 8*, 43–48.—Practical article for dermatological nurses that gives suggestions for assessment practice in clinical settings.

Thompson, A. R., Clarke, S. A., Newell, R., Gawkrodger, G., & The Appearance Research Collaboration. (2010). Vitiligo linked to stigmatisation in British South Asian women: A qualitative study of the experiences of living with vitiligo. *British Journal of Dermatology, 163*, 481–486.—Describes nuances of cultural factors influencing body image concern.

Thompson, A., & Kent, G. (2001). Adjusting to disfigurement. Processes involved in dealing with being visibly different. *Clinical Psychology Review, 21*, 663–682.—A clinically oriented review of the literature on disfigurement and interventions likely to be helpful.

CHAPTER 38

Body Image Issues in Oncology

CRAIG A. WHITE
CAROLINE HOOD

Introduction

Cancer diagnosis and survival is rising as a result of an aging population, earlier diagnosis, and new and different treatments. Individuals diagnosed with cancer frequently commence treatment within a couple of weeks of receiving their diagnosis. Treatment pathways are often more complex and can result in greater symptom burden over a prolonged period of time. Many treatments are also now being delivered within an outpatient setting that reduces periods of contact with health care professionals. Recently there has been an increased focus on the needs of individuals who are living with and beyond cancer and on the quality of care that these individuals experience. The importance of explicitly assessing psychological needs at key points in the patient pathway and providing psychological care as part of routine care planning is now being acknowledged.

Cancer–Related Body Image Concerns

Appearance and Functional Changes

Cancer and cancer treatments can significantly change appearance and body integrity, particularly in some cancers. For some people the distress associated with cancer centers on appearance-related changes that may act as persistent reminders of the disease. Such distress can trigger preexisting vulnerabilities to psychological disorders and adjustment problems. Appearance changes are particularly traumatic when accompanied by functional changes (e.g., loss of speech) because multiple stressors may trigger appearance-related cognitions more frequently.

Some cancers have visible appearance effects (e.g., disfigurement from head and neck cancer). Less observable appearance changes, for example, lymphedema (swelling caused by drainage failure in the lymphatic system), can also have a significant negative impact on appearance and can influence many aspects of an individual's life.

The speed with which appearance changes occur can also influence psychological adjustment. A patient who experiences gradual loss (e.g., hair) has some time to adjust, whereas the surgical loss of a body part happens suddenly. The degree to which the change in appearance is permanent can also affect patients' responses. Some patients cope well only because they are told that the changes are temporary (e.g., temporary ileostomy) and may operate in denial therefore failing to adapt in the short term. Many appearance changes are reversible or can be minimized. Some patients now undergo immediate surgical reconstruction, thus avoiding the need to adjust to dramatically altered appearance. For example, approximately one-third of women who undergo mastectomy opt for immediate breast reconstruction.

Sensory Changes

In addition to appearance changes, cancer and its treatment may result in sensory changes, including auditory (e.g., changes in speech production for patients with laryngeal cancer, or the noises produced by an artificial limb used to replace an amputated limb due to osteosarcoma), olfactory (e.g., colorectal tumors result in placement of a stoma), or tactile changes (e.g., alterations in breast sensation in patients with breast reconstruction). These sensory changes can also influence how others respond to the patient and may be viewed as important as appearance-related changes to both patient and close others.

Treatment and Decision Making

Surgery may involve removal of a body part in addition to the tumor. This is mostly associated with short-term effects, although it may involve longer-term reductions in body satisfaction (such as with cystectomy for bladder cancer) or increases in body image discomfort (such as that experienced by some women for up to 2 years after mastectomy). Surgery to an internal body part, although not publicly visible, can cause significant body image distress because of its particular psychological importance (e.g., the removal of a testicle). Scarring resulting from surgery, as occurs when a bowel resection is done, can also be distressing. Interestingly, a small portion of patients consider themselves to be "incomplete" as a result of cancer surgery, a factor associated with increased risk of psychopathology.

Body image concerns may also be focused on external devices, such as when a stoma or an external feeding device is needed. Some women who undergo mastectomy without reconstruction report having difficulty adjusting to breast prostheses. Indeed, many women report more problems adjusting to the prostheses than to the surgical change in appearance (e.g., mastectomy scars).

Chemotherapy can also affect appearance, for example, by causing hair loss or by requiring the presence of catheters. Additionally, corticosteroids may cause changes in facial appearance, and cancer may result in pallor or postural changes associated with fatigue. Women with breast cancer may experience weight gain because of treatment-induced menopause, hormone treatments, changes in endocrine function, overall activity level, and possibly overeating. Radiotherapy can be associated with visible dermatological changes. Moreover, the body marking used for treatment planning concerns some patients.

These appearance-related changes resulting from treatment are often ranked as more severe than side effects such as nausea, insomnia, breathlessness, and fatigue. Patients' responses to such changes, though not always apparent, can significantly affect their self-confidence and overall well-being and therefore warrant careful consideration. In some instances, diminished self-confidence does not return to pretreatment levels, even when prior appearance is restored.

People with decisions to make about appearance-changing cancer treatment need support when evaluating how their thoughts, beliefs, and feelings about appearance may influence these decisions. For example, women who choose lumpectomy over mastectomy usually have more anticipatory anxiety concerns about appearance, and breast-conserving surgery does seem to have fewer negative body image effects. Although women are likely to place more importance on survival when it comes to deciding about cancer treatments, there may be a minority for whom appearance is so important that they opt for a medically less desirable alternative. Some patients may refuse any treatment rather than undergo extremely disfiguring surgery, such as radical vulvectomy.

Surgery may also be offered to women who have a high genetic risk of developing cancer (e.g., risk-reducing mastectomy or oophorectomy). Women considering this form of surgery are often quite concerned about the potential impact on appearance and subsequent reactions of their partner. Although the majority of women who undergo risk-reducing mastectomy and breast reconstruction experience positive psychological benefits, a proportion report negative effects on appearance and feelings of femininity. Some patients experience skin necrosis, nipple loss, infection, and pain, as well as the perception that the breast feels unnatural when touched, which increases the likelihood of dissatisfaction. In gen eral, body image outcomes are hard to predict. For example, patients who undergo reconstruction surgery may still experience dissatisfaction with body change(s) to an extent that influences their daily living.

In summary, there is no demonstrable relationship between size, severity or visibility of change, and level of psychological distress. The effect of body change(s), such as hair loss, should also not be overlooked in men who often experience similar feelings to women.

Children and Adolescents

Fan and Eiser (2009) have published an informative systematic literature review on body image of children and adolescents. Overall there is currently insufficient evidence to support the hypothesis that children and adolescents with cancer have poorer body image than healthy peers. Adolescents appear to have more concerns than younger children, and males appear to cope better than females with appearance change. Appearance change is more important particularly after treatment, during remission, or following discharge due to the impact in relation to social interaction. Subjective perception of physical appearance is important and cognitive appraisal of physical appearance-related characteristics affects overall psychosocial adjustment.

While difficulties with body image can result in higher levels of anxiety and depression and more behavioral problems, social support can reduce the overall impact and enhance adjustment. Social networks, such as friends, partners, or family, play an important role by allowing the individual (child, adolescent, or adult) to test the reactions of others, reintegrate their experience, and regain confidence in different situations. Additionally, some individuals benefit from formal or informal support from other individuals with the experience of cancer. Adolescents with cancer may be less inclined to report difficulties, and this is an important point to consider when evaluating body image concerns in this population.

Conceptualization of Body Image in Oncology

Prevailing models of body image in cancer have been overly simplistic (e.g., focusing on negative/positive or secure/insecure dimensions) and limiting. However, a heuristic, multidimensional model of body image in oncology was developed in 2000 by White (see Figure 38.1). From the perspective of this model, clinicians and researchers need to understand the value attached to the body part affected by cancer. Patients should be asked about appearance concerns, and if these exist, be given the opportunity to describe their thoughts, feelings, behaviors, life experiences, and beliefs related to appearance.

People who have greater levels of investment in body parts affected

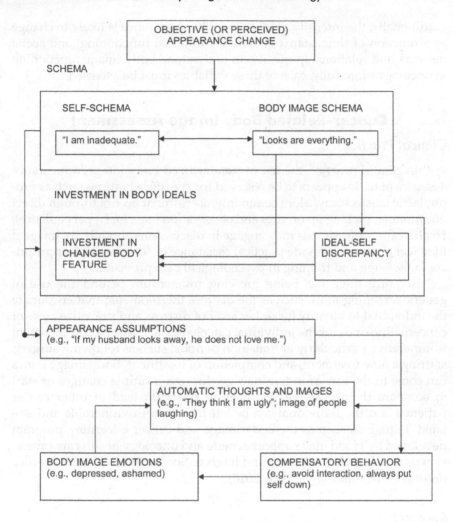

FIGURE 38.1. A heuristic model of important body image dimensions.

by cancer are more likely to experience psychological problems related to appearance change. However, Carver and colleagues demonstrated that patients with greater investment in appearance were more resilient when it came to self-perceptions of general attractiveness, femininity, and sexual desirability. They also found that investment in body integrity or intactness had an adverse effect on social and recreational functioning and produced greater self-alienation. Although these findings are limited by the use of an nonvalidated measure, they reinforce the critical observation that we should not assume that high levels of appearance investment invariably have a globally deleterious effect on other psychological variables.

Additionally, the intensity of investment in appearance is likely to change as a function of time, status of cancer, emotional functioning, and social network and relationship quality. To understand body image functioning in oncology more fully, each of these variables must be assessed.

Cancer-Related Body Image Assessment

Clinical Practice

Within clinical practice, the use of standardized body image/appearance assessment tools appears to be reserved for specific situations such as prophylactic mastectomy. More commonly, assessment occurs through direct questioning, picking up on cues and observation (e.g., for hypervigilance). Health care professionals may engage in discussions about body image if they feel unable to provide practical assistance or feel they lack appropriate knowledge and training in psychological care provision.

Recently there has being growing momentum behind the use of generic screening tools, such as the distress thermometer, that encourage the individual to identify his or her level of distress and prioritize areas of concern. Priorities for the individual can change and therefore assessment is imperative particularly at transition periods, such as following surgery, starting a new treatment, and completion of treatment. Body image issues can come to the fore as individuals go through multiple changes or start to compare themselves against healthy peers (instead of other cancer patients) and the individual can be left feeling both vulnerable and isolated. Initiatives such as the body image and cancer e-learning program developed by Hood may support generic and oncology health care professionals to improve assessment and intervention(s) within clinical practice (*learnzone.macmillan.org.uk*; July 2010).

Research

Body image assessment within oncology is still primitive. Assessment methods have included open-ended questions, semistructured interviews, and self-report measures. Some assessments consist of single-item evaluations, and most questionnaires lack adequate standardization, have poor psychometric properties, and/or are insufficiently validated. Some measurement strategies may have variable sensitivity to assessing body image change. The content of many currently available and well-validated body image measures is not suitable for use in oncology because the focus is on weight-related appearance. However, some measures, such as Cash's Appearance Schemas Inventory—Revised (ASI-R) and his Situational Inventory of Body-Image Dysphoria (SIBID), are readily applicable with little or no modification (see Chapters 5, 15, and 18). More recently, Carr and colleagues have developed a short form of the Derriford Appearance

Scale (DAS24) that measures appearance-related self-consciousness and social anxiety. The DAS24 has been validated in both clinical and nonclinical populations and can be used in a wide variety of clinical settings.

Additionally, a few oncology-specific measures have emerged, such as the Body Image Scale (BIS) that, although not tumor-site specific, evaluates behavioral and satisfaction variables as well as self-consciousness, physical attractiveness, and physical integrity. The BIS was developed by Hopwood and colleagues and is compatible with the quality of life assessments developed by the European Organization for Research and Treatment of Cancer Quality of Life Group. Kopel and colleagues developed the Body Image Instrument for use with adolescents; it evaluates patient perception of appearance, reactions of others to appearance, and the value placed on appearance. Furthermore, Carver and colleagues devised the Measure of Body Apperception to assess attitudes reflective of investment in appearance and body integrity.

Delivering Sensitive Care

Delivery of psychological care for people with cancer would be greatly enhanced if all clinical staff were knowledgeable and competent in assessing body image (e.g., body satisfaction and level of investment in appearance), providing basic intervention, and recognizing problems requiring assessment by specialists in psychosocial oncology. These specialists can evaluate a range of related psychosocial variables (e.g., appearance schemas and compensatory behaviors) and provide appropriate intervention at the level required. There should be equitable access to specialist services and this is particularly important for those professionals who treat cancers that have a major negative impact on appearance and function.

Conclusions and Future Directions

There is an urgent need for consensus on what constitutes clinically significant body image disturbance in cancer survivors. Through understanding cancer patients' experiences the true impact of body image change(s) can be appreciated. Given their intensive patient contact, oncology nurses may be in a particularly advantageous position to apply an improved understanding of body image variables in cancer assessment and treatment.

Further research needs to be performed to demonstrate the effectiveness of interventions for body image problems among persons with cancer. For example, Cash's cognitive-behavioral program for body image self-help or therapy can be tailored to assist this population (see Chapter 47). More work is also needed to apply mainstream body image research to cancer. In general, taking a multidimensional approach to research and clinical practice that is informed by current body image theory is essential. Fortunately, some of these developments are occurring. Recent publication of cancer-specific body image assessment tools will likely assist in establishing validated models that can be used to guide assessment, psychological and medical treatment, and outcome evaluation within cancer care settings.

Informative Readings

Bessell, A., & Moss, T. (2007). Evaluating the effectiveness of psychosocial interventions for individuals with visible differences: A systematic review of the empirical literature. *Body Image: An International Journal of Research, 4,* 227–238.—An overview identifying methodological limitations of studies and lack of evidence to support the effectiveness of existing interventions.

Carr, T., Moss, T., & Harris, D. (2005). The DAS24: A short form of the Derriford Appearance Scale DAS59 to measure individual responses to living with problems of appearance. *British Journal of Health Psychology, 10,* 285–298.—A description of the development, validity, and psychometric properties of a short body image questionnaire assessing self-consciousness and social anxiety in both clinical and nonclinical populations.

Carver, C. S., Pozo-Kaderman, C., Price, A., Noriegs, V., Harris, S., Derhagopian, R. P., et al. (1998). Concern about aspects of body image and adjustment to early breast cancer. *Psychosomatic Medicine, 60,* 168–174.—A prospective evaluation of the role of appearance investment and body image integrity in a group of women with early-stage breast cancer.

Cash, T. F. (2008). *The body image workbook: An 8-step program for learning to like your looks* (2nd ed.). Oakland, CA: New Harbinger Publications.—A structured, empirically supported cognitive-behavioral approach to body image improvement.

DeFrank, J. T., Bahn Mehta, C. C., Stein, K. D., & Baker, F. (2007). Body image dissatisfaction in cancer survivors. *Oncology Nursing Forum, 34,* 36–41.—A quantitative study identifying factors associated with body image dissatisfaction and comparing results across six different cancer types.

Fan, S.-Y., & Eiser, C. (2009). Body image of children and adolescents with cancer: A systematic review. *Body Image: An International Journal of Research, 6,* 247–256.—A narrative review and discussion of research on body image and psychosocial functioning of youth with cancer.

Hood, C. (2010). Project to improve care for people coping with changes in body image. *Cancer Nursing Practice, 9,* 26–32.—An overview of the development of a body image tool kit incorporating an e-learning program for general health care professionals and a workbook for individuals with cancer.

Hopwood, P., Fletcher, I., Lee, A., & Al Ghazal, S. (2001). A body image scale for use with cancer patients. *European Journal of Cancer, 37,* 189–197.—A description of the development and psychometric properties of a brief assessment scale for body image variables in cancer.

Kopel, S. J., Eiser, C., Cool, P., Grimer, R. J., & Carter, S. R. (1998). Assessment of body image in survivors of childhood cancer. *Journal of Pediatric Psychology, 23*, 141–147.—An outline of the development of the Body Image Instrument, a 28-item measure of general appearance, body competence, others' reaction to appearance, value of appearance, and self-consciousness.

Rumsey, N., Clarke, A., White, P., Wyn-Williams, M., & Garlick, W. (2004). Altered body image: Appearance-related concerns of people with visible disfigurement. *Journal of Advanced Nursing, 48*, 443–453.—A cross-sectional study using qualitative and quantitative methodology to identify the extent and type of psychosocial needs of outpatients with visible disfigurement.

Varni, J. W., Katz, E. R., Colegrove, R., & Dolgin, M. (1995). Perceived physical appearance and adjustment in children with newly diagnosed cancer: A path analytic model. *Journal of Behavioral Medicine, 18*, 261–277.—A well-executed study that tests a conceptual model of the contribution of perceived physical appearance to depressive symptoms, self-esteem, and social anxiety.

Wallace, M. L., Harcourt, D., Rumsey, N., & Foot, A. (2007). Managing appearance changes resulting from cancer treatment: Resilience in adolescent females. *Psycho-oncology, 16*, 1019–1027.—A study using semistructured interviews to explore the experience of appearance change during and after cancer treatment.

White, C. A. (2000). Body image dimensions and cancer: A heuristic cognitive behavioural model. *Psycho-oncology, 9*, 183–192.—A review that argues for integration of mainstream body image research with body image research in cancer care.

CHAPTER 39

Body Image Issues
in Obstetrics and Gynecology

HELEN SKOUTERIS

Introduction

Body image issues in obstetrics and gynecology impact negatively on
women's health and well-being. Yet, alarmingly, a recent survey by Leddy
and colleagues, of 458 Fellows of the American College of Obstetricians
and Gynecologists, revealed that less than one-third of physicians assessed
for body image concerns during routine gynecological and obstetrical
care. This is surprising for two reasons: (1) obstetricians and gynecologists often act as primary care physicians for women over the life cycle,
and (2) body dissatisfaction is often associated with negative psychological functioning, such as depression and maladaptive behaviors (e.g.,
unhealthy eating and extreme weight loss behaviors) that have serious
negative implications for women's health and well-being, and potentially
also for the unborn fetus during pregnancy. This chapter extends the one
on this topic in the previous edition of this handbook, reviewing literature
published since January 2000, and concluding with future directions for
research in this area.

Obstetrics

The reproductive phase, which includes both pregnancy and the early
postpartum, is a period of significant developmental transition compris-
ing numerous physiognomical and psychosocial changes, including, but

342

not limited to, hormonal fluctuations, the experience of pregnancy-related physical symptoms and changes to appearance (e.g., nausea, backache, varicose veins, stretch marks, acne, and swollen ankles and feet), changes to one's interactions and relationships with others, and the adaptation to being a new mother. In addition, the rapid physical changes that occur in body and shape over a relatively short (40-week) period make pregnancy an ideal time to examine body image prospectively. There can be significant psychological and emotional sequelae as a result of these changes. One such sequel is a concern about body image. During pregnancy, women are likely to reevaluate their body image over time as their size increases, body shape changes, and pregnancy-related physical symptoms become more pronounced. This potentially allows for a more powerful test of the factors leading to body dissatisfaction than at other times in women's lives when body shape remains relatively stable.

Prior to 2005, research in the area of body image issues during the reproductive phase was either cross sectional, or if focused on pregnancy, prospective to the end of the second trimester only, and if focused on the postpartum, prospective only to 6 weeks postbirth. In 2005, two prospective studies that tracked women longitudinally from the first or early to mid-second trimester to the mid-late third trimester in pregnancy were published. Rocco and colleagues investigated the effect of pregnancy on eating disorders, dietary habits, and body image perception using the Body Attitudes Test at 12-, 22-, and 34-weeks gestation, and at 2 days and 4 months postbirth. They showed that eating disorder symptomatology, subthreshold eating disturbance, and body satisfaction improved during the middle phase of the pregnancy, 22-weeks gestation, with a return to previous poorer levels in the postpartum. It appears that pregnancy is a time of increased body acceptance for women with eating disorder symptoms, as well as for women with no history of dieting or disordered eating, suggesting that the health of the developing fetus takes priority over women's body image. More recently Clark and her colleagues provided qualitative data from interviews conducted with perinatal women who also spoke about placing the well-being of their developing fetus above their body aesthetics; women noted that this increased functionality of their body helped them cope with the body changes and physical symptoms associated with pregnancy.

The other study published in 2005, by Skouteris and her colleagues, was the first of a series of studies that resulted from a program of research with two main aims. The first aim was to examine body image changes in women as they progress through pregnancy and the postpartum. Two key aspects of body image were examined: (1) body dissatisfaction as assessed by attitudes using the four subscales of the Body Attitudes Questionnaire most suitable to pregnant women: feeling fat, strength and fitness, salience of weight and shape, and attractiveness; and (2) discrepancies between current and ideal body size as measured by figural stimuli.

Pregnancy Figure Rating Scales (PFRS), one version for *current* body size and the other for *ideal* body size, were developed with ratings from 1 (very small) to 10 (very large) for depictions of three body parts: bust, stomach, and buttocks. Findings in relation to the first aim revealed that women felt less fat at late pregnancy than at any other time point during pregnancy and prior to pregnancy. Conversely, women reported feeling more fit and strong prior to the pregnancy than they did during the pregnancy, and feeling more attractive prior to pregnancy than they did during early to mid-second trimester and late pregnancy. Women also adapted to body changes over the course of their pregnancy, choosing a more realistic ideal body size on the PFRS as their pregnancy progressed.

The second aim of this program of research was to determine predictors of body image concerns during pregnancy and the postpartum. Skouteris and colleagues found that depressive symptoms, physical appearance comparisons, and perceived sociocultural pressure to be thin at early to mid-second trimester (16–23-weeks gestation) predicted feeling less attractive in late pregnancy (32–39-weeks gestation), and that perceived sociocultural pressure, depressive symptoms, and public self-consciousness, at early to mid-second trimester, were significant univariate predictors of feeling fat late in pregnancy. Moreover, the experience of weight-related teasing at 24–31-weeks gestation predicted feeling less attractive in late pregnancy. Skouteris and colleagues were the first to show that factors noted in the general body image literature as predictors of body image also appeared to impact on body dissatisfaction during pregnancy.

As an extension of this research reported in 2005, Clark and colleagues conducted a prospective longitudinal study from early to mid-second trimester to 12-months postbirth. The findings of both studies revealed that the dissipation of feeling fat during late pregnancy does not continue into the postpartum. Women told Clark and her colleagues, in their qualitative study, that there is no longer an excuse to be large when the baby is born: "Now I look at my stomach and think 'well, now she's not in there it's not so good' ... you have a baby and then you're left with a big stomach and then you've got to try to get rid of it" (p. 338). Moreover, feeling fatter in the postpartum and having a higher salience of weight and shape may also be related to unrealistic expectations that women have about the speed and ease with which their body will return to its prepregnancy shape after the birth.

Clark and colleagues also reported, with prospective data, that depressive symptoms appear to be more strongly predictive of body image disturbance (BID) than are body image concerns predicting later increases in depression. Given that depression involves negative appraisals of the self, body dissatisfaction may follow, as body dissatisfaction too is a negative appraisal of the self. However, Walker and colleagues showed that body image after birth was both a significant concurrent and prospective predictor of depressive symptoms 2 days after delivery and 6 weeks postbirth, in a low-income, ethnically diverse sample of women. Similarly, Symons Downs and colleagues reported that body image concerns earlier on in pregnancy were predictive of higher depressive symptoms later on in pregnancy and the postpartum. Further research is needed to clarify the causal relationship between depressive symptoms and body image concerns through pregnancy and the postpartum.

Given the established links between depressive symptoms and body dissatisfaction in both nonpregnant and pregnant women, and between maternal attachment and antenatal depressive symptoms, Haedt and Keel were recently prompted to examine the cross-sectional associations between maternal attachment, depressive symptoms, and body dissatisfaction during pregnancy. Contrary to previous findings, there was no association between maternal attachment and depression here; nor were maternal attachment and body dissatisfaction associated. Maternal attachment was only positively correlated with number of weeks gestation and, interestingly, body dissatisfaction, *not* depression, moderated this association, suggesting that screening for high levels of body dissatisfaction during pregnancy may be as important as screening for depression.

Finally, Kamysheva and colleagues extended previous research by showing that greater body dissatisfaction was associated not only with increased depressive symptoms but also with lower self-esteem during pregnancy (15–25-weeks gestation); indeed, self-esteem mediated the relationships between depression and feeling fatter, less attractive, and having greater salience of shape and weight. Their findings further extended previous research by also revealing, for the first time, that pregnancy-related physical symptoms were related to body image concerns, specifically to feeling less strong and fit (frequency of symptoms, level of discomfort of symptoms, and effects of symptoms on life) and to greater salience of weight and shape (level of discomfort of symptoms, and effects of symptoms on life). Physical symptoms were related to the pregnancy but not the prepregnancy strength/fitness scores, suggesting that the pregnancy-related fatigue and nausea may play a role in how strong and fit women perceive themselves to be earlier on in pregnancy.

Gynecology

At the outset of this chapter, the fact was highlighted that gynecologists often act as primary care physicians for women over the life cycle. Gynecological care ranges from the routine Pap smear to polycystic ovary syndrome (PCOS) to the more serious genital, cervical, and breast cancers. There is now an established literature that reveals that breast, cervical, and genital cancers can impact negatively on women's body image (see Chapter 38). Just as public self-consciousness, depressive symptoms, poor self-esteem, and physical symptoms are associated with BIDs in pregnant and nonpregnant women, these associations can also be present in women with breast cancer and other forms of cancer. In relation to breast cancer specifically, prophylactic mastectomy has been shown to reduce the risk of breast cancer in women who are genetically predisposed. However, the body image concerns pertaining to mastectomy have not been studied extensively in women who have undergone bilateral prophylactic mastectomy (BPM). An integrative review of the literature by McGaughey revealed that only 13 studies have examined body image after BPM; 11 of these used a retrospective design that ignored women's body image prior to BPM, and only two studies have evaluated body image before and after BPM. The findings of her review revealed that up to 50% of women who undertake a BPM suffer a negative effect on body image after the surgery. As genetic testing for breast cancer risk and BPM become more widely used, it is imperative that potential negative effects of BPM, including BIDs, should be discussed at length with women who are considering the procedure.

Another gynecological disorder that has been associated in recent times with body image concerns is premenstrual dysphoric disorder (PDD), a severe form of premenstrual syndrome. De Berardis and colleagues found that alexithymic women with PDD exhibited significantly greater body dissatisfaction than nonalexithymics. Alexithymia is characterized by the inability to express one's emotions and feelings in words. Moreover, De Berardis argued that, given that body dissatisfaction appears to be related to severity of premenstrual depressive symptoms, the combination of mood and BIDs may increase the risk for developing eating disorders, especially bulimia nervosa. Further research that is longitudinal in design is needed to evaluate this hypothesis.

We also know that body image concerns are common among overweight and obese women, and recent evidence provided by Liao and colleagues suggests that this is especially the case for women with PCOS. PCOS is the most common endocrine disorder in women of childbearing age, and women who have this disorder are typically large in terms of weight status. Hence, designing interventions that target reduction of body dissatisfaction, such as the implementation of exercise programs, and evaluating the effectiveness of such programs is essential in order to combat the distress with body size and shape that is prevalent among women with PCOS.

Finally, there is some evidence, albeit limited, that suggests that the physical changes associated with menopause may result in some women feeling less attractive than their premenopausal self and that the symptoms women experience during menopause may influence body image. Deeks and McCabe showed that although menopausal women revealed lower ratings of attractiveness and fitness compared to premenopausal women, they were slightly more accepting of a larger body size. They concluded that changes brought on by both age and menopause may influence how a woman feels during this transition in her life; moreover, women during menopause may feel that society accepts that they will no longer be as thin as premenopausal women. More recently, McKinley and Lyon extended these findings by showing that anxiety related to women's appearance and aging was found to be related to women's body surveillance and body shame, and that positive menopausal attitudes, specifically related to appearance, were related to a more positive self-esteem. Given the surprisingly limited research in this area, a better understanding of how both aging and menopause influence body image changes later on in women's lives is clearly warranted.

Conclusions and Future Directions

This chapter focused on the correlates, both cross sectional and prospective, of body image issues in obstetrics and gynecology. An emerging area of research that will have further implications for body dissatisfaction during pregnancy and the postpartum is excessive gestational weight gain. The importance of childbearing in the development of body image concerns in women has been recognized for over a decade; in particular, it is a time at which many women are at risk of gaining excessive weight. Given the distress that many women experience with the change in their bodies during pregnancy and the postpartum, this is a time where interventions to address overweight/obesity and body dissatisfaction in women are likely to be successful. However, the prevention of high levels of body dissatisfaction and, potentially, obesity during the reproductive phase will only be effective when models of risk factors during these years have been examined systematically and rigorously and the interplay between risk factors is well understood. Clearly, further research is needed to foster the development of evidence-based models and related clinical interventions for promoting psychological, social, and physical well-being during the perinatal period. This is also the case for body image concerns in gynecology. It is important that women have available assistance while they cope with changes that are necessarily associated with gynecological disorders and that might lead to BID. Screening for body dissatisfaction, extreme weight loss behaviors, and/or a history of eating disorders during routine obstetrical and gynecological visits should be considered by the physicians and other allied health professionals who care for women during the different stages in their lives.

Informative Readings

Clark, A., Skouteris, H., Wertheim, E., Paxton, S., & Milgrom, J. (2009). My baby body: A qualitative insight into women's body-related experiences and mood during pregnancy and the postpartum. *Journal of Reproductive and Infant Psychology, 27,* 330–345.—A qualitative analysis of women's body image and mood through pregnancy and the early postpartum.

Clark, A., Skouteris, H., Wertheim, E., Paxton, S., & Milgrom, J. (2009). The relationship between depression and body dissatisfaction across pregnancy and the postpartum: A prospective study. *Journal of Health Psychology, 14,* 23–31.—A longitudinal prospective study that examined the relationship between depressive symptoms and body dissatisfaction through pregnancy and the first year postbirth.

De Berardis, D., Campanella, D., Gambi, F., Sepede, G., Carano, A., Pelusi, L., et al. (2005). Alexithymia and body image disturbances in women with premenstrual dysphoric disorder. *Journal of Psychosomatic Obstetrics and Gynaecology, 26,* 257–264.—A cross-sectional evaluation of alexithymia and body image in women with PDD.

Deeks, A. A., & McCabe, M. P. (2001). Menopause stage and age and perceptions of body image. *Psychology and Health, 16,* 367–379.—A cross-sectional analysis of perceptions of appearance, health, fitness, body image, and preoccupation with weight in pre-, peri-, and postmenopausal women.

Haedt, A., & Keel, P. (2007). Maternal attachment, depression, and body dissatisfaction in pregnant women. *Journal of Reproductive and Infant Psychology, 25,* 285–295.—A cross-sectional evaluation of psychological factors that influence maternal attachment during pregnancy, including body image.

Kamysheva, E., Skouteris, H., Wertheim, E., Paxton, S., & Milgrom, J. (2008). Examination of a multi-factorial model of body-related experiences during pregnancy: The relationships among physical symptoms, sleep quality, depression, self-esteem, and negative body attitudes. *Body Image: An International Journal of Research, 5,* 152–163.—A cross-sectional assessment of the relationships among several body experiences/attitudes during pregnancy, including four aspects of body image—feeling fat, attractiveness, salience of shape and weight, and strength and fitness.

Leddy, M. A., Jones, C., Morgan, M. A., & Schulkin, J. (2009). Eating disorders and obstetric–gynecologic care. *Journal of Women's Health, 18,* 1395–1401.—An evaluation of obstetrician–gynecologists' eating disorder-related knowledge, attitudes, and practices.

Liao, L. M., Nesic, J., Chadwick, P. M., Brooke-Wavell, K., & Prelevic, G. M. (2008). Exercise and body image distress in overweight and obese women with polycystic ovary syndrome: A pilot investigation. *Gynecological Endocrinology, 24,* 555–561.—A pilot study evaluating the effect of a self-directed walking program on body image in obese women with PCOS.

McGaughey, A. (2006). Body image after bilateral prophylactic mastectomy: An integrative literature review. *Journal of Midwifery and Women's Health, 51,* e45–e49.—Reviews research that has examined the effect of prophylactic mastectomy on women's subsequent body image.

McKinley, N. M., & Lyon, L. A. (2008). Menopausal attitudes, objectified body consciousness, aging anxiety, and body esteem: European American women's body experiences in midlife. *Body Image: An International Journal of Research,*

5, 375–380.—Shows that menopausal attitudes and menopausal appearance attitudes are related to body surveillance.

Rocco, P., Orbitello, B., Perini, L., Pera, V., Ciano, R., & Balestrieri, M. (2005). Effects of pregnancy on eating attitudes and disorders: A prospective study. *Journal of Psychosomatic Research, 59*, 175–179.—A longitudinal evaluation of how pregnancy influences the course of eating disorders, and body image perception and satisfaction in normal women and in women with a history of disordered eating.

Skouteris, H., Carr, R., Wertheim, E., Paxton, S., & Duncombe, D. (2005). A prospective study of factors that lead to body image dissatisfaction during pregnancy. *Body Image: An International Journal of Research, 2*, 347–361.—A longitudinal analysis of the social and psychological factors earlier on in pregnancy that might impact on body dissatisfaction during late pregnancy.

Symons Downs, D., DiNallo, J. M., & Kirner, T. L. (2008). Determinants of pregnancy and postpartum depression: Prospective influences of depressive symptoms, body image satisfaction, and exercise behavior. *Annals of Behavioral Medicine, 36*, 54–63.—A prospective analysis of women's exercise and psychological health behaviors across each trimester of pregnancy and 6 weeks postbirth.

Walker, L., Timmerman, G., Kim, M., & Sterling, B. (2002). Relationships between body image and depressive symptoms during postpartum in ethnically diverse, low income women. *Women and Health, 36*, 101–121.—A prospective analysis during the first 6 weeks postbirth examining the influence of ethnicity, sociodemographic factors, and psychological factors on body dissatisfaction.

CHAPTER 40

Body Image Issues in Rheumatology

MEENAKSHI JOLLY

Introduction

Rheumatic diseases are conditions that cause inflammation, swelling, and pain in the joints and/or muscles. These diseases may severely impair movement and result in visible alterations in the body's appearance. Over 21% of U.S. adults (46 million people) acknowledge that they have doctor-diagnosed arthritis. Because arthritis is the leading cause of disability in adults, it is not surprising that they account for over 77 million ambulatory care visits annually. Nearly 27 million have clinical osteoarthritis. Of the other rheumatic diseases, rheumatoid arthritis affects 1.3 million, spondylo-arthropathies 0.6–2.4 million, systemic lupus erythematosus 161,000–322,000, and systemic sclerosis 49,000 U.S. adults.

Pain, fatigue, and decreased range of motion at the joints may lead to functional or role impairment and disability. Furthermore, patients with rheumatologic diseases may develop inflammation in other organs, causing impairment and/or damage, visible or invisible disfigurement, depression, and fibromyalgia. Side effects of medications are frequently visible. Therefore, quality of life may be reduced. Some of these diseases preferentially afflict women and do so at a younger age than most chronic diseases. All these factors may lead to body image concerns.

Patients with rheumatic diseases are concerned about changes in their body, function and appearance, and call it an "unmet need." Physicians tend to focus on the physical manifestations of rheumatic diseases (e.g., pain, swelling) and less on how the disease affects patients' perception of their body; and how these changes may affect their psychosocial health. Studies of body image in patients with rheumatic diseases are scant despite an obvious need for them. This chapter discusses patients with rheumatic diseases, their unique body image concerns, and the body image literature.

Osteoarthritis

Osteoarthritis (OA) is the most common joint disease, is due to the "wear and tear" of joints, and is degenerative. It more often affects middle- to older-aged groups, and women. It results in joint swelling, pain, limited mobility, and loss of independence. Body image concerns are a central theme in those with severe OA. Among patients with a history of congenital hip dislocation, development of OA is common. During childhood these patients may limp, develop leg length differences, disability, feel inferior, and may not want to be seen in public.

Changes in posture with increasing disability are a concern for some patients with OA whose efforts to camouflage their disfigurement with clothing have been unsuccessful. In various studies, these patients reported difficulties doing activities of daily living that can promote a poor body image. For example, a woman with severe OA reported having to remain half-standing while urinating. Others have indicated body image distress after total hip replacement surgery for severe OA. They felt a strong sense of loss of their leg or strangeness regarding the artificial joint, but this sensation decreased with time. Only one study has quantitatively examined body image among patients with OA. Carr compared 106 patients with OA and 458 with rheumatoid arthritis and found body image to be significantly worse among those with OA.

Patients with hip OA experience adverse effects on their sexual and marital health due to hip pain, stiffness, and loss of libido. Assistive devices, such as walking sticks, have not been universally accepted by patients with arthritis despite acknowledgment of the possibility of improving their mobility. Some of the reported barriers to their use include self-consciousness, lost pride, and fear of losing independence.

Rheumatoid Arthritis

Rheumatoid arthritis (RA) is a chronic, systemic autoimmune condition that usually affects people between 40 and 50 years of age. It is three times more prevalent among women. Joints are often involved; however, lungs, eyes, and blood cells are also at risk. Joint inflammation manifests as pain, swelling, and stiffness in multiple joints, most frequently involving hands and wrists. Cervical spine, shoulders, hips, knees, and ankles may be involved, causing mobility problems and functional restrictions. Lung or eye involvement and anemia may also contribute to these functional restrictions. Hand disfigurement, rheumatoid nodules on the hands and elbows, loss of independence, side effects of medications (corticosteroids and immuno-suppressives), effects on sexual activity, and depression may lead to or worsen body image concerns.

Research has indicated that 34% of patients with early RA and 30% with chronic RA feel unattractive due to their disease. In a qualitative study, Williams and Barlow explored body experiences within the context of arthritis. Patients' principal concerns related to body parts most affected by their disease that include visibly swollen and disfigured hands, knees, and feet. One patient described her fingers as all twisted and having a gargoyle appearance. Side effects of treatment, especially cortisone-induced weight gain, worsened how patients with RA perceived their weight and shape. Women felt a step behind their peer group in social circumstances, and that the "arthritis had robbed them of 20 years of life." Some women felt that their femininity was adversely affected. They were "self-conscious," "uncomfortable," and "embarrassed" about their appearance and mobility in social situations; and felt less attractive to their partner and potential partners. Their body changes provoked negative emotions and isolation.

Concern about physical appearance was also evident from a study by Vamos and colleagues, who examined the perceptions of hand appearance among 80 women with RA. Results indicated that the objective appearance of hands predicted negative emotions; body image factors and negative emotions predicted the desire for reparative hand surgery. Among women with RA and visibly abnormal feet, loss of femininity, frustration, anger, and anxiety may occur. Wearing therapeutic footwear has been viewed unfavorably, causing similar negative emotions and concerns about how others would perceive the footwear, their sexuality, and femininity. Talking about patients' feelings about changes in their body due to their arthritis may be seen as a taboo area that is avoided by their partner and friends, as well as by health professionals.

Although there is some evidence that, at the time of presentation, patients with early RA report perceptions of lower attractiveness, Cornwell and Schmitt found that body image among 26 patients with RA was similar to healthy controls. In contrast, other studies have found that self-perceived body attractiveness was lower among patients with RA than college women, and that juvenile RA patients were intensely disparaging about their own body, felt fatter, and they had a poorer body image than matched, healthy controls. Moreover, Ben Tovim and Walker found the intensity of both body disparagement and weight/shape concerns to be inversely correlated with the age of RA onset. Monaghan and colleagues found that disability and self-perceived appearance predicted 31% of the variance in depression among patients with RA. In research by the present author, poorer self-reported body image was found among women with

RA than among healthy age-matched controls, and body image correlated inversely with depression and directly with overall mental health. Body image in RA did not correlate with the presence of rheumatoid factor (an antibody present among patients with RA), disease activity, functional status, irreversible bone damage, or visible disfigurement.

Systemic Lupus Erythematosus

Systemic lupus erythematosus (SLE) is a systemic autoimmune disease that disproportionately affects young women; women are affected nine times more frequently than men. It is usually more prevalent in ethnic minorities. Health outcomes including health-related quality of life are poor among patients with SLE, and especially worse among ethnic minorities. SLE can cause inflammation and damage in any organ. About two-thirds of patients develop cutaneous manifestations that may be visible, transient, or permanent rashes, scars, dyspigmentation, skin dimpling, photosensitivity, and hair loss. Arthritis, serositis, nephritis, and hematological and neuropsychiatric problems are common. Patients may experience pregnancy losses, thromboembolic events, skin ulcers, and fibromyalgia. Patients with lupus nephritis and end-stage renal disease may additionally have dialysis port/shunts and calciphylaxis that may add to visible body changes. Hence, the disease may lead to significant functional impairment and disability, along with visible disfigurement.

The most common problems reported by patients with SLE include depressed feelings, reduced activity, stress, and changes in body image. In a study by Stein et al., 96% of patients with SLE had polyarthritis and 88% had cutaneous manifestations. Eighty-three percent had used corticosteroids and 68% were currently using them. Most reported a poor self-image due to the effects of the disease or its treatment on their physical appearance, work status, and sexuality. These effects included fatigue (90%), rash (68%), mood swings (67%), alopecia (63%), and pain (26%). Corticosteroids were identified as contributing to poor self-image due to associated moon faces, weight gain, low sexual desire, bruising, and sleeping difficulties.

Hale's qualitative study documented the appearance-related concerns of 10 women with SLE. All of the women experienced skin rashes; some were severely affected. Venturing out in public with visible skin disease incited stares and remarks from strangers. Efforts to conceal rashes were sometimes unsuccessful, and at times disfigured women preferred to stay indoors. During summer months, appearing in public was especially difficult while wearing a hat, long-sleeved shirts, and long skirts. Dressing this way to prevent sun exposure to their photosensitive skin at times brought unwanted attention as it set them apart from others. Moreover, concern about sun exposure, fatigue, pain, need for frequent rest, unpredictability of flares, and depression frequently resulted in women avoiding social and family activities, thus becoming isolated. More than 80% of patients with SLE identify "changes in body appearance" as "an area of unmet need." Indeed, body image recently has been recognized as an important domain for disease-targeted patient-reported outcome measures in SLE.

Research by Cornwell et al. found a poorer body image among 23 subjects with SLE than among 26 with RA and 28 healthy persons. Of women with SLE, 53% felt unattractive due to their disease. Furthermore, Curry and colleagues measured body image among 100 women with SLE and 71 disease-free controls; body image was worse in the SLE group. The present author's research group has found significant body image concern among patients with SLE and its association with disease activity, depression, and health-related quality of life. Significant sexual health concerns were reported in younger patients with greater disease activity and worse health status. Use of corticosteroids correlated with body image concerns. Body image may mediate the effects of disease activity on health-related quality of life.

In Monaghan's cross-sectional study, self-perceived appearance mediated the relationship between physical health-related quality of life and depression. In our own prospective pilot study, body image predicted health-related quality of life over time. In a recent pilot intervention study by the present author aimed at improving body image in patients with SLE, we determined that a cognitive-behavioral program (see Chapter 47) resulted in significant improvements in body image, as well as associated decrease in depression and increase in quality of life.

Systemic Sclerosis

Systemic sclerosis (SS), or scleroderma, is a multisystemic autoimmune disease characterized by fibrosis of the skin that leads to visible or invisible skin tightness. SS may also involve esophagus, stomach, bowels, lungs, kidneys, and vasculature. SS causes functional limitations and may cause facial and acral disfigurement. SS is four times more prevalent in women, and usually occurs between 30 and 50 years of age. Visible disfigurement may include hair loss, small mouth aperture, tight facial skin (giving the face a pinched appearance and causing tight skin elsewhere), dyspigmentation, coup en saber, telengectasias, morphea, digital pits, raynauds, ischemic ulcers, contraction flexures, loss of fingers or toes, and calcinosis. Weight loss may cause concern and remind patients of their disease, leading to fears that they will visibly deteriorate and not be able to recognize themselves.

According to Benrud-Larson's research with 121 patients with SS, their body image dissatisfaction, sometimes greater than that found among severe burn injury patients, was associated with age, skin tightness above the elbows, and functional disability. Depression mediated the relationship between body image dissatisfaction and psychosocial functioning.

Ankylosing Spondylitis

Ankylosing spondylitis (AS) is an inflammatory, multisystemic, autoimmune disease that occurs between 18 and 30 years of age and is three times more common among men. The most common presentation is from inflammation and damage of the spine and pelvis, which causes low-back pain, stiffness, and decreased range of motion. Other joints may also be inflamed. Posture and mobility may become visibly altered as ankylosis of the spine progresses. Eyes and blood vessels may also be involved.

Patients with AS are concerned with spinal curvature, and pain and stiffness in the neck, shoulders, back, and legs. Some perceive that their stooped posture and impaired mobility due to pain make their bodily appearance "age" beyond that expected for their chronological age. Most self-presentation concerns among men with AS involve loss of body fitness, which may motivate them to do daily physical exercises.

Other Rheumatic Diseases

Sarcoidosis is a multisystem granulomatous disease that tends to occur among young adults. It usually affects lungs but may also affect eyes, skin, joints, vasculature, lymph nodes, and blood counts. Skin involvement may range from rashes and painful nodules to disfiguring lupus pernio lesions. Dermatomyosistis and polymyositis are inflammatory myopathic conditions seen more often in women than in men, and typically in persons between 40 and 50 years of age. Proximal muscle weakness is the hallmark, which may impose major mobility restrictions. However, when it involves respiratory muscles it may be life threatening. Other organs involved frequently include lungs, which can be debilitating. An association with malignancies is known. Muscle weakness when accompanied with skin involvement suggests dermatomyositis. Various types of visible skin rashes and nail bed changes may be evident. Vasculitis is a heterogeneous set of vascular inflammatory disorders that may be accompanied by skin rashes, skin ulcers, and kidney and lung involvement. All these rheumatic conditions adversely affect body weight and functional capabilities, and are associated with visible bodily changes. Furthermore, the medications utilized to treat these disorders may cause visible bodily alterations (weight, acne, striae, hair loss, cushingoid faces), and may also cause premature ovarian failure. Thus, loss of perceived femininity may be a real concern for these patients. Unfortunately, at this time there are no published body image studies on persons with these diseases.

Conclusions and Future Directions

Rheumatic diseases cause significant adverse changes in the body, some visible, some not. These diseases can occur at a young age, especially in women. Because body image is important to one's psychosocial functioning, compliance with care, and quality of life, interdisciplinary research on these chronic disease conditions is greatly needed. Early detection and interventions may not only rehabilitate the patient and their loved ones, but also may improve overall health outcomes and reduce the direct and indirect costs of his or her medical care. Discussions on changes in body image and the effects it has or may have on patients with rheumatic conditions need to be encouraged from both sides, by the patient and the physician. This requires a major shift in the way we assess and provide medical care for these patients. Patients' beliefs that "doctors care for your body but don't care how you feel about your body" should challenge our approach toward the care of these patients. This requires interdisciplinary health care research, clinical collaboration, and above all, shifting from a biomedical model to a biopsychosocial model.

Informative Readings

Ben Tovim, D. I., & Walker, M. K. (1995). Body image, disfigurement and disability. *Journal of Psychosomatic Research*, *39*, 283–291.—Compares attitudes toward body among women with disabling and/or disfiguring disorders and compares with controls.

Benrud-Larson, L. M., Heinberg, L. J., Boling, C., Reed, J., White, B., Wigley, F. M., et al. (2003). Body image dissatisfaction among women with scleroderma: Extent and relationship to psychosocial function. *Health Psychology*, *22*, 130–139.—Examines body image dissatisfaction and its relationship to psychosocial functioning in women with scleroderma.

Carr, A. J. (1999). Beyond disability: Measuring the social and personal consequences of osteoarthritis. *Osteoarthritis and Cartilage*, *7*, 230–238.—Examines the measurement of handicap in patients with OA and RA.

Cornwell, C. J., & Schmitt, M. H. (1990). Perceived health status, self-esteem and body image in women with rheumatoid arthritis or systemic lupus erythematosus. *Research in Nursing and Health*, *13*, 99–107.—Study reporting poor body image in SLE as compared to healthy controls and patients with RA.

Curry, S. L., Levine, S. B., Corty, E., Jones, P. K., & Kurit, D. M. (1994). The impact of systemic lupus erythematosus on women's sexual functioning. *Journal of Rheumatology*, *21*, 2254–2260.—Study reporting poor body image in SLE as compared to disease-free controls.

Erkolahti, R. K., Ilonen, T., & Saarijärvi, S. (2003). Self-image of adolescents with diabetes mellitus type-I and rheumatoid arthritis. *Nordic Journal of Psychiatry*, *57*, 309–312.—Describes body image and vocational and educational goals in adolescent patients with chronic illness.

Fujita, K., Makimoto, K., & Hotokebuchi, T. (2006). Qualitative study of osteoarthritis patients' experience before and after total hip arthroplasty in Japan. *Nursing and Health Sciences, 8,* 81–87.—Qualitative study exploring the perspectives of patients with OA undergoing total hip replacement surgery before and after the surgery.

Hale, E. D., Treharne, G. J., Norton, Y., Lyons, A. C., Douglas, K. M. J., Erb, N., et al. (2006). "Concealing the evidence": The importance of appearance concerns for patients with systemic lupus erythematosus. *Lupus, 15,* 532–540.—Examines the concerns of patients with SLE about their appearance and the recognition of this by health care professionals using semistructured interviews.

Joachim, G., & Acorn, S. (2003). Life with a rare chronic disease: The scleroderma experience. *Journal of Advanced Nursing, 42,* 598–606.—Focus group study of the perspective of patients with scleroderma to understand the experiences of living with this disease.

Jolly, M., Mikolaitis, R. A., Cornejo, J., Sequeira, W., Cash, T. F., et al. (2011). Body image in patients with systemic lupus erythematosus. *International Journal of Behavioral Medicine.* Advance online publication doi:10.1007/s12529-011-9154-9.—Study indicating poorer body image quality of life in SLE patients relative to healthy controls.

MacSween, A., Brydson, G., & Fox, K. (2004). Physical self-perceptions of women with rheumatoid arthritis. *Arthritis Care and Research, 51,* 958–963.—Determines the psychometrics of the Physical Self-Perception Profile and Perceived Importance Profile in RA.

Monaghan, S. M., Sharpe, L., Denton, F., Levy, J., Schrieber, L., & Sensky, T. (2007). Relationship between appearance and psychological distress in rheumatic diseases. *Arthritis and Rheumatism, 57,* 303–309.—Examines levels of appearance concerns and illness-specific measures and their relation with psychological distress in SLE and RA.

Plach, S. K., Stevens, P. E., & Moss, V. A. (2004). Corporeality: Women's experiences of a body with rheumatoid arthritis. *Clinical Nursing Research, 13,* 137–155.—Examines how 20 women with RA experience life in their body.

Stein, H., Walters, K., Dillon, A., & Schulzer, M. (1986). Systemic lupus erythematosus—A medical and social profile. *Journal of Rheumatology, 13,* 570–576.—Assesses social functioning in SLE including self-image and sexual functioning.

Vamos, M., White, G., & Caughey, D. (1990). Body image in rheumatoid arthritis: The relevance of hand appearance to desire for surgery. *British Journal of Medical Psychology, 63,* 267–277.—Investigates the importance of body image concerns relating to hand appearance in determining the desire to have surgery in patients with RA.

Williams, B., & Barlow, J. (1998). Falling out with my shadow. In S. Nettleton & J. Watson (Eds.), *The body in everyday life* (pp. 125–142). New York: Routledge.—Explores lay perceptions of the body in the context of arthritis.

CHAPTER 41

Body Image Issues Associated with Burn Injuries

JOHN W. LAWRENCE
JAMES A. FAUERBACH

Introduction

A severe burn is a devastating injury that can have a life-long physical, psychological, social, occupational, and financial impact on a burn survivor's life. Despite substantial improvements made over the last half century in acute care, burn injuries involve long recovery periods and result in less than optimal functional and cosmetic outcomes for many individuals. Many long-term physical complications can develop secondary to a major burn injury, including hypertrophic or keloidal scarring, limitations in range of motion across scarred joints, impaired skin integrity and sensation, and damaged or amputated body parts. The psychosocial challenges of recovering from a severe burn include posttraumatic stress, depression, grieving the loss of one's own physical integrity, grieving the loss of loved ones who may have died in the burn incident, chronic pain, chronic itching, new physical limitations, adapting to dramatic change in one's appearance, coping with social stigmatization and discrimination, and staying engaged in a long physical rehabilitation process. This chapter provides an overview of the research on the psychosocial recovery process from severe burns with an emphasis on the psychological and social challenges of adapting to permanent changes in one's appearance. The reader is also encouraged to consult Chapter 29, which focuses on congenital conditions that result in visible difference.

The Epidemiology of Burns

Globally, approximately 300,000 people die from fire-related burns annually. In the United States, burn injuries result in approximately 1 million emergency room visits, 50,000 hospitalizations, and 5,000 deaths every year. According to Edelman, in the United States, the lifetime cost of a burn death is four times greater than cancer and six times greater than heart disease.

Risk factors for burns include socioeconomic status (SES), age, gender, and mental health status. In both developed and nondeveloped countries, SES is perhaps the most frequently reported risk factor for both burn morbidity and mortality. Ninety-five percent of all fire-related burns occur in low- to middle-income countries. SES influences both environmental and behavioral variables that increase the likelihood of being burned. For example, low-SES people tend to live in inadequate housing stock and have more dangerous jobs. Also, irregular heat, electricity, or water in a household increases the likelihood a family will have an open fire in the home.

Children, particularly those below age 5, have a higher risk of being burned. Most commonly, children incur scald burns when they spill a hot liquid on themselves; however, about 10% of all child abuse cases in the United States are burn related. In regard to gender, males are more likely to be burned in industrialized countries due to an increased likelihood of engaging in high-risk work and behavior. In developing countries, especially in East Asia, women are burned more often due to the frequent practice of cooking over an open fire while wearing loose-fitting, highly flammable clothing.

In retrospective studies, burn survivors, as a group, have been found to have higher levels of psychopathology—in particular, mood disorders and substance abuse—than the general population. Some researchers have posited that deficits in executive functioning related to preexisting psychopathology can lead to higher risk-taking and lower precaution-taking behaviors, causing accidents that may lead to burns.

Body Image

Severe burns result in permanent scarring. Even after reconstructive surgery, burn scars are often rough in texture, discolored, dry, and relatively less pliable than noninjured skin. Approximately 50% of burn scars have areas of hypertrophic scarring, in which the skin is raised, lumpy, and easily irritated. These scars are often painful and itchy for months or years after the burn injury.

This permanent change in appearance is often a challenge to many burn survivors' body image. Burn survivors must cope with their own emotional response to the change in appearance, as well as the social reactions of others. Partridge hypothesized that adjustment to the change in one's appearance following a burn happens in three stages. In the first 6 months after injury, the survivor is focused on survival and physical recovery. In the second stage, between 6 months and 2 years, the person turns to adjusting to the permanent changes in his or her appearance, the social ramifications of those changes, and the common feelings of grief, anger, and depression. In the third stage, the person develops a new acceptance of his or her body, rejects the cultural norm of body perfection, and through his or her actions implicitly or explicitly advocates tolerance for appearance diversity.

In regard to assessing body image among burn survivors, two burn-specific body image measures have been developed. First, the Burn Specific Health Scale is a multifactor measure of burn adjustment that has been refined over the years. Its subscales include body image, sexuality, and social adjustment. Second, the Satisfaction with Appearance Scale is a 14-item questionnaire measuring both self-appraisal and social-behavioral components of body image. Both these instruments are designed to be used with adults. To date, no burn-specific body image measure has been developed to use with children.

There have been relatively few studies on the prevalence and predictors of body image disturbance among burn survivors. Most have been completed in the United States or Europe, so any generalizations about the phenomenon are tentative. The studies that have compared burn survivors, both adults and children, to nonburned comparison groups have not found group differences on body image measures. One possible explanation for this surprising finding is that body image dissatisfaction is normative in industrialized countries. In regard to predictors, severity of burn scarring has tended to have a modest relationship with body image; the correlation between the two variables has ranged from 0 to .40, depending on how severity was measured. A major limitation of these studies has been that there is no gold standard for measuring scar severity, so proxy variables such as total body surface area burned or numbers of burn-related surgeries have been used. In regard to scar location, some researchers have hypothesized that it is more difficult to adapt to socially visible scars, such as scars on the face, because of the stigmatizing reactions of others. Other researchers have argued that it is more difficult to cope with hidden scars because the person has fewer opportunities to learn how to deal with the reactions of others, so he or she lives in fear of the scar being revealed. The research to date has not provided strong support for either hypothesis. The presence of a facial scar has tended to have a low correlation with body image measures, ranging from 0 to .20. In comparison to men, women burn survivors have tended to have poorer body image; however, the gender difference in burn survivors has not been as great or as consistent across studies as it has been in the general population. Across studies the strongest correlates of body image among burn survivors has been social and emotional variables such as social support, perceived social stigmatization, importance of appearance, and depression (ranging from .30 to .60).

Social Integration and Social Stigmatization

As described in other chapters in this book, body image is greatly influenced by one's social environment. Like obesity, scars are highly stigmatized in Western culture. Scarring is used in many horror movies and video games to dehumanize villains, such as Two-Face in the *Batman* series. Burn survivors frequently describe experiencing a variety of stigmatizing behaviors such as an absence of friendliness and courtesy, staring, pointing, startled and disgusted reactions, ignoring, avoidance, confused behavior, teasing, bullying, and discrimination. In Lawrence et al.'s recently developed measure of perceived stigmatization, these stigmatizing behaviors reflect three factors: (1) absence of friendly behavior, (2) staring and confused behavior, and (3) hostile behavior. These behaviors communicate to the burn survivor a lack of social acceptance, social discomfort, and social rejection, respectively.

A number of experimental studies have demonstrated that people are prone to engage in nonhostile stigmatizing behavior when confronted with a person with a visible difference. For example, several studies compared social reactions to actors with and without mock facial scars. When exposed to a "scarred individual," participants maintained a greater social distance from, were less likely to offer help to, and minimized their social interaction with the actor. A variety of hypotheses have been posited to explain why people are prone to react to people with visible differences with stigmatizing behavior. An evolutionary theory conjectures that startled and disgusted reactions to scarring are due to an innate reflexive reaction, the goal of which is to protect oneself from disease. A second theory speculates that because severe scarring is relatively rare in the general population, confused and startled behavior is due to a lack of knowledge about how to act in a novel social situation. Third, it is often hypothesized that stigmatizing behavior, in particular, hostile behavior such as teasing and bullying, is culturally determined based in the overvaluation of "perfect appearance" and the denigration of appearances that deviate from the ideal.

Similar to body image, there has been little research on the epidemiology of stigmatizing experiences among people with burn scars or other visible differences. In regard to the prevalence of stigmatizing behavior, several studies have compared the peer victimization experiences of children with and without craniofacial conditions and found no differences between groups. Among adults with visible differences, there have been no studies investigating the frequency of victimizing experiences or job discrimination. In the studies that have been done, difference severity, cognitive deficits, and social skills deficits have tentatively been identified as risk factors for experiencing stigmatization.

Interventions

For the past half-century, burn treatment research has focused on improving survival rates, and more recently, on improving physical functioning. There has been relatively little research on interventions to improve psychosocial outcomes. Fortunately, a number of programs aimed at improving the body image and social integration of burn survivors have been developed and are often available through regional burn centers; however, to date, few randomized controlled trials testing their efficacy have been completed.

As discussed further in Chapter 46, perhaps the most common intervention aimed at improving body image is reconstructive surgery. Though there has been a good deal of excitement about possible improvements in surgical and skin regeneration interventions at conferences held by organizations such as the American Burn Association, there has been little research evaluating the aesthetic outcomes of these interventions or their effects on the psychosocial functioning of burn survivors. Reconstructive surgery does not restore the preburn appearance of most survivors of severe burns, and the survivor must learn to live with the fact that he or she is visibly different.

In regard to psychosocial interventions, both psychotherapy and social-level interventions have been developed. Cognitive-behavioral therapy (CBT) with a strong social skills component has been hypothesized by a number of burn researchers to be a potentially effective intervention. The model posits that social interactions between a person without a disfigurement and a person who has a visible distinction have a high probability of being awkward because they are novel situations for most people. Anticipating negative reactions from others, the burn survivor may engage in a range of avoidance and escape behaviors (e.g., refusing to go to social events, wearing clothing that hides his or her appearance, avoiding eye contact, minimizing conversations, or launching preemptive hostile attacks) that increase the likelihood of a negative social interaction. Moreover, after becoming socially disengaged, the burn survivor spends a good deal of time ruminating about his or her visible distinction, thus leading to depression. Several studies have found poor body image to be highly related to depression among burn survivors. In an effort to mitigate the emotionally painful rumination, the burn survivor might engage in distraction strategies, such as drug and alcohol abuse or excessive television watching, that make both emotional regulation and social integration more difficult.

The CBT model proposes to teach the burn survivor a variety of skills to break the repetitive cycle of social isolation, rumination, and depression. Most importantly, burn survivors are taught specific social skills to manage social interactions. These social skills include exuding confident body language, making eye contact, having a prepared brief explanation of the injury, positively reinforcing others' behaviors with a smile or playful comment, guiding the topic of the conversation, and assertively asking people to stop rude behavior. In addition, cognitive therapy techniques aimed at questioning the dominant culture's distorted values about appearance and engendering self-acceptance (see Chapter 47) can be used with burn survivors.

There have also been a variety of efforts to intervene in the social environment of burn survivors. For example, many burn centers have school reentry programs. In these programs a burn professional first consults with the burn survivor and his or her family to develop a plan and agree on what information will be shared with the school and how the burn survivor's story will be told. Usually, the burn professional visits the school and speaks to the burn survivor's teachers and classmates with the goal of telling the burn survivor's story, demystifying the burn healing process, and engendering empathy and social support for the burn survivor. Though burn reentry programs are very popular in the burn treatment community, there have been no controlled studies demonstrating their effectiveness.

There are several nonprofit organizations working to provide social support for burn survivors and others with visible distinctions and advocating public policy to alter societal norms that devalue people with visible distinctions. Based in the United States, the Phoenix Society for Burn Survivors is "a nonprofit organization dedicated to empowering anyone affected by a burn injury." They provide a range of services to burn survivors. For example, in coordination with over 30 burn centers across the United States, the Phoenix Society coordinates and provides training for peer support groups. In addition, they host the annual World Burn Congress, a conference that brings together burn survivors, their families, firefighters, and burn care professionals to address the aftercare and reintegration issues of burn survivors.

Changing Faces is a charity based in the United Kingdom dedicated to supporting and representing people with visible distinctions. This organization provides group and individual counseling, supports research, works with schools and employers to "ensure a culture of inclusion for people with disfigurement," and leads campaigns to change public policies and the attitudes that are espoused in the media, society, and government. Changing Faces recently initiated the "face equality" campaign with the goal of challenging "media, advertisers, and the film industry [to] adopt more factual and unbiased portrayals of people with disfigurements, actively avoiding language and imagery that creates prejudice."

In addition, the campaign has asked politicians and policy makers to "ensure that facial prejudice and discrimination are effectively outlawed by improving anti-discrimination law and promoting best practice."

Conclusions and Future Directions

The study of body image and the social integration of burn survivors is a new field in rehabilitation psychology. Many of the existing studies have methodological limitations. For the field to progress, several logistic issues need to be addressed. First, doing quality psychosocial research is a complex process requiring extensive training and time. Few burn centers have faculty dedicated to conducting psychosocial research. Professional research positions and training must be funded to improve the quality of research being completed. Second, for a variety of reasons, burn survivors are a difficult group to study. Burns are relatively rare. Burn centers serve geographically extended regions. Burn survivors often have multiple stressors in their life making participation in longitudinal research difficult. Thus, the samples of survivors reported in many studies in the burn literature are small, not random, and have high attrition rates. In order to address these issues the field needs to engage in more coordinated multisite research, employ epidemiological research strategies for difficult-to-follow populations, and develop valid assessment instruments. Finally, randomized controlled trials must be implemented to test the effectiveness of interventions such as CBT and school reentry programs.

Informative Readings

Bessell, A., & Moss, T. P. (2007). Evaluating the effectiveness of psychosocial interventions for individuals with visible differences: A systematic review of the empirical literature. *Body Image: An International Journal of Research, 4,* 227–238.—A detailed review of the methodological limitations of the intervention studies in the visible distinctions literature.

Blakeney, P., Partridge, J., & Rumsey, N. (2007). Community integration. *Journal of Burn Care and Research, 28,* 598–601.—A review of the issues related to community integration of burn survivors.

Changing Faces. (2010, April 15). Available at *www.changingfaces.org.uk/Home*—The website for the advocacy group Changing Faces for people with visible distinctions.

Dissanaike, S., & Rahimi, M. (2009). Epidemiology of burn injuries: Highlighting cultural and socio-demographic aspects. *International Review of Psychiatry, 21,* 505–511.—A review of the causes and risk factors of burn injuries around the world.

Edelman, L. S. (2007). Social and economic factors associated with the risk of burn injury. *Burns, 33*, 958–965.—A review of risk factors related to SES and burn injuries.

Klinge, K., Chamberlain, D. J., Redden, M., & King, L. (2009). Psychological adjustments made by post-burn injury patients: An integrative literature review. *Journal of Advanced Nursing, 65*, 2274–2292.—A review of risk factors for psychological maladjustment following a burn injury.

Lawrence, J. W., Fauerbach, J. A., Heinberg, L., Doctor, M., & Thombs, B. D. (2006). The reliability and validity of the Perceived Stigmatization Questionnaire (PSQ) and the Social Comfort Questionnaire (SCQ) among an adult burn survivor sample. *Psychological Assessment, 18*, 106–111.—Presents the psychometric evaluation of questionnaires measuring perceived stigmatization and social comfort among adult burn survivors.

Lawrence, J. W., Fauerbach, J. A., & Thombs, B. D. (2006). A test of the moderating role of importance of appearance in the relationship between perceived scar severity and body-esteem among adult burn survivors. *Body Image: An International Journal of Research, 3*, 101–111.—Tests the hypothesis that importance of appearance interacts with scar severity to predict body image.

McKibben, J. B. A., Ekselius, L., Girasek, D. C., Gould, N. F., Holzer, C., III, Rosenberg, M., et al. (2009). Epidemiology of burn injuries II: Psychiatric and behavioural perspectives. *International Review of Psychiatry, 21*, 512–521.—A review of risk factors and prevention opportunities related to psychiatric and behavioral variables for burn injuries.

Partridge, J. (2006). From burns unit to boardroom. *British Medical Journal, 332*, 956–959.—Describes the author's journey from being a burn survivor to founding the advocacy group Changing Faces. The article gives a personal perspective of the psychosocial challenges faced by burn survivors.

Phoenix Society for Burn Survivors. (2010, April 15). Available at *www.phoenix-society.org/*—The website for the burn survivor advocacy group Phoenix Society for Burn Survivors.

Thompson, A., & Kent, G. (2001). Adjusting to disfigurement: Processes involved in dealing with being visibly different. *Clinical Psychology Review, 21*, 663–682.—Reviews the literature on the psychosocial challenges faced by people with visible distinctions and describes the CBT model of adaptation.

PART VII

CHANGING THE BODY
Medical, Surgical, and Other Approaches

CHAPTER 42

Weight Loss and Changes in Body Image

DAVID B. SARWER
REBECCA J. DILKS
JACQUELINE C. SPITZER

Introduction

This chapter provides an overview of the changes in body image that occur with weight loss. Most of the research in this area has focused on changes in body image that occur with conventional treatments such as diet, exercise, and behavioral modification. Other studies have looked at changes in body image in persons with obesity who receive cognitive-behavioral interventions that do not focus on changing eating behavior and activity levels (see Chapter 47). Within the past decade, a number of studies have investigated changes in body image that occur with the massive weight losses seen in persons who undergo bariatric surgery. Unfortunately, some of these individuals experience loose, hanging skin in different areas of the body that leads many to consider and some to undergo body contouring procedures performed by plastic surgeons.

The Obesity Problem

Obesity is a serious medical condition and is believed to be one of the world's most pressing health problems. Obesity is defined by an individual's body mass index (BMI) that evaluates a person's weight relative to his or her height. Individuals with a BMI ≥ 30 kg/m^2 are clinically obese, whereas those who have a BMI ≥ 40 kg/m^2 are extremely (or morbidly) obese. In the United States, approximately one-third of the adult population is obese. Another third is overweight (BMI between 25 and 30 kg/m^2) and, as a result, at risk of developing obesity in the future. Other Westernized countries report similar rates of obesity and a growing number of non-Westernized countries are seeing an increase in the rate of obesity. While obesity is often seen as an aesthetic issue, it is a major medical condition. The presence of obesity increases the risk of a number of medical conditions, including cardiovascular disease, type II diabetes, hypertension, sleep apnea, musculoskeletal problems, and several forms of cancer.

Obesity and Body Image

As discussed in detail in Chapters 20 and 21, overweight and obese individuals tend to be more dissatisfied with their bodies and outward appearance than their normal-weight counterparts. This issue has been most frequently studied in women; men are underrepresented in obesity and weight loss treatment literatures. The degree of dissatisfaction seems to be directly related to the amount of excess weight a person has. The association between BMI and body image dissatisfaction (BID) may even be stronger than the current research suggests, given that many of the studies of this issue have not included persons with extreme obesity. In addition to reporting dissatisfaction with their overall size and weight, many persons with obesity also report dissatisfaction with discrete body features. Regardless of the focus of concern, BID is related to lower self-esteem and increased symptoms of depression in obese individuals, and, therefore is believed to be a marker for other psychological problems. Another factor that may contribute to psychosocial distress is weight-related stigma. Bias against obese individuals has been found in social, educational, occupational, and medical settings and may be associated with discriminatory treatment.

Some persons with obesity are motivated to lose weight to improve their health and reduce their risk for weight-related health problems in the future. For most individuals, however, the motivation to lose small or large amounts of weight is to improve their physical appearance. When patients are asked about their expectations for their lives after weight loss, many will report that they are looking forward to wearing a wider range of smaller sized and more fashionable clothes. Very few patients, even those with severe obesity and significant health problems, speak as enthusiastically about lowering their blood sugar or high blood pressure.

Obesity Treatments

There is a wide range of treatments recommended for weight loss. Behavioral and/or lifestyle interventions include self-directed diets, commercial weight loss programs, Internet-based programs, nutritional counseling, physical activity, hospital-based programs, residential weight loss facilities, and low-calorie diets. Both over-the-counter and U.S. Food and Drug Administration (FDA)-approved weight loss medications are appropriate for some individuals. For those with extreme obesity, bariatric surgery is an option.

Behavioral or lifestyle interventions typically focus on decreasing caloric intake and increasing physical activity. These programs come in a myriad of forms, ranging from self-help programs and books to commercial programs. Clinical investigations of these programs indicate that they typically produce a weight loss of 7–10% of initial body weight. Similar weight losses are seen with weight loss medications. The modest weight losses with both lifestyle modification and pharmacotherapy rarely meet patients' expectations; most patients hope to lose significantly more weight. While some patients do lose more weight, others fail to lose even 5% of their initial weight, particularly if they struggle to make the dietary and behavioral changes necessary for weight loss. Nevertheless, weight losses of even 5% of initial body weight often are associated with improvements in a number of weight-related health problems.

Improvements in Body Image with Weight Loss

Several studies have found that body image improves with even modest weight reduction. For example, Foster and colleagues found that women who lost an average of 19 kg (42 pounds) in 24 weeks reported significant improvements in body image. Over the next 24 weeks, women regained approximately 3 kg (6.6 pounds) on average, a change that was associated with a slight, yet significant worsening in body image. Nevertheless, body image remained significantly improved compared to baseline.

Other studies, particularly one by Annis and colleagues, have made cross-sectional comparisons of overweight/obese, formerly overweight/ obese, and never-overweight women. Currently overweight women report greater BID, overweight preoccupation, and dysfunctional appearance investment as compared to never-overweight women. Although formerly and never-overweight women did not differ on overall body satisfaction (indirectly suggesting improvement in body satisfaction with weight loss), formerly overweight women scored worse than never-overweight women with regard to overweight preoccupation and dysfunctional appearance investment and were more similar to currently overweight women on these domains. Collectively, these findings support the concept of "phantom fat" or "vestigial body image," in which some of the body image cognitions associated with excess body weight may not fully change with weight loss.

Many individuals report that weight loss leads to an increase in the number of compliments on their physical appearance, often from loved ones or more distant acquaintances. Although many women find these comments flattering, others find the increased attention on their physical appearance uncomfortable and disconcerting. This may be particularly true for persons with a history of sexual abuse, who may have become used to being "invisible" to others and whose excess body weight has deflected sexual attention from them. As a result, weight loss has the potential to impact both body image, as well as the dynamics of romantic and sexual relationships. Although these issues have received little formal study to date, our observations of them suggest that they are worthy of clinical attention and further study.

Improvements in Body Image without Weight Loss

Other studies have investigated improvements in psychosocial status and body image in overweight and obese women in the absence of weight loss. Such interventions have been called "undieting" or "anti-dieting" approaches and developed, in large part, out of the concern that dieting and weight loss promotes the development of eating disorders and other untoward psychological symptoms (a hypothesis that has not been supported in subsequent studies). These programs, largely based on cognitive-behavioral principles, are designed to improve eating behavior and maladaptive cognitions about eating, body image, and other psychosocial domains without inducing weight loss.

The findings of these studies have varied. Some have found that these interventions lead to improvements in body image, self-esteem, and depression. Others have shown improvements in self-esteem and depression, but no impact on body image. Given the growth of the obesity problem and the increasing emphasis on the importance of weight loss and maintenance to improve physical health, these interventions, to some extent, have fallen out of favor. Nevertheless, most behavioral weight loss interventions include a "body image module" as part of treatment. This module typically encourages patients to identify and modify their distorted cognitions and maladaptive body image behaviors related to their weight and shape.

"Anti-dieting" and body image interventions may hold promise during the weight maintenance phase of weight loss treatment. Weight regain is the Achilles' heel of most behaviorally based and pharmacological treatments for weight loss. As noted above, it is associated with a worsening in body image. Some researchers have suggested that combining a behavioral weight loss program with a cognitive-behavioral body image intervention (see Chapter 47) delivered during the weight maintenance phase of treatment may be one approach to promote successful weight maintenance.

Extreme Obesity and Bariatric Surgery

Approximately 5% of the adult population in the United States suffers from extreme obesity, defined by a BMI ≥ 40 kg/m². The health consequences of extreme obesity are often far more serious than those seen with less severe obesity, with a number of studies demonstrating a strong relationship between BMI and mortality. Bariatric surgery appears to be the most effective treatment for extreme obesity. Estimates suggest that approximately 200,000 Americans undergo surgery annually. The surgery typically is recommended for patients with a BMI ≥ 40 kg/m² or those with a BMI > 35 kg/m² in the presence of significant comorbidities. The most common surgical procedures are the gastrointestinal bypass and laparoscopic adjustable gastric banding. With both procedures food intake is limited by the creation of a gastric pouch at the base of the esophagus. Although this restriction promotes weight loss in both procedures, the gastrointestinal bypass is also thought to induce weight loss through favorable effects on gut peptides. Patients typically lose 50–60% of excess body weight with gastric bypass procedures and 40–50% with gastric banding procedures 2 years postoperatively.

The significant health problems associated with extreme obesity motivate many individuals to pursue bariatric surgery. Many extremely obese persons also pursue bariatric surgery for its anticipated effects on their psychosocial well-being, including body image. In the past few years, several comprehensive reviews of the literature on the psychosocial and behavioral aspects of bariatric surgery have been published. The reader is referred to the article by Sarwer, Wadden, and Fabricatore in the Informative Readings section.

Body Image and Massive Weight Loss

The massive weight loss following bariatric surgery is associated with significant improvements in both physical and psychosocial functioning. Self-esteem, depressive symptoms, health-related quality of life, and body image improve substantially in the first year after surgery. These psychosocial benefits, however, appear to be limited to the first few postoperative years and may regress when patients begin to regain weight.

Although body image typically improves after bariatric surgery, some patients report residual BID associated with loose, sagging skin of the breasts, abdomen, thighs, and arms following massive weight loss. Most patients consider the development of excess skin to be a negative consequence of surgery. This dissatisfaction likely motivates some individuals to seek body contouring procedures to address these concerns. These are considered to be reconstructive procedures, as they are designed to return the patient to a "normal" appearance and address functional issues related to physical discomfort and pain. However, in the United States these procedures are rarely covered by insurance.

To date, the psychosocial and physical outcomes of these procedures, as well as the factors that motivate the decision to seek them, have received little empirical attention. The breast-reduction surgery literature provides a framework from which to conceptualize these issues for postbariatric surgery patients. The experience of having very large breasts is associated with heightened self-consciousness, low self-esteem, and BID. Similar to bariatric surgery patients, women who seek breast reduction report reduced quality of life and increased depressive symptoms and anxiety, as well as lower self-esteem. Most women who undergo breast-reduction surgery also report that the physical discomfort and pain associated with large breasts motivates them to seek surgical treatment. More than 80% of women with large breasts report that they interfere with their ability to engage in physical activity, and almost half report a period of sick leave from work secondary to their symptoms. These symptoms are positively associated with body mass.

Encouragingly, most women who undergo breast reduction report satisfaction with their postoperative result. The most common reason for dissatisfaction is scarring, which is also a significant issue with patients who undergo body contouring surgery. Studies have repeatedly found that women report improvements in health-related quality of life, self-esteem, and body image following breast reduction. Patients also typically report significant reductions in pain and increases in physical activity. At least one study, conducted by Song and colleagues, has suggested similar improvements in body image following body contouring surgery.

Clinical Considerations for Patients Who Undergo Body Contouring

Chapter 45 and other resources provide detailed recommendations on the psychological assessment and management of individuals who seek plastic surgery. Some of the unique clinical issues of the patient who presents for body contouring surgery are highlighted here.

Patients who experience massive weight loss may hold unrealistic expectations about the aesthetic results of body contouring surgery. Some may incorrectly anticipate that surgery will result in a total body transformation that makes their body comparable to persons who never experienced excessive body weight. Others may not fully understand that body contouring surgery often produces large and visible scars and skin irregularities, as well as residual deformities in body shape.

The patients' subjective perception of the postoperative result is at the heart of the body image concerns of these, and all, plastic surgery procedures. It is possible that some body contouring patients may develop a preoccupation with their physical appearance similar to that seen with body dysmorphic disorder (BDD; see Chapters 35 and 45). The rate of BDD among persons with extreme obesity or those who undergo body contouring surgery is unknown. As the physical deformities found in most patients with massive weight loss are neither slight nor imagined, the diagnosis technically cannot be applied to them. However, studies of patients undergoing other reconstructive surgical procedures suggest that they often report a level of preoccupation with their appearance consistent with BDD.

Although the magnitude and durability of the weight losses seen with bariatric surgery are quite impressive, between 20 and 30% of patients experience suboptimal weight losses or weight gain in the first 2–3 years after surgery. Many patients present for body contouring within the first 2 years of the bariatric procedure and when they have not experienced a period of prolonged weight stability. Others may be malnourished from poor adherence to the recommended postoperative diet, which may compromise wound healing. Weight gain following body contouring surgery may affect postoperative satisfaction and potentially compromise the aesthetic result. Thus, candidates for body contouring ideally should remain weight stable for approximately 3–6 months prior to surgery.

Conclusions and Future Directions

The past two decades have brought an increased understanding of the changes in body image that occur with weight loss. In general, a reduction in body weight leads to an improvement in body image. However, this conclusion is not universal and the complete picture of this area of research is somewhat more complicated. Although most individuals who lose weight experience improvement in body image, this improvement often diminishes with weight regain. Others may report little change in body image following weight loss, in part because they had a relatively positive body image and were motivated to lose weight to improve their health. For persons with extreme obesity, the massive weight loss typically seen with bariatric surgery often improves body image. However, some of those patients report dissatisfaction with their resulting appearance and turn to body contouring surgery with a plastic surgeon with the hope of further improving their appearance and body image.

The extant research literature includes a number of additional nuances. Most studies have focused on women; few have investigated changes in body image in men who lose weight, in part because they present for weight loss treatment infrequently as compared to women. Similarly, little focus has been paid to the body image changes that occur for children and adolescents who enter into weight loss treatment (see Chapter 20). Perhaps one of the few "silver linings" in the currently unchecked worldwide obesity problem is that it will provide ample opportunity to investigate these and other issues in the future.

Informative Readings

AACE/TOS/ASMBS. (2008). Metabolic and bariatric surgery medical guidelines for clinical practice for the perioperative nutritional and nonsurgical support of the bariatric surgery patient. *Endocrine Practice, 14*(Suppl. 1). Available at *www.aace.com/pub/pdf/guidelines/Bariatric.pdf.*—A detailed overview and decision-making guidelines about bariatric surgery for health care professionals.

Annis, N. M., Cash, T. F., & Hrabosky, J. I. (2004). Body image and psychosocial differences among stable average-weight, currently overweight, and formerly overweight women: The role of stigmatizing experiences. *Body Image: An International Journal of Research, 1,* 155–167.—Cross-sectional study supporting the concept of "phantom fat," in which body image cognitions associated with excess body weight may not fully change with weight loss.

Buchwald, H., Avidor, Y., Braunwald, E., Jensen, M. D., Pories, W., Fahrbach, K., et al. (2004). Bariatric surgery: A systematic review and meta-analysis. *Journal of the American Medical Association, 292,* 1724–1737.—A review of the literature on bariatric surgery focusing on weight loss and postoperative resolution of obesity-related comorbidities.

Foster, G. D., Wadden, T. A., & Vogt, R. A. (1997). Body image before, during, and after weight loss treatment. *Health Psychology, 16,* 226–229.—Study finding that body image improves with weight loss but also worsens with modest weight regain.

Matz, P. E., Foster, G. D., Faith, M. S., & Wadden, T. A. (2002). Correlates of body image dissatisfaction among overweight women seeking weight loss. *Journal of Consulting and Clinical Psychology, 70,* 1040–1044.—Research illustrating relationships between body image, self-esteem, and depressive symptoms.

Mitchell, J. D., & deZwaan, M. (Eds.). (2005). *Bariatric surgery: A guide for mental health professionals.* Routledge, New York.—Overview of pre- and postoperative psychosocial issues of individuals who undergo bariatric surgery.

Ramirez, E. M., & Rosen J. C. (2001). A comparison of weight control and weight control plus body image therapy for obese men and women. *Journal of Consulting and Clinical Psychology, 69,* 440–446.—An experiment investigating improvements in body image between two groups that received either a weight control intervention or a weight control intervention plus cognitive-behavioral body image therapy.

Sarwer, D. B., Thompson J. K., & Cash T. F. (2005). Body image and obesity in adulthood. *Psychiatric Clinics of North America, 28,* 69–87.—An overview of the relationship between body image and obesity, with a specific focus on the assessment and treatment of BID.

Sarwer, D. B., Thompson, J. K., Mitchell, J. E., & Rubin, J. P. (2008). Psychological considerations of the bariatric surgery patient undergoing body contouring surgery. *Plastic and Reconstructive Surgery, 121,* 423e–434e.—A detailed review of the pre- and postoperative psychosocial issues of patients who undergo bariatric surgery and present for body contouring surgery.

Sarwer, D. B., Wadden, T. A., & Fabricatore, A. N. (2005). Psychosocial and behavioral aspects of bariatric surgery. *Obesity Research, 13*, 639–648.—Review paper that details the research on the preoperative characteristics of persons who present for bariatric surgery and the psychological changes that occur postoperatively.

Sarwer, D. B., Wadden, T. A, & Foster, G. D. (1998). Assessment of body image dissatisfaction in obese women: Specificity, severity, and clinical significance. *Journal of Consulting and Clinical Psychology, 66*, 651–654.—A study investigating the differences in body image between obese women seeking weight loss treatment and nonobese women.

Song, A. Y., Rubin, J. P., Thomas, V., Dudas, J. R., Marra, K. G., & Fernstrom, M. H. (2006). Body image and quality of life in post massive weight loss body contouring patients. *Obesity, 14*, 1626–1636.—One of the first studies to investigate changes in body image and quality of life following body contouring surgery.

Young, V. L., & Watson, M. E. (2006). Breast reduction. In D. B. Sarwer, T. Pruzinsky, T. F. Cash, R. M. Goldwyn, J. A. Persing, & L. A. Whitaker (Eds.), *Psychological aspects of reconstructive and cosmetic plastic surgery: Clinical, empirical, and ethical perspectives* (pp. 189–206). Lippincott, Williams & Wilkins: Philadelphia.—A detailed review of research on the psychological issues in breast reduction surgery.

CHAPTER 43

Exercise and Changes in Body Image

KATHLEEN A. MARTIN GINIS
REBECCA L. BASSETT

Introduction

Exercise is defined as planned, structured, and repetitive physical movement that is performed in order to improve or maintain physical fitness. Countless studies have demonstrated the physical health benefits of regular exercise, such as reduced risk for chronic disease and increased longevity, as well as psychological benefits such as reduced symptoms of anxiety and depression. Given the potential for exercise to improve both physical and psychological well-being, researchers and interventionists have become increasingly interested in the utility of exercise for improving body image.

Three separate meta-analyses have examined the effects of exercise training interventions on body image. These meta-analyses include studies that varied tremendously in terms of body image outcome measures, the types and intensities of exercises prescribed, and the populations sampled. Despite such variability, the results of the meta-analyses have been very consistent: Exercise has significant positive effects on body image.

This chapter begins with a discussion of the mechanisms that may account for the positive effects of exercise on body image. An understanding of mechanisms is necessary so that researchers can develop models and theories that explain the exercise–body image relationship and interventionists can design exercise programs that maximize body image improvements. Subsequently, we discuss individual and exercise program factors that could moderate the effects of exercise on body image. The chapter concludes with recommendations for developing exercise-focused body image interventions and for advancing research in this area.

Mechanisms Underlying the Effects of Exercise on Body Image

Within the exercise and body image literature, there seems to be an inherent assumption that exercise-induced improvements in physical fitness are responsible for improvements in body image. Fitness reflects one's level of cardiorespiratory endurance (or aerobic fitness), muscular strength and endurance, flexibility, body composition (e.g., body fat, lean muscle mass), and ability to perform functional activities such as those associated with daily living. In their literature review, Martin Ginis, Bassett, and Conlin identify 13 studies that examined potential mechanisms by which exercise improves body image. Changes in body composition were the most studied fitness mechanism (11 studies), followed by aerobic fitness (6 studies), and muscular strength (4 studies).

Martin Ginis and colleagues' review showed that body composition change is inconsistently related to exercise-induced body image change. Only six of the 11 studies found a significant relationship between these variables. Thus, greater decreases in body weight, body fat, and body circumference do not necessarily lead to greater improvements in body image. Of the studies that did find a significant relationship, changes in body composition accounted for less than 15% of the variance in body image change. Likewise, improvements in aerobic fitness and muscular strength were not reliably related to body image change. Less than a third of studies reported significant relationships between these variables. When significant, changes in aerobic fitness and strength accounted for only modest variance in body image change (typically < 20%). Taken together, these findings suggest that, at best, fitness changes play only a minor role in explaining the effects of exercise on body image. Thus, the assumption that exercise-induced fitness changes are responsible for improvements in body image is challenged by the evidence.

It is possible, however, that *perceived* changes in fitness (e.g., perceived improvements in weight loss, muscle tone, strength, and endurance) might trigger improvements in body image, rather than objective changes in fitness per se. Only one study has examined this possibility. In that 2005 study, by Martin Ginis and colleagues, men and women participated in a 5-day/week strength-training program for 12 weeks. Among the men, body image improvements were associated with perceived, but not actual, increases in muscularity and strength, and perceived, but not actual, decreases in body fat. Among women, body image improvements were associated with perceived and actual increases in strength, and perceived, but not actual, changes in muscularity and body fat. These findings suggest that the extent to which people believe their body has changed as a result of their exercise behavior has a greater impact on body image than the extent to which their body has actually changed. Presumably, unlike objective measures of fitness, measures of perceived fitness capture the meaningfulness of the change to the exerciser. When exercisers perceive a meaningful transformation in their body, body image is more likely to improve.

According to Sonstroem and colleagues' expanded Exercise and Self-Esteem Model, increased physical self-efficacy is another mechanism by which exercise may improve body image. Physical self-efficacy refers to beliefs about one's capabilities to perform *specific* physical tasks (e.g., confidence in one's ability to run 5 miles or to lift 100 pounds), as well as beliefs about one's physical fitness and functioning *in general* (e.g., beliefs about strength, agility, and physical condition). Exercise-related changes in self-efficacy reflect the sense of personal control, physical mastery, and competence that is gained from exercise participation.

Of three studies that examined self-efficacy as a mechanism, all found significant relationships between exercise-induced change in self-efficacy and changes in body image. Interestingly, these studies show that self-efficacy is a significant predictor of body image change even after controlling for objective changes in physical fitness. Once again, the evidence suggests that when it comes to exercise and body image, actual changes in one's physical abilities are not nearly as important as the experience and interpretation of those changes.

Who Benefits from Exercise Interventions?

The positive effects of exercise training on body image have been demonstrated in both men and women and in people young and old. Meta-analyses have been used to test whether the magnitude of body image change varies as a function of sex or age, but the results have been equivocal. With regard to sex differences, the average effect size in studies involving women tends to be larger than the average effect size for studies involving men. However, these differences are not statistically significant. Given that there are nearly five times as many studies of women than men, it is not clear whether nonsignificance is due to a lack of statistical power or a true absence of meaningful differences. With regard to age differences, two of the meta-analyses reported that younger people derived greater body image improvements than older people, whereas the third meta-analysis showed the opposite pattern of results. Differences in the strategies used to create and compare age categories across the meta-analyses make it difficult to draw any firm conclusions regarding the role of age as a moderator.

It does seem clear, however, that people with the poorest initial body image benefit most from exercise interventions because they have the most room for improvement. Likewise, people who are unaccustomed to exercise tend to reap greater body image improvements from a training program than those who are used to exercise. This is because improvements in the mechanism variables—objective and perceived fitness, and self-efficacy—can be quite drastic for out-of-shape beginner exercisers who have negative perceptions of their fitness and doubts about their physical abilities. In support of this notion, Campbell and Hausenblas's meta-analysis shows that people who are overweight or obese tend to derive greater improvements in body image from exercise interventions than people who are normal weight.

If those with the poorest body image have the most to gain from exercise interventions, then it follows that exercise training could be particularly beneficial to people whose body image may be threatened by disease or disability. Although few controlled studies have examined the effects of exercise interventions on body image among such persons, the extant data are promising. For example, exercise training has been shown to increase body satisfaction among people with chronic conditions such as cancer, heart disease, multiple sclerosis, and spinal cord injury. Exercise training has also been associated with better body image during pregnancy and postpartum and among people undergoing treatment for eating disorders. These findings speak to the robustness of exercise for improving body image across various populations.

What Types of Exercise Are Most Effective for Body Image Change?

Exercise prescriptions typically consist of four components: frequency, intensity, time, and type (commonly referred to as the "FITT principles" of exercise prescription). Frequency refers to the number of exercise sessions prescribed over a given period (e.g., five sessions per week). Intensity refers to the level of effort required during the exercise (e.g., mild, moderate, or heavy intensity). Time is the prescribed duration of exercise for a given session (e.g., 30 minutes). Type refers to the specific mode of exercise (e.g., aerobic exercise such as jogging or swimming vs. resistance exercise such as lifting weights). Very few studies have compared the effects of different types of exercise prescriptions on changes in body image. As a result, what is known about exercise prescription is derived from meta-analyses that have statistically compared effect sizes across studies with different FITT characteristics.

Campbell and Hausenblas have published the most recent and comprehensive meta-analysis of the effects of exercise interventions on body image. Their meta-analysis includes 57 studies that have both an exercise intervention and a control condition. Drawing from Campbell and Hausenblas's findings, the following preliminary recommendations can be made for prescribing exercise to improve body image:

- *Frequency*: Exercise frequency is positively associated with body image change. People will derive greater improvements in body image when they exercise on more days per week.
- *Intensity*: Earlier meta-analyses showed that mild-intensity exercise had essentially no effect on body image change. Campbell and Hausenblas found that moderate- and strenuous-intensity exercise yield similar, positive effects on body image. Therefore, exercise must be performed at least at a moderate intensity in order to produce body image change.
- *Type*: The type of exercise does not moderate body image change. Aerobic exercise, strength-training, and combined aerobic/strength-training interventions are equally effective.
- *Time*: There is no relationship between the duration of exercise sessions and body image change. Exercise that is performed for shorter or longer durations will produce similar improvements in body image.

Recommendations for Developing Exercise Interventions

There are at least three programmatic elements that should be taken into account when designing an exercise intervention to improve body image. First, regarding prescription, exercise should be performed frequently (public health guidelines recommend exercising on most days of the week) and at a moderate-to-strenuous intensity. If changes in self-efficacy do indeed mediate the effects of exercise on body image, then successful workouts at a challenging intensity should result in greater self-efficacy and body image change than successful, easier, low-intensity workouts. Likewise, if changes in fitness account for the effects of exercise on body image, then frequent, intense exercise will generate greater improvements in actual fitness and, potentially, perceived fitness. With regard to exercise type, meta-analytic evidence indicates that all types of exercise are equally effective. However, we suspect that the exerciser's goals and body ideals could moderate the effectiveness of different types of exercise. For instance, a man who wants to be stronger and more muscular would likely derive greater body image benefits from a strength-training program than from a jogging intervention. Hence, we urge interventionists to consider exercisers' objectives and preferences when developing exercise interventions to improve body image.

Second, interventionists should ensure that they prescribe exercise activities that are enjoyable. Some evidence suggests that exercise enjoyment is positively associated with body image change. People who enjoy their workouts may exercise harder and more effectively than those who don't enjoy exercising, thus reaping greater improvements in objective and perceived fitness as well as self-efficacy. Enjoyable workouts may also elicit better postexercise mood states that could subsequently lead to more positive feelings about oneself and one's body. Exercise programmers can enhance enjoyment by creating opportunities for exercisers to socialize with one another, by adding variety to workouts, and by ensuring that the program's fitness leaders are positive and encouraging.

Third, we suggest that exercise programmers emphasize the physical and mental health benefits of exercise, rather than touting exercise as a strategy for changing appearance. Programs that help people set realistic and attainable goals and that teach people how to monitor progress in terms of functional fitness improvements should have a more positive impact on body image than programs emphasizing "building buns of steel" and "fighting flabby abs." Furthermore, people who come to realize the intrinsic benefits and pleasures of exercise are more likely to adhere to a long-term exercise regimen than people who are motivated primarily by the desire to lose weight and resculpt their body. By helping exercisers shift the focus away from appearance, interventionists can contribute to body image improvements and encourage people to find more enduring reasons for exercise adherence.

Future Research Directions

To date, most experimental investigations of exercise and body image have examined the effects of exercise *training* interventions (i.e., exercise programs that are carried out for several weeks or months) on *trait* measures of body image. In addition, preliminary evidence indicates that single, *acute* bouts of exercise can lead to significant improvements in *state* body image. For example, in a 2010 study, LePage and Crowther had female exercisers complete measures of state body dissatisfaction at random times and immediately postexercise over a 10-day study period. State body dissatisfaction was lower after exercise than at random time points, indicating that acute exercise can result in acute improvements in body image. Additional research is needed to determine whether improvements in trait body image may be achieved as the result of accumulated, individual bouts of state body image-enhancing exercise. There may also be factors that mediate or moderate the acute effects of exercise on state body image. Other issues and questions that warrant research attention are summarized below:

• An understanding of the mechanisms by which exercise improves body image has been hindered by a lack of theory-driven research. Bandura's self-efficacy theory and the Exercise and Self-Esteem Model are potential frameworks in which future research might be couched. Researchers must begin looking beyond objective fitness change as a potential mechanism. Furthermore, appropriate statistical methods (e.g., mediational analyses, structural equation modeling) should be used when testing these models and examining variables that mediate and moderate the effects of exercise on body image.

• Exercise should be explored as a preventive measure against the development of body dissatisfaction. For example, can exercise provide a buffer against the negative effects of minor weight gain, aging, and other potential threats to body image? Healthy levels of exercise may also play a role in the prevention of body image disturbance associated with eating disorders. However, compulsive exercise to compensate for binge eating or to achieve excessive weight loss serves to maintain eating pathology.

• Research is needed to determine how long exercise-related improvements in body image persist, and whether the duration differs for aerobic versus strength training.

• The role of personality factors should be considered. For instance, do individual differences along dimensions such as perfectionism, neuroticism, extroversion, and gender-role orientation influence the exercise–body image relationship?

• The relationship between exercise-induced changes in mood and changes in body image needs to be examined. The exercise-related biochemical changes that improve mood (e.g., increased neurotransmitter production) may also play a role in body image enhancement.

• Investigators have just begun to examine whether characteristics of the exercise physical environment (e.g., presence of mirrors) and social environment (e.g., coexercisers of the other sex) moderate the effects of exercise on body image. Identification of environmental moderators would be valuable for those who design and implement exercise programs.

• Most research has focused on exercise-related changes along cognitive and affective dimensions of body image (e.g., satisfaction with appearance, social physique anxiety). Additional studies are needed to determine the effects of exercise on perceptual aspects of body image (e.g., effects on self-estimates of one's body size) and on behavioral aspects (e.g., effects on the type of clothing one chooses to wear).

• The role of body image in determining exercise initiation and persistence is not yet fully understood. The study of body image variables within broader exercise motivational frameworks would help to shed light on this issue.

Conclusions

Exercise can be an effective intervention for improving body image among both men and women. Those with the lowest baseline levels of body satisfaction tend to reap the largest gains from exercise training. Changes in objective indices of physical fitness play a minor role in body image change, whereas improvements in perceived fitness and self-efficacy appear to be important mechanisms by which exercise improves body image. The body image benefits of an exercise training program can be maximized by exercising more frequently and intensely. It is also important that people find exercise activities that they enjoy. Exercise enjoyment may not only lead to greater improvements in body image but may also help people adopt a life-long exercise habit. Of course, as Chapter 23 reveals, some sports or athletic activities entail risks to favorable body image functioning.

Informative Readings

Bane, S. M., & McAuley, E. (1998). Body image and exercise. In J. Duda (Ed.), *Advances in sport and exercise psychology measurement* (pp. 311–322). Morgantown, WV: Fitness Information Technology.—A review of body image measures used in exercise and other research.

Campbell, A., & Hausenblas, H. A. (2009). Effects of exercise interventions on body image: A meta-analysis. *Journal of Health Psychology, 14,* 780–793.—A meta-analysis of 57 exercise training studies that concludes that exercise interventions produce greater improvements in body image than control conditions.

Fox, K. R. (1997). *The physical self: From motivation to well-being.* Champaign, IL: Human Kinetics.—A discussion of the importance of the physical self (1) as a determinant or motivator of behaviors including exercise, and (2) as a contributor to mental health and well-being.

Hausenblas, H. A., & Fallon, E. A. (2006). Exercise and body image: A meta-analysis. *Psychology and Health, 21,* 33–47.—A meta-analysis of 121 exercise and body image studies and potential moderators of the exercise–body image relationship.

LePage, M. L., & Crowther, J. H. (2010). The effects of exercise on body satisfaction and affect. *Body Image: An International Journal of Research, 7,* 124–130.—An observational study of the effects of exercise on young women's state body image and the moderating roles of trait body image and motivations for exercise.

Lindwall, M., & Lindgren, E. C. (2005). The effects of a 6-month exercise intervention programme on physical self-perceptions and social physique anxiety in non-physically active adolescent Swedish girls. *Psychology of Sport and Exercise, 6,* 643–658.—A randomized controlled trial demonstrating the effectiveness of twice-weekly exercise in improving social physique anxiety among young girls.

Martin Ginis, K. A., Bassett, R. L., & Conlin, C. (in press). Body image and exercise. In E. Acevedo (Ed.), *Oxford handbook of exercise psychology*. Oxford, UK: Oxford University Press.—A comprehensive review of the experimental exercise–body image literature and a commentary regarding possible mechanisms and future research directions.

Martin Ginis, K. A., Eng, J. J., Arbour, K. P., Hartman, J. W., & Phillips, S. M. (2005). Mind over muscle? Sex differences in the relationship between body image change and subjective and objective physical changes following a 12-week strength-training program. *Body Image: An International Journal of Research, 2,* 363–372.—A study of the relationships between body image change and real and perceived changes in physical fitness among men and women in a strength-training program.

Sonstroem, R. J. (1997). The physical self-system: A mediator of exercise and self-esteem. In K. R. Fox (Ed.), *The physical self: From motivation to well-being* (pp. 3–26). Champaign, IL: Human Kinetics.—A chapter that outlines the expanded Exercise and Self-Esteem Model.

Tucker, L. A., & Maxwell, K. (1992). Effects of weight training on the emotional well-being and body image of females: Predictors of greatest benefit. *American Journal of Health Promotion, 6,* 338–371.—A seminal study of factors related to body image improvements following a strength-training program.

Tucker, L. A., & Mortell, R. (1993). Comparison of the effects of walking and weight training programs on body image in middle-aged women: An experimental study. *American Journal of Health Promotion, 8,* 34–42.—An exercise training study that shows that weight training leads to greater improvements in women's body image than does walking.

Williams, P. A., & Cash, T. F. (2001). The effects of a circuit weight training program on the body images of college students. *International Journal of Eating Disorders, 30,* 75–82.—A controlled study confirming the effectiveness of weight training, independent of aerobic activity, in the improvement of body image, social physique anxiety, and physical self-efficacy.

CHAPTER 44

Body Art and Body Image

LEEANA KENT

> The body is the physical link between ourselves, our souls, and the outside world.
>
> —Ebin (1979, p. 1)

Introduction

The physical body has a long history of being the focus of both considerable personal and social scrutiny, with an individual's appearance being one of the first and most salient characteristics noticed by others. Physical appearance is associated with people's self-concept and identity, and it impacts their social interactions with others. Consequently, the body and its aesthetics is a fundamental resource in a person's attempt to form a sense of identity and to interact with and derive meaning from the social environment. Indeed, as a way of contributing to their sense of self, many people choose body art to manage their appearance. Regardless of the purpose for temporarily or permanently modifying the body, all forms are ultimately undertaken to cultivate personal and social identity. This chapter explores the concept of body art and the contemporary practice of both provisional and enduring forms of body modification. It summarizes aspects of mainstream and less conventional modes of body art, followed by an overview of personality correlates and motivations for engaging in body modification, and an examination of gendered body art practices.

Forms of Body Art

Temporary Forms

Many individuals use body art to momentarily modify their appearance. Such techniques generally utilize the skin or hair as the medium for modification. Cosmetics applied to the skin, such as makeup and body paint, are employed as a means to comply with (or reject) societal appearance norms. Evidence suggests that use of makeup increases social perceptions of attractiveness, femininity, and sensuality. Body painting, on the other hand, is predominantly utilized within certain cultures (e.g., Indigenous Australians) to mark a specific event, as the body paint signifies departure from the individual's everyday self. Although often symbolic in nature, body paint is also used to enhance one's physical attractiveness, which contributes to increased positive body image and social confidence.

Hair, while remaining a temporary form of body art, is somewhat more permanent than cosmetics. In Western society, both sexes routinely cut, color, curl, style, and depilate their hair. For example, male facial hair has historically been modified and styled to indicate one's social positioning, whereas punks of the 1970s used the Mohawk to symbolize group affiliation. Women tend to remove hair from the armpits and legs, which is associated with femininity and has become a normative practice in many societies. Conversely, in non-Western cultures people tend to adorn (rather than routinely remove) their hair using various ornaments such as shells, feathers, or beads.

Permanent Forms

Methods of body art that are more enduring include scarification (cutting), branding (burning), infibulation (piercing), and tattooing (insertion of indelible pigment). Permanent body art is generally associated with the prevailing characteristics of the individual (e.g., gender), robust social alliances, and appreciable intergenerational continuity. However, unlike the less permanent cosmetics and coiffure practices that are subject to fashion trends, enduring forms of body art are less transitional in nature.

Permanent body art can be categorized as nonmainstream and mainstream. Scarification and branding fall within the nonmainstream category. Scarification, or cicatrization, is a particularly painful process whereby the skin is lifted and incised, followed by application of an irritant designed to enhance the formation of cicatrices. Scarification is also symbolic of developmental status, and is used to augment the individual's physical attractiveness and body image. Like scarification, branding is a form of self-expression. It involves the skin being given a third-degree burn designed to create a permanent scar. Techniques include laser, chemicals, electrocautery, freezing, or hot metal branding irons. Traditionally, both modes have been associated with tribal membership and rites of passage, as well as announcing one's social role and status. Although predominantly restricted to indigenous cultures, scarification and branding have recently emerged within Western societies as a nonmainstream form of body art.

Conversely, piercing and tattooing are very much part of contemporary mainstream society. Research suggests that although the prevalence of body piercing seems to have stabilized during the last decade, its popularity remains high. The frequency of body piercing within the general Western population remains at more than one in 10, whereas among more specific populations (i.e., university students) it is as high as one in two. Despite the commonality of piercing as a form of body art, multiple facial piercings or piercing of genitalia are still regarded as being at the periphery of mainstream society. Tattooing has experienced a sharp rise in prevalence in the last 10 to 15 years and has become increasingly popular among all social sectors. Recent estimates indicate that between 10 and 25% of the Western population are now tattooed.

Personality Correlates and Motivations

Associated with the greater social acceptance of piercing and tattooing, scientific research into the personality correlates of those who acquire body art has begun to shift. Prior to this swing in the late 1990s, the dominant focus of scientific research examining personality characteristics associated with body art was on the deviant personality profile of the tattooed person. Such examination was generally achieved using institutionalized or incarcerated populations. These sampling methods pose serious limitations on the generalizability of the findings, which predominantly indicate psychopathology or personality disorder present. More recent research engaging broader participant samples suggest few significant differences in the personality profiles of tattooed and nontattooed individuals. Forbes and others, however, argue that an extraverted personality and a need for stimulation may have indirectly contributed to earlier research that found that tattooees have a significantly greater risk of psychological illness. Cash and others' found modest but significant associations between the excitement-seeking facet of extraversion and both piercing and tattooing among college women. Moreover, among those women without body art, excitement seeking predicted more favorable attitudes and intentions regarding body art.

Recent investigations by Tiggemann and others have built on this contention, showing that tattooees have a higher "need for uniqueness" regarding appearance than nontattooed individuals. Although the need for uniqueness is more important for tattooees, there appears to be no difference between tattooed and nontattooed individuals in their appearance investment or body satisfaction. However, the measurement of appearance investment has typically been in relation to the "normative" appearance ideals, and not in relation to having a unique appearance. As striving for uniqueness is associated with positive self-esteem, examination of aesthetic investment in relation to a unique appearance may provide a previously untapped insight into the body image of those with body art. In sum, the need for uniqueness and distinctive appearance investment are important motivators for becoming tattooed.

An extensive body of literature on the motivations for obtaining body art exists. In their review of this literature, Wohlrab and colleagues outlined 10 overarching motivational categories. They identified self-identity and self-beautification as being the two most commonly cited reasons for becoming pierced or tattooed. The quest for identity is clearly central, with body art being a visual expression of an individual's self-identification. It allows the wearer to articulate an aesthetic uniqueness to self and others, thus increasing the wearer's sense of individuality. The self-identification motivation is closely associated with the drive to aesthetically improve one's physical appearance. As a way of embellishing the body, tattoos are often described as works of "living art." The perception of physical beautification, however, may be unique to the wearer and not held by others. Indeed, negative stereotypes of individuals with body art continue despite the increased popularity of permanent body art across all age groups and social classes. As a consequence, negative appraisals from others tend to be harmful and may negate some of the pleasure derived from the acquisition of the body art. This is particularly so for women, with tattooed women being judged as less physically attractive and having more negative characteristics than tattooed males or nontattooed individuals.

Gendered Body Art

Male and female bodies are viewed and valued differently. This contention is supported by the occurrence of gender-oriented forms of body art. For example, tattoos have historically been associated with males and masculinity. However, tattooing has recently begun to cross traditional gender boundaries, with women representing approximately half of the tattoo artist's clientele. Despite the growing incidence of women acquiring a tattoo, the tattooed female body is considered by some to be a gender role violation. Nonetheless, the modified female body has profoundly gendered meaning, with the tattooed female body representing sexuality and exhibitionism. Conversely, the tattooed male body signals strength and power.

In keeping with society's gendered appearance expectations and traditions, males and females tend to choose different styles and bodily locations for their body art. For example, males tend to place their tattoo(s) on more visible areas of the body, with the majority displaying a preference for placement on the arm, followed by the back, and upper and lower legs.

In contrast, females generally place their tattoo(s) on parts of the body that are less visually salient, demonstrating a predilection for the breast, shoulder blade, lower back, hip, and ankle as a tattoo site. The penchant for different bodily locations and degrees of visibility may be in part due to tattoos historically being associated with males and therefore until now more socially acceptable as a male form of body modification.

Conclusions and Future Directions

Body art in its various forms is clearly infiltrating contemporary mainstream society. As such, reliance on earlier psychological research investigating the personality profile of the modified individual is problematic. This is due to the possible confounding effects associated with the sampling methods employed in these foundation studies. Despite the questionable applicability of much of the earlier research to mainstream society, the findings seem to have nevertheless perpetuated the negative social perceptions and attributions regarding individuals sporting body art (particularly permanent forms) as social deviants. In the past decade, a stream of research (e.g., Armstrong and her colleagues) on individual differences and motivations in obtaining body art was largely grounded in concerns that tattooing and piercing were health-risking behaviors. Examination of recent empirical evidence on the personality profiles of people with body art indicates few differences between those with modified bodies and their unmodified counterparts. Moreover, motivations for engaging in body art unmistakably signify body modification to be closely associated with the desire for social inclusion, rather than social exclusion.

In light of the prosocial motivations for obtaining body art, and the increasing popularity of piercings and tattoos in contemporary society, an exploration of the "social" determinants influencing the decision-making process leading to the acquisition of (or intention to acquire) body art is overdue. Indeed, psychology's traditionally pathology focus of body modification research is no longer appropriate for a behavior that is contemporarily prosocial in nature. In addition, our knowledge base would benefit from a change in research focus from examining stereotypes of persons with body art to a focus on perceptions of the form and content of the body art per se. Present and future research ought to center on individual differences and the sociopsychological factors that may influence perceptions of body art. Thus, future research would benefit from examining attitudes toward the body art itself as opposed to attitudes toward the wearer.

Given the paucity of knowledge about appearance-related motivations for acquiring body art, as well as the body image of individuals sporting body art, future research would benefit from such empirical examinations. For example, considering that Western society places a premium on bodily appearance, does evaluating one's physical appearance from a third-person's perspective impact motivations to acquire body art? That is, does engaging in self-objectifying behaviors influence the likelihood of permanently modifying the body's appearance? And if so, in what way? (See Chapter 6 on self-objectification theory.) Furthermore, although we know that tattoos have historically been associated with males and masculinity, experimental research has yet to examine the impact of gender typing and gendered role on body art practices. Indeed, what roles do masculinity and femininity have in the decision-making process associated with obtaining body art in its different forms? Is it different for males and females? These questions need to be addressed. Overall, current scientific knowledge about the individual and sociopsychological aspects of body art as they relate to body image is minimal at best, clearly indicating the need for broader examination of this topic.

Informative Readings

Ames, D. R., & Iyengar, S. S. (2005). Appraising the unusual: Framing effects and moderators of uniqueness-seeking and social projection. *Journal of Experimental Social Psychology, 41,* 271–282.—An experimental study on the need for uniqueness, social projection, and perceived similarity to a target group.

Armstrong, M. L., Owen, D. C., Roberts, A. E., & Koch, J. R. (2002). College tattoos: More than skin deep. *Dermatology Nursing, 14,* 317–323.—An examination of the physical and psychological correlates of tattooing, and the associated need for health-related education.

Copes, J. H., & Forsyth, C. J. (1993). The tattoo: A social psychological explanation. *International Review of Modern Sociology, 23,* 83–89.—An examination of personality correlates of tattoos.

Forbes, G. B. (2001). College students with tattoos and piercings: Motives, family experiences, personality factors, and perception by others. *Psychological Reports, 89,* 774–786.—A study examining social psychological factors associated with tattoos and piercings.

Hawkes, D., Senn, C. Y., & Thorn, C. (2004). Factors that influence attitudes toward women with tattoos. *Sex Roles, 50,* 593–614.—An examination of contemporary attitudes toward women with and without tattoos.

Laumann, A. E., & Derick, A. J. (2006). Tattoos and body piercings in the United States: A national data set. *Journal of the American Academy of Dermatology, 55,* 413–421.—Information on the prevalence of tattoos and body piercing, and the incidence of subsequent health concerns.

Pitts, V. (2003). *In the flesh: The cultural politics of body modification.* New York: Palgrave Macmillan.—A review and critique of the modified body and self-identity within contemporary culture.

Sanders, C. (1989). *Customizing the body: The art and culture of tattooing.* Philadelphia: Temple University Press.—A comprehensive review of body modification from historical, sociological, and contemporary art perspectives.

Swami, V., & Furnham, A. (2007). Unattractive, promiscuous and heavy drinkers: Perceptions of women with tattoos. *Body Image: An International Journal of Research, 4*, 343–352.—A study indicating that negative perceptions of tattooed women continue in contemporary society.

Tate, J. C., & Shelton, B. L. (2008). Personality correlates of tattooing and body piercing in a college sample: The kids are alright. *Personality and Individual Differences, 45*, 281–285.—A comparison between tattooed and pierced individuals and their nonmodified counterparts, highlighting negligible differences and cautioning against pathologizing body modifiers.

Tiggemann, M., & Golder, F. (2006). Tattooing: An expression of uniqueness in the appearance domain. *Body Image: An International Journal of Research, 3*, 309–315.—A study exploring motivations for becoming tattooed, including the need for a unique appearance.

Wohlrab, S., Fink, B., Kappeler, P. M., & Brewer, G. (2009). Perception of human body modification. *Personality and Individual Differences, 46*, 202–206.—An examination of the modified body in relation to perceived health and mate selection.

Wohlrab, S., Stahl, J., & Kappeler, P. M. (2007). Modifying the body: Motivations for getting tattooed and pierced. *Body Image: An International Journal of Research, 4*, 87–95.—A literature review that culminates in the identification of 10 broad motivations for body art.

CHAPTER 45

Cosmetic Surgery and Changes in Body Image

DAVID B. SARWER
CANICE E. CRERAND
LEANNE MAGEE

Introduction

According to the American Society of Plastic Surgeons, approximately 13.1 million cosmetic surgical and minimally invasive cosmetic treatments were performed in the United States in 2010. The top five cosmetic and minimally invasive procedures performed in 2010 can be seen in Table 45.1. Females were the recipients of 91% of these procedures. The vast majority of these treatments were minimally invasive procedures such as Botox injections, soft tissue fillers (e.g., Restalyne), and chemical peels. Among the 1.5 million cosmetic surgical procedures performed, breast augmentation was the most popular with 296,203 procedures. These statistics, although well known to individuals within the plastic surgery community, are often staggering to lay persons who have little idea about the number of Americans who use cosmetic medical treatments to enhance their appearance. The estimated cost of these cosmetic treatments was $10 billion in 2009.

As the popularity of cosmetic medical treatments has grown, so has the interest in the psychological aspects of these procedures. This chapter provides an overview of psychological studies of cosmetic surgery patients, with a particular emphasis on the relationship between body image and cosmetic surgery. The chapter also reviews studies that have investigated changes in psychosocial status and body image following

TABLE 45.1. Number of Top Five Cosmetic Surgical and Minimally Invasive Procedures Performed in 2010 in the United States

Surgical cosmetic procedures	
1. Breast augmentation	296,203
2. Nose reshaping	252,261
3. Eyelid surgery	208,764
4. Liposuction	203,106
5. Tummy tuck	116,352

Minimally invasive cosmetic procedures	
1. Botox	5,379,360
2. Soft tissue fillers	1,773,328
3. Chemical peel	1,144,865
4. Laser hair removal	937,602
5. Microdermabrasion	824,706

Note. Data courtesy of the American Society of Plastic Surgeons (ASPS), National Clearinghouse of Plastic Surgery Statistics, 2011 Report of the 2010 Statistics. Available at *www.plasticsurgery.org/Media/Statistics.html.*

cosmetic surgery. This literature is used to offer recommendations to the mental health professional for the psychological assessment and management of cosmetic surgery patients.

Psychosocial Considerations in Cosmetic Surgery

The growth in cosmetic surgery and minimally invasive procedures can be understood from a number of theoretical perspectives that are reviewed in this handbook, including sociocultural development of beauty standards and practices (Chapter 2), evolutionary theories of attractiveness (Chapter 3), cognitive-behavioral perspectives (Chapter 5), and feminist and objectification theories (Chapter 6). The development of minimally invasive procedures and advances in wound care that allow procedures to be performed more safely and with less recovery time than in the past have also likely contributed to the growth. In addition, the general public's exposure to cosmetic surgery through the mass media has greatly influenced its popularity as well. Recent studies have shown that greater vicarious experience of cosmetic surgery is associated with greater approval of cosmetic surgery, as well as a greater likelihood of considering surgery for oneself. Two studies of undergraduate women demonstrated that 3–5% had undergone cosmetic procedures themselves, and one-half to two-thirds had friends or family members who had undergone cosmetic surgical procedures. It may not be media or vicarious exposures alone that influence attitudes toward cosmetic surgery, but rather the internalization of the unattainable ideals of beauty perpetuated by the mass media and messages about cosmetic surgery that are also thought to be reflected in these findings.

Several chapters throughout this text refer to research investigating the relationship between body image dissatisfaction (BID) and the pursuit of appearance-enhancing behaviors. Both the degree of investment in physical appearance and the degree of dissatisfaction have been thought to shape attitudes and behaviors related to cosmetic surgery. BID is considered to be a primary motivation for cosmetic surgery. Studies of cosmetic surgery patients have found that patients report heightened BID preoperatively. In many of these investigations, patients did not report greater global BID, but rather a more specific dissatisfaction with the feature being considered for surgery.

Although elevated levels of BID appear to be common among persons who seek cosmetic procedures, a substantial minority of individuals present for cosmetic surgery with a degree of dissatisfaction and preoccupation consistent with body dysmorphic disorder (BDD; see Chapter 35). In cosmetic surgery populations, 5–15% of patients appear to have some form of the disorder. Although persons with BDD typically report concerns with the appearance of their skin, hair, and nose, any body part can become a source of preoccupation. BDD is characterized by repetitive, intrusive, and uncontrollable thoughts about a perceived appearance flaw. These thoughts are typically accompanied by ritualized and time-consuming behaviors (e.g., excessive grooming behaviors), which are performed in an effort to improve or camouflage the perceived defect, and ultimately, to reduce appearance-related distress. However, these behaviors only lead to increased preoccupation and distress about appearance. Significant emotional distress, impairment in social and occupational functioning, including social avoidance and decreased quality of life, frequently result from BDD symptoms.

Persons with BDD frequently seek cosmetic medical treatments as a means of improving their perceived defects. In contrast to most patients, individuals with BDD are typically dissatisfied with the outcome of such treatments. Furthermore, two retrospective studies have found that greater than 90% of persons with BDD report either no change or a worsening in their BDD symptoms following cosmetic treatments. Of even greater concern, studies have documented high rates of suicidal ideation, suicide attempts, and self-harm behaviors (e.g., "do-it-yourself" surgery) among patients with BDD. There are also reports of patients with BDD who have threatened to sue or physically harm their treatment providers. In light of these issues, there is growing consensus that cosmetic treatments should be contraindicated for persons with BDD, for the safety of both patients and the surgical team.

Psychosocial Status Following Cosmetic Surgery

A great majority of cosmetic surgery patients report satisfaction with their postoperative results. Studies also suggest that most women report improvements in body image postoperatively, although most of these studies have followed these women for no longer than 2 years. The impact of cosmetic surgery on other areas of functioning, such as self-esteem, depressive symptoms, and quality of life, is less well understood. While some studies have shown improvements in these domains postoperatively, other studies have found no significant improvements. The occurrence of postoperative complications also may negatively impact psychosocial outcomes, but this issue has received little study to date.

In the past decade, seven epidemiological studies that investigated silicone gel-filled breast implants and all-cause mortality have found an association between cosmetic breast implants and suicide. Women who have undergone cosmetic breast augmentation exhibit a two- to three-fold increased rate of suicide compared to the general population, a rate that is greatest among women receiving implants after age 40. Although one study suggested that the occurrence of suicide among women with breast implants was more frequent than among women who underwent other forms of cosmetic surgery, a subsequent investigation with a larger sample found no difference in the rate of suicide among breast augmentation and other cosmetic surgery patients.

Research indicates that breast implants do not directly increase mortality in women. Rather, potential explanations of this relationship largely have focused on the preoperative functioning and psychosocial status of the patients. Women who undergo breast augmentation exhibit a number of characteristics that are, in and of themselves, risk factors for suicide, including more lifetime sexual partners and a greater use of oral contraceptives, younger age at the time of their first pregnancy, a history of terminated pregnancies, more frequent alcohol and tobacco use, and below-average body weight. Some studies have also suggested that women with breast implants have greater rates of mental illness than women in general. One epidemiological study has documented a higher rate of previous psychiatric hospitalizations among women with breast implants when compared with women who received other cosmetic procedures and women who underwent breast reduction, but information on diagnosis, history of illness, or other psychiatric treatments for the women was not reported. A history of mental illness requiring psychiatric hospitalization is one of the strongest risk factors for suicide. Other studies have also shown that women with breast implants report a higher rate of outpatient psychological or psychiatric treatment compared with other women.

Nevertheless, the relationship between preoperative psychopathology and subsequent suicide following cosmetic breast augmentation remains inconclusive. In a review of these studies identifying a relationship between breast implants and suicide, an alternative explanation for the epidemiological findings suggested that improvements in body image following breast augmentation may actually produce a protective effect for women who may have otherwise been at increased risk for suicide due to other preexisting demographic and psychosocial risk factors. This hypothesis, although intriguing, has yet to receive any direct empirical study.

Psychological Assessment and Management of Cosmetic Surgery Patients

This literature can be used to inform the psychological assessment and management of cosmetic surgery patients. Psychologists and other mental health professionals may encounter individuals interested in cosmetic surgery in several contexts. Mental health professionals may be asked by a plastic surgeon or other physician to conduct an evaluation to determine a patient's psychological appropriateness for surgery. A plastic surgeon may refer a patient to a mental health professional if the patient is having an untoward psychological response to a postoperative outcome. Providers who have a more general psychotherapy practice, and particularly those who focus on body image, may encounter new or existing patients who have had or who are considering cosmetic surgery. The section below focuses on patients referred to the mental health professional by a plastic surgeon or other professional.

Psychological Assessment of the Preoperative Patient

In general, the vast majority of patients interested in cosmetic surgical and nonsurgical procedures are thought to be psychologically appropriate for treatment. Most patients typically have specific appearance concerns, internal motivations for surgery, and realistic postoperative expectations. Thus, most do not need a psychological evaluation prior to undergoing a cosmetic procedure. Few, if any, cosmetic surgeons require such evaluations. Patients who display symptoms of psychopathology during their initial consultation with the cosmetic surgeon, as well as those with a history of psychopathology, are most likely to be referred to a mental health professional. Nevertheless, many surgeons will elect not to perform procedures on patients who are thought to have a significant and untreated psychiatric problem.

Many of the early descriptions of cosmetic surgery patients are complete with elaborate interpretations of the role of unconscious conflicts and poor parental relationships in the decision to seek surgery. There is no evidence, however, to suggest that such interpretations are necessarily valid or useful in determining patients' appropriateness for surgery. Rather, a more straightforward evaluation of current psychosocial functioning, as found in a general cognitive-behavioral assessment, is recommended.

An evaluation of a prospective patient should focus on the thoughts, behaviors, and experiences that have contributed to appearance dissatisfaction and the decision to seek treatment. This involves the assessment of the "ABCs" of a patient's interest in surgery—the (A) antecedents to the decision to seek a cosmetic treatment; the (B) behavioral responses to appearance concerns; and the (C) consequences of surgery, or how the person expects surgery will impact his or her life. The evaluation should determine whether the patient's thoughts and behaviors are maladaptive or reflect psychopathology that would contraindicate treatment. In addition, the assessment should focus on the patient's motivations and expectations for cosmetic surgery, appearance and body image concerns, and psychiatric history and current status.

In assessing motivations for surgery, the mental health professional may want to begin by asking, "When did you first think about changing your appearance with cosmetic surgery?" Similarly, it may be instructive to ask, "What other things have you done to improve your appearance?" In addition to providing historical information, these questions may also reveal the presence of some obsessive or delusional thinking, as well as compulsive or bizarre behaviors related to physical appearance. It is not uncommon for cosmetic surgery patients to report that they have tried several "do-it-yourself" treatments in an attempt to improve their appearance. Many of these were most likely not helpful and some potentially dangerous.

The role of social relationships in the decision to seek surgery should be assessed. Patients should be asked how romantic partners, family members, and close friends feel about their decision to change a physical feature. Patients who seek treatment specifically to please a current partner or to attract a new one are thought to be less likely to be satisfied with their postoperative outcomes. Thus, the mental health professional should inquire about patients' general expectations about how a change in appearance, which may be subtle and possibly unnoticed by others, will influence their lives.

Cash's model of the historical and proximal influences on body image (see Chapter 5) provides a useful framework to assess the appearance and body image concerns of surgical candidates. Patients should be able to articulate specific concerns about their appearance that should be visible with little effort. Patients who are markedly distressed about slight or imagined defects may be suffering from BDD. The nature of the appearance defect may be difficult for mental health professionals to assess for at least two reasons. First, appropriate ethical care would prohibit these professionals from asking patients to remove clothing to view the defect. Second, the judgment of an appearance feature is highly subjective. What a mental health professional judges to be a feature well within the range of normal may be an appearance defect that a cosmetic surgeon judges as treatable. As a result, the degree of emotional distress and impairment, rather than the specific nature of the defect, may be more accurate indicators of BDD in these patients.

Although heightened BID is considered typical for individuals interested in cosmetic surgery, some of the thoughts and behaviors that contribute to both the development and maintenance of this dissatisfaction may be maladaptive. Many patients believe that others take notice of their appearance defects. Others report anxiety or avoidance of specific social situations because of self-consciousness about their appearance. Asking about the amount of time spent thinking about a feature or the activities missed or avoided may indicate the degree of distress and impairment a person is experiencing and help determine the presence of BDD.

The assessment of psychiatric history and current status, as would be done in any mental health consultation, is a central part of the evaluation. Given the number of persons who undergo surgery each year, it is likely that all of the major psychiatric diagnoses can be found in this patient population. Particular attention should be paid to disorders with a body image component, such as eating disorders, as well as mood and anxiety disorders. The presence of a psychiatric disorder, however, may not be an absolute contraindication for cosmetic surgery, with the exception of BDD (as detailed above). In the absence of sound data on the relationship between psychopathology and surgical outcome, appropriateness for surgery should be made on a case-by-case basis and include careful collaboration between the mental health professional and the referring surgeon.

Approximately 20% of patients who seek cosmetic medical treatment report using a psychiatric medication. As mental health professionals frequently observe, patients who receive these medications from primary care physicians often do not experience complete relief from their symptoms. Thus, a psychopharmacological evaluation should be considered if symptoms do not appear to be well controlled. If the patient is in treatment with another mental health professional, the consultant should contact this professional and discuss the patient's appropriateness for cosmetic treatment.

At the conclusion of the evaluation, the mental health professional should share his or her clinical impressions with the patient, as well as his or her recommendation to the referring physician about the appropriateness for surgery. Though referring physicians will make the ultimate determination about the decision to go forward with surgery, it is good practice to share the results of the consultation with the patient.

Psychological Management of the Postoperative Patient

Mental health professionals may be referred patients who already have undergone surgery and are dissatisfied with a technically successful procedure or experiencing an exacerbation of psychopathology that was not detected preoperatively. The initial assessment of these patients should be similar to that described above. Cognitive-behavioral therapy to improve body image (see Chapter 47) may be useful with these individuals, although more diagnosis-specific treatments also may be indicated.

Cosmetic surgery patients can represent an interesting and unique experience for the mental health professional. Before agreeing to accept these consultations, the professional should examine his or her own beliefs about cosmetic surgery and its ability to positively impact persons' lives. Though cosmetic surgical treatments are not beneficial to everyone, consulting professionals should be open to the belief that changing the outward appearance can improve internal perceptions of the self and result in psychological benefits for appropriate patients.

Conclusions and Future Directions

As cosmetic surgery continues to increase in popularity, so too does interest in understanding why individuals seek to change their physical appearance. Body image appears to play an integral part in both the motivation to seek cosmetic surgery as well as the psychological outcomes observed in those who undergo these procedures. Future research should continue to investigate how factors associated with body image, such as cognitive and behavioral investment in appearance, the tendency to engage in appearance-based social comparisons, and appearance-based rejection sensitivity, may influence the motivation to seek cosmetic surgery and satisfaction with surgical outcome. Mental health professionals are likely to encounter patients who seek to alter their appearance through cosmetic surgery and should be aware of disorders, such as BDD, which may contraindicate surgery, as well as anxiety, depression, substance abuse, and other psychological disorders. Additional investigation is also needed to accurately assess base rates of psychopathology in cosmetic surgery populations, the relationships between such psychopathology and body image, and the effects of psychopathological symptoms on the pursuit of and satisfaction with cosmetic surgery.

Informative Readings

American Society of Plastic Surgeons. (2011). *National Clearinghouse of Plastic Surgery Statistics, 2011 Report of the 2010 Statistics*. Arlington Heights, IL: Author. Available at *www.plasticsurgery.org/Media/Statistics.html*.—A web-based resource providing educational information for medical professionals, patients, and the media, as well as statistics on the number of plastic surgery procedures performed by members of the American Society of Plastic Surgeons.

Cash, T. F., Duel, L. A., & Perkins, L. L. (2002). Women's psychosocial outcomes of breast augmentation with silicone gel-filled implants: A 2-year prospective study. *Plastic and Reconstructive Surgery, 109,* 2112–2121.—A prospective study of the psychosocial status of 360 breast augmentation patients that demonstrated postoperative satisfaction with body image and appearance, stable psychosocial outcomes, and an overall perception that the benefits outweighed the risks of augmentation surgery.

Crerand, C. E., Franklin, M. E., & Sarwer, D. B. (2006). Body dysmorphic disorder and cosmetic surgery. *Plastic and Reconstructive Surgery, 118,* 167e–180e.— Provides an overview of BDD and its relationship to aesthetic medical treatments.

Crerand, C. E., Phillips, K. A., Menard, W., & Fay, C. (2005). Non-psychiatric medical treatment of body dysmorphic disorder. *Psychosomatics, 46,* 49–55.—Empirical study detailing the frequency, types, and outcomes of cosmetic medical treatments sought and received by 200 individuals with BDD.

Honigman, R., Phillips, K. A., & Castle, D. J. (2004). A review of psychosocial outcomes for patients seeking cosmetic surgery. *Plastic and Reconstructive Surgery, 113,* 1229–1237.—A review of 37 studies of psychosocial outcomes of cosmetic surgery that concludes that patients are generally satisfied with surgical outcomes and that identifies psychosocial risk factors for poor surgical outcomes and postoperative dissatisfaction.

Phillips, K. A., Menard, W., Fay, C., & Weisberg, R. (2005). Demographic characteristics, phenomenology, comorbidity, and family history in 200 individuals with body dysmorphic disorder. *Psychosomatics, 46,* 317–325.—Empirical study that examines the clinical and demographic characteristics of BDD in the largest sample of persons with the disorder including those who had and had not received psychiatric treatment.

Sarwer, D. B. (2006). Psychological assessment of cosmetic surgery. In D. B. Sarwer, T. Pruzinsky, T. F. Cash, R. M. Goldwyn, J. A. Persing, & L. A. Whitaker (Eds.), *Psychological aspects of reconstructive and cosmetic plastic surgery: Clinical, empirical, and ethical perspectives* (pp. 267–283). Philadelphia: Lippincott, Williams & Wilkins.—Offers recommendations for clinical assessments of pre- and postoperative cosmetic surgery patients, including suggestions for evaluating body image concerns and symptoms of BDD.

Sarwer, D. B., Brown, G. K., & Evans, D. L. (2007). Cosmetic breast augmentation and suicide. *American Journal of Psychiatry, 164,* 1006–1113.—Reviews the literature regarding the relationship between suicide and cosmetic breast augmentation and offers suggestions for research as well as clinical care.

Sarwer, D. B., & Crerand, C. E. (2004). Body image and cosmetic medical treatments. *Body Image: An International Journal of Research, 1,* 99–111.—Reviews historical and contemporary research on the psychosocial status of cosmetic surgery patients, with a focused exploration of the role of BID and disturbance in the pursuit of specific types of plastic surgery.

Sarwer, D. B., & Crerand, C. E. (2008). Body dysmorphic disorder and appearance enhancing medical treatments. *Body Image: An International Journal of Research, 5,* 50–58.—Reviews the relationship between BDD and cosmetic treatments and provides suggestions for the clinical management of BDD in cosmetic medical settings.

Sarwer, D. B., & Magee, L. (2006). Physical appearance and society. In D. B. Sarwer, T. Pruzinsky, T. F. Cash, R. M. Goldwyn, J. A. Persing, & L. A. Whitaker (Eds.), *Psychological aspects of reconstructive and cosmetic plastic surgery: Clinical, empirical, and ethical perspectives* (pp. 23–36). Philadelphia: Lippincott, Williams & Wilkins.—A review of the evolutionary and sociocultural influences on appearance and their role in the pursuit of plastic surgery.

Sarwer, D. B., Wadden, T. A., Pertschuk, M. J., & Whitaker, L. A. (1998). The psychology of cosmetic surgery: A review and reconceptualization. *Clinical Psychology Review, 18,* 1–22.—Provides a historical review of the literature and proposes a model of the relationship between body image and cosmetic surgery.

Veale, D. (2004). Advances in a cognitive-behavioural model of body dysmorphic disorder. *Body Image: An International Journal of Research, 1,* 113–125.—A revision of a cognitive-behavioral model concerning the etiology, maintenance, and treatment of BDD, with updated empirical evidence and a discussion of risk factors for BDD.

Body Image and Biomedical Interventions for Disfiguring Conditions

DIANA HARCOURT
NICHOLA RUMSEY

Introduction

A sizeable body of research has demonstrated the potential psychosocial impact of living with a condition resulting in disfigurement (see Chapters 29 and 41). This work has repeatedly shown that individuals are not equally affected, and although some can manage the challenges presented to them very well, others are less successful in doing so. Most people with a disfiguring condition will undergo some form of biomedical intervention. This chapter reviews the extent to which these interventions address the psychosocial needs of adults with visible differences. It focuses on interventions for people affected by facial disfigurement or breast cancer, but the issues are relevant to a broad range of disfiguring conditions.

Biomedical Interventions

Developments in biomedical interventions over recent years have meant that many people now survive conditions or trauma (e.g., cancer, burns) that would have previously proven fatal. However, they are likely to be left with an altered appearance or visible difference, and may undergo further biomedical interventions that seek to restore their looks. Likewise, people living with congenital conditions are likely to be offered, or seek, treatment in a quest to change their physical appearance. These interventions include plastic surgery to modify existing body tissue, reconstructive surgery to restore the shape or appearance of a body part that is missing, and laser surgery to alter the appearance of the skin.

There can be a tendency to assume that biomedical interventions that alter a person's objective appearance will offer psychosocial benefits, essentially through improved body image and quality of life and reduced distress, including lower levels of social anxiety. However, although they might shift an individual's appearance toward "the norm" and could thereby benefit psychosocial functioning, they are not a universal panacea.

Laser Treatment

Laser treatment aims to improve the objective appearance of skin conditions such as birthmarks. However, this can be a very painful and prolonged intervention. Research by Hansen and colleagues found that, although patients reported improvements in the color of their port-wine stain, the size and texture tended not to improve. Importantly, although most patients worried less about their appearance after treatment, it did not affect their perceptions of how they were viewed by other people or their social interactions with them. In summary, laser treatment altered their objective appearance to an extent, but had limited impact on psychosocial issues and body image.

Surgical Interventions

The term *surgical interventions* encompasses a vast range of procedures that vary in the extent of invasiveness involved, the degree to which the decision for the type and timing of surgery is made by the individual or his or her health care team, and whether it is an established component of routine care or a more pioneering procedure. Although some procedures may be elected solely by the individual and are available at any time (e.g., breast reconstruction after mastectomy), others (e.g., surgery for young people born with a cleft lip and palate) are typically provided in line with rigid treatment protocols that allow little leeway for individual differences in social and personal factors. Some involve a single procedure but many involve a succession of operations before an acceptable aesthetic result is achieved.

Breast Reconstruction

The American Society of Plastic Surgeons reported over 86,000 breast-reconstruction procedures were performed in the United States in 2009.

The national audit of mastectomy and breast reconstruction in the United Kingdom reported that more than 3,200 immediate reconstruction procedures took place during a 15-month period to March 2009, representing around 18% of those who underwent mastectomy during this time. In addition, more than 1,500 women underwent delayed reconstruction during the audit period, and many of these women underwent, or were planning, additional procedures such as reduction of the contralateral breast, scar revisions, and nipple reconstruction. The number of women electing to undergo breast reconstruction will continue to increase as the procedure becomes more widely available.

Reconstruction is typically believed to offer benefits to women whose body image has altered following mastectomy. Likewise, it is often assumed that undergoing reconstructive surgery in the same operation in which the mastectomy is carried out (immediate reconstruction) is preferrable to living with a mastectomy and then undergoing reconstruction at a later date (delayed reconstruction). However, research to date has failed to definitively support these assumptions, partly because of limitiations with study design (e.g., small samples and retrospective designs). A prospective study of 103 women who chose mastectomy alone, or mastectomy with immediate or delayed reconstruction, reported improved body image among those having delayed reconstruction but no significant difference between the other two groups. This study concluded that immediate reconstruction still entails a woman having to adjust to an altered body image and that this surgery is not a panacea for the disfigurement and distress associated with mastectomy.

Women's decisions about whether to undergo breast reconstruction and the type and timing of surgery have been explored at considerable length. They are likely to be informed by many factors, including a woman's attitude toward using a breast prosthesis, the opinions of significant others, how the options are presented to her, the importance she places on appearance, and her attitude toward the specific risks associated with each procedure (e.g., implants run the risk of infection and needing to be replaced).

Adjustment to a reconstructed breast takes time and the final aesthetic outcome is not immediately evident. Some research suggests that women undergoing transverse rectus abdominus myocutaneous (TRAM) flap procedures (which use abdominal tissue to recreate a breast shape) report higher levels of longer-term satisfaction with outcome than their peers who elect reconstruction using implants. However, rather than encouraging the view that any particular type or timing of breast reconstruction is preferrable to any other (or to no reconstruction at all), it is more important to ensure that each woman is able to make the decision that is best for her. Nevertheless, some women find making these decisions very difficult. This is partly because of the range of options and the need to consider complex information, often in a relatively short period of time around the time of diagnosis of cancer, when their ability to consider all the options in detail is typically impaired.

Sheehan and collaborators found that 47% of the 123 patients who had undergone breast reconstruction in their study reported some degree of regret about their decision. Regret was associated with levels of depressive symptoms, unrealistic expectations of the outcome of reconstruction, and inadequate presurgical information. This highlights the importance of ensuring prospective patients have access to information that meets their individual needs, the opportunity to meet others who have previously made the decision, and sufficient time and support to consider their options fully. Easily accessible interventions to support patients faced with this decision need to be developed and rigorously evaluated.

Full Face Transplantation

In recent years, the potential for full face transplantation has been seen, by some, as the ultimate surgical intervention for people with extensive facial disfigurement. Although surgeons have felt confident that the necessary surgical expertise has been available for some time, the debate around the psychological and ethical implications of this radical procedure is ongoing. Partial face transplants have taken place in France, China, and the United States, with the most high-profile case being that of Isabelle Dinoire in 2005. In early 2010, surgeons in Spain conducted the world's first full face transplant on a farmer who had extensive disfigurement after a gunshot wound to the face. Alex Clarke, a clinical psychologist and member of the U.K. Face Transplant Team, has written extensively on the psychosocial aspects of facial transplantation and the need for carefully planned psychological support before and after any such procedure. Her work highlights the complex challenges facing transplant teams and patients, notably how to screen potential recipients, manage their expectations, ensure they understand risk information, and help them assimilate their new face into their body image and sense of identity.

The psychological and social implications of having a face that previously "belonged" to somebody else are still unknown, but they can be extrapolated on the basis of the existing research into adjustment to acquired disfigurement. Recipients must adjust to a change in facial appearance and its movement and functional ability. They must also manage the reactions of other people to the change in their appearance and they may become a focus of attention by those who are intrigued by the novelty of their situation.

Further challenges include the demands of an intensive, life-long regimen of immune-suppressive drugs to reduce the risk of the donated face being rejected. However, side effects of these drugs include increased risk of infections and cancers. Nonadherence to immune-suppressive drugs (which is typically around 15–20% among other types of transplant patients) increases the likelihood of rejection and the need for either a further transplant or a large graft of the recipient's own tissue (an option that would have already been pursued, before a face transplant, if sufficient tissue was available). Furthermore, lifestyle and behavior changes will be needed. These could include dietary changes to reduce the risk of postoperative diabetes and avoidance of sun exposure to reduce the increased risk of skin cancers.

The potential irony is that those who are most psychologically resilient to the challenges of such invasive surgery, its uncertain outcome, and the demanding postoperative regimen may be more able to cope with the demands of living with a visible difference, and therefore less likely to seek a face transplant. In contrast, those who volunteer for this procedure are likely to be more distressed by their appearance and psychologically vulnerable.

The notion of full face transplantation also raises issues and consequences for the recipient's and donor's families (e.g., complex support and decision making), as well as for society in general. For example, does the availability of full face transplantation indicate society's lack of acceptance of visible difference and imply that people who have a disfiguring condition should go to any length to make their appearance more acceptable to the wider public?

Limitations of Biomedical Interventions

Although biomedical interventions may improve objective aspects of a disfiguring condition, they do not remove it entirely and may result in additional scarring on parts of the body that were previously unaffected. For example, reconstructive procedures that involve moving tissue from another part of the body create scarring at the previously unscarred donor site.

Patients' and health professionals' expectations of the outcome of biomedical interventions and their motivations for pursuing such options may not correspond. Although they may both want to "improve" appearance and body image, their understanding of what constitutes "improvement" may differ considerably. A surgeon may define it in terms of a neater scar, but patients may anticipate this to mean the visible difference is removed entirely and their appearance is ostensibly "normal." Recent research examined the notion of "normality" among women seeking breast reconstruction. They described their motivation for surgery in terms of *appearing normal* (e.g., "looking normal to others"; "looking like I used to"), *behaving as normal* (i.e., fulfilling everyday activities), *restoring normality* (in terms of self-image and identity), and *normal health* (i.e., anticipating that reconstruction would improve their emotional well-being and remove the visible reminder of the cancer). If a patient's understandings do not concur with those of his or her surgical team, there may be confusion as to what the surgery is trying to achieve. If his or her expectations are unrealistic, the potential for disappointment and requests for further corrective surgery is high.

Biomedical interventions typically involve a succession of procedures over time and patients may feel as if they are on a surgical treadmill. For example, repair of a cleft lip and palate entails multiple invasive procedures, but the impact of each operation on body image remains unclear. Deciding not to pursue further surgical intervention can be difficult, but could indicate that the individual has successfully incorporated his or her appearance into his or her body image.

Clearly, biomedical interventions offer benefits to many patients, but they do not address all the psychosocial needs of people faced with a disfiguring condition. Since psychosocial factors determine adjustment to disfigurement, it follows that body image and appearance-related concerns among these populations should be addressed through psychosocial interventions, either independently or alongside biomedical interventions.

Psychosocial Interventions and Provision of Care

Psychosocial interventions can usefully be considered in terms of tiers ranging from relatively simple information provision offered by any member of a health care team, through to specialist interventions delivered by trained psychosocial experts to people identified as warranting individual, targeted support. A challenge remains in how to ensure that those who may benefit from tailored, specialist support are identified and referred.

Specialist interventions have tended to be based around social interaction skills training (SIST) or cognitive-behavioral therapy (CBT) approaches. SIST, delivered as a group or one-to-one intervention, can improve individuals' confidence and ability to initiate, engage in, and manage social interactions with other people. Likewise, CBT-based interventions can be effective when they are specific to body image and appearance-related concerns. As Chapter 47 discusses, CBT facilitates change in how persons process information (thoughts) about their looks, how they feel about themselves (emotions), and how they engage or avoid others (behaviors).

Group psychosocial interventions can be beneficial because they enable an individual to practice social interaction skills among others who have a personal understanding of the challenges he or she faces, yet they can be difficult for those with high levels of social anxiety. A flexible use of both individual and group interventions may provide the most effective support, and research should identify which interventions are most suited to whom.

A current concern is the lack of specialist psychosocial services for people with disfiguring conditions. In the United Kingdom, there is only one specialist unit, Outlook, which means potential clients may have to travel long distances to access this level of intervention. In response, Bessell and others developed a computer-based CBT and SIST intervention that was found to be as acceptable and effective as face-to-face delivery of the same intervention. This suggests potential for online interventions, and work now focuses on the development of a web-based intervention for young people. Online discussion boards have also shown potential to offer effective support. However, despite positive outcomes, a systematic review has criticized existing evaluations of psychosocial interventions on the basis of poor design and inadequate sample sizes.

Conclusions and Future Directions

Although research in this area has increased in recent years, much still needs to be done. Advances in surgical interventions will continue, so it is imperative that their impact upon psychological well-being and body image is evaluated. Meanwhile, psychosocial interventions must be designed, evaluated, and implemented, including support for complex cases (e.g., those experiencing posttraumatic stress disorder, as well as changes to appearance after traumatic injury).

Clinicians and researchers are faced with important challenges, including the choice of appropriate measures of outcomes and mediating and moderating factors. Given the complexity of issues involved in adjustment, a combination of measures is recommended, including body image, appearance-related anxiety, and the role of appearance in the individual's self-schema.

The longer-term impact on body image of biomedical and psychosocial interventions needs to be examined through longitudinal research. The extent to which interventions meet the needs of people from differing cultural and ethnic backgrounds needs to be examined, and attention should also focus on the needs of young people with disfiguring conditions.

Not everyone who has a visible difference or disfiguring condition will want biomedical and/or psychosocial interventions. Many are able to manage the challenges they face very well. However, others may benefit from appropriate support. Biomedical interventions are unlikely to address fully an individual's appearance and body image concerns in isolation. There is a need for readily available psychosocial interventions that can meet individuals' changing needs over time. As the number of people living with a disfiguring condition continues to increase, so does the need for effective body image interventions.

Informative Readings

Bessell, A., & Moss, T. P. (2007). Evaluating the effectiveness of psychosocial interventions for individuals with visible differences: A systematic review of the empirical evidence, *Body Image: An International Journal of Research, 4*, 227–238.—A review of 12 self-help, CBT, counseling, and SIST interventions.

Brill, S. E., Clarke, A., Veale, D. M., & Butler, P. E. M. (2006). Psychological management and body image issues in facial transplantation. *Body Image: An International Journal of Research, 3*, 1–15.—Proposes a detailed framework for the anticipation and management of psychological change to ensure adjustment among face transplant recipients.

Clarke, A., & Butler, P. E. M. (2004). Face transplantation: Psychological assessment and preparation for surgery. *Psychology, Health and Medicine, 9*, 315–326.—Written before the first full face transplantation had taken place, an examination of the potential psychological impact of face transplantation and consideration of the issues needing to be addressed.

Denford, S., Harcourt, D., Rubin, L., & Pusic, A. (in press). Understanding normality: A qualitative analysis of breast cancer patients' concepts of normality after mastectomy and reconstructive surgery. *Psycho-Oncology*, DOI: 10.1002/pon.1762.—A qualitative study of interviews with 35 women who chose to undergo breast reconstruction.

Hansen, K., Kreiter, C. D., Rosenbaum, M., Whitaker, D. C., & Arpey, C. J. (2003). Long-term psychological impact and perceived efficacy of pulsed-dye laser therapy for patients with port-wine stains. *Dermatologic Surgery, 29*, 49–55.—A retrospective survey of 55 children and adults who underwent laser therapy to treat a port-wine stain (birthmark).

Harcourt, D., Rumsey, N., Ambler, N., Cawthorn, S. J., Reid, C., Maddox, P., et al. (2003). The psychological impact of mastectomy with or without immediate breast reconstruction: A prospective, multi-center study. *Plastic and Reconstructive Surgery, 111*, 1060–1068.—A quantitative study of 103 women undergoing mastectomy with or without immediate or delayed breast reconstruction.

Hu, E. S., Pusic, A. L., Waljee, J. F., Kuhn, L., Hawley, S. T., Wilkins, E., et al. (2009). Patient-reported aesthetic satisfaction with breast reconstruction during the long-term survivorship period. *Plastic and Reconstructive Surgery, 124*, 1–8.—A survey of longer-term satisfaction among 250 women who had breast reconstruction with TRAM flap or implants, conducted using the BREAST-Q (a patient-reported outcome measure specifically for women undergoing breast surgery).

Rumsey, N. (2004). Psychological aspects of face transplantation: Read the small print carefully. *American Journal of Bioethics, 4*, 10–13.—Considers the psychosocial implications of face transplantation.

Rumsey, N., & Harcourt, D. (2004). Body image and disfigurement: Issues and interventions. *Body Image: An International Journal of Research, 1,* 83–97.—An overview of the psychosocial impact of visible difference.

Rumsey, N., & Harcourt, D. (2005). *The psychology of appearance,* Maidenhead, UK: Open University Press.—An overview of issues around appearance research and provision of care, including biomedical and psychosocial interventions for people with a visible difference.

Sheehan, J., Sherman, K. A., Lam, T., & Boyages, J. (2008). Regret associated with the decision for breast reconstruction: The association of negative body image, distress and surgery characteristics with decision regret. *Psychology and Health, 23,* 207–219.—A study of factors influencing regret among 123 women who had undergone immediate or delayed breast reconstruction following mastectomy.

PART VIII

CHANGING BODY IMAGES
Psychosocial Interventions for Treatment and Prevention

CHAPTER 47

Cognitive-Behavioral Approaches to Body Image Change

JOSÉE L. JARRY
THOMAS F. CASH

Introduction

Body image cognitive-behavioral therapy (BI-CBT) is clearly established as an effective treatment for body image disturbance (BID). This chapter reviews the evidence for this claim. BI-CBT aims at modifying dysfunctional thoughts, feelings, and behaviors through interventions such as psychoeducation, self-monitoring, cognitive restructuring, desensitization, and exposure and response prevention. This review examines which components of body image particularly benefit from BI-CBT and which seem relatively unimproved. Moreover, what is the impact of BI-CBT on nontargeted psychosocial concomitants of body image (e.g., eating attitudes, self-esteem)? Evidence for the effectiveness of self-help BI-CBT is reviewed, with a discussion of its most beneficial components. We then consider BI-CBT for persons with obesity, an eating disorder, or body dysmorphic disorder (BDD). Finally, an eight-step body image intervention suitable for self-help and therapist-assisted, or therapist-directed, work is presented.

Outcomes of BI-CBT

Improvement in Body Image Dimensions

In a descriptive review of the empirical literature examining the effectiveness of stand-alone body image therapy published in 2004, Jarry and

415

Berardi found that overwhelmingly, these interventions included a CBT component and were conducted with non-eating-disordered, nonclinical samples. Most frequently, participants were college women. Jarry and Berardi found that all dimensions of body image improved significantly after treatment. In 2005, Jarry and Ip published a meta-analysis examining the effectiveness of stand-alone BI-CBT. Overall, Jarry and Ip found this therapy to be highly effective at improving the attitudinal and behavioral dimensions of body image, with the latter improving the most. However, body image investment did not significantly ameliorate. Jarry and Ip speculated that this may be attributable to the fact that although CBT effectively addresses the manifestations of overinvestment, it does not truly target the origins of this investment, thus possibly leaving the fundamental motivation to overinvest relatively intact. Furthermore, much of the outcome research with body image investment has used measures that tap more benign investment (i.e., valuing one's appearance and its self-management) rather than dysfunctional investment (i.e., schemas that emphasize appearance as a pivotal determinant of self-worth).

Although the perceptual component of body image does improve after BI-CBT, size overestimation improves equally whether the intervention includes size estimation accuracy training or not. Thus, overestimation may be the expression of body image dissatisfaction and when the latter is addressed with attitudinal interventions, its perceptual expression subsides.

Improvements in Eating Pathology and Psychological Functioning

In their review, Jarry and Berardi found that eating attitudes and behaviors significantly improved after BI-CBT. This was attributed to the fact that body image overvaluation and dissatisfaction are core elements of disordered eating. Therefore, improving the former should, and does, result in improvements in the latter. These authors also found that general psychological well-being variables such as anxiety, depression, and self-esteem improved after BI-CBT. With the finer-grain analysis afforded by meta-analysis, Jarry and Ip were able to demonstrate that, in controlled experimental designs, eating-related and general psychological variables improved equally and just as much as did body image variables. Moderators of the impact of BI-CBT on the generalization of change to psychological variables have seldom been tested. However, Strachan and Cash tested several individual differences such as presence/absence of obesity and self-reported history of an eating disorder and found none to affect the outcome of treatment. Similarly, Jarry and Ip concluded that the impact of BI-CBT on psychological variables was unaffected by moderators such as participants' initial level of BID, treatment focus (e.g., attitudinal, behavioral), or extent of therapist availability. Together, these findings speak to the very close association between body image distress, eating pathology, and general psychological discomfort, and suggest that intervening on one of these dimensions is likely to benefit the others.

The Effectiveness of Self-Help BI-CBT

Self-help BI-CBT has been investigated in several studies conducted by Cash and his colleagues, all examining the impact of components of his self-help program. In their reviews, Jarry and Berardi as well as Hrabosky and Cash found that self-directed BI-CBT with minimal therapist contact reliably ameliorates body image. However, the complete absence of therapist contact was associated with changes on fewer dimensions of body image. This more limited impact of completely self-directed BI-CBT was attributed to lower compliance, which may result in fewer positive changes. In their meta-analysis, Jarry and Ip found that therapist-assisted BI-CBT was more effective than was self-directed work.

Hrabosky and Cash closely examined what components of self-help BI-CBT appear most beneficial. In their review, they showed that an intervention consisting of psychoeducation combined with systematic self-monitoring was as effective as one consisting of these two components plus a cognitive-restructuring component. They also found that components such as cognitive restructuring and mirror exposure are associated with either low compliance from participants or actual treatment drop-out. This is not surprising as such components are either emotionally trying, cognitively complex, or both. Thus, it appears that entirely self-directed BI-CBT is most appropriate for its less emotionally and cognitively challenging components, whereas therapeutic assistance may be necessary for its more personally demanding components.

BI-CBT for Individuals with Obesity

Obesity interventions often do not include direct body image work, as weight reduction is assumed to be the essential means by which body image will improve. When present, body image work usually is combined with a weight loss and exercise program. Two studies have systematically examined BI-CBT in individuals with obesity. In 1995, Rosen, Orosan, and Reiter found that BI-CBT with no weight loss component resulted in significant improvement in body image, eating behavior, and psychological variables and that these gains were maintained at a 4.5-month follow-up. In 2001, Ramirez and Rosen compared a weight loss and BI-CBT intervention to a weight loss intervention alone. Both groups showed equivalent improvements in body image and psychological variables. However, as participants regained the lost weight over the 1-year follow-up, their body image satisfaction decreased. Taken together, these results suggest that BI-CBT effectively improves body image in individuals with obesity (see Chapter 42). Furthermore, during the weight loss maintenance phase of treatment, focusing on improving body image may help sustain body image improvements in the likely event of some weight regain.

BI-CBT for Individuals with Eating Disorders

Historically, body image seldom has been directly and systematically addressed in the treatment of individuals with eating disorders (see Chapters 32–34). When it is, it most often is a component of a larger CBT intervention that aims primarily to normalize eating behavior and to restore weight for underweight patients. Although body image concerns may get more attention in the treatment of patients with anorexia nervosa because of the crucial need for weight gain, some have aptly pointed out the importance of addressing these concerns before attempting weight gain, given that they motivated weight loss to begin with and are an impediment to weight gain during treatment.

Body image dissatisfaction improves moderately after CBT for eating disorders, even when it is not a target of treatment, as demonstrated by Rosen's 1996 review. Importantly, elevated body image concerns predict relapse and treatment drop-out. Nevertheless, no research has examined the additive efficacy of systematic BI-CBT to standard CBT for eating disorders.

The importance of advanced work on body image in the treatment of eating-disordered patients is reflected in cognitive-behavioral therapy–enhanced (CBT-E) recently proposed by Christopher Fairburn. CBT-E is predicated on the development of a tailor-made formulation of the factors maintaining the eating pathology for each patient regardless of his or her specific eating disorder diagnosis. In this formulation, the overvaluation of appearance occupies a central place. The work on body image is initiated after an initial focus on achieving regular eating. The components of this work are reviewed briefly below.

First, therapist and patient identify the overvaluation of shape and weight and its consequences, determining what proportion of the patient's self-worth rests on shape and weight relative to other domains of the self such as relationships and career. The social and behavioral consequences of this overinvestment are elucidated including excessive dieting, which creates a vulnerability to bingeing. The second step consists of enhancing previously underdeveloped areas of self-worth and addresses developmental delays due to excessive focus on shape and weight during formative years. The third step consists of addressing shape checking and avoidance. Self-monitoring of checking and avoidance is followed by the development of strategies for reducing these behaviors such as intercepting checking and exposure exercises for avoidance. The fourth step consists of addressing "feeling fat" as not being a true emotion but rather, a mask for other emotions that are then discovered through self-monitoring. The fifth step consists of identifying the proximal and distal origins of appearance overvaluation to provide the patient with some insight into the sources of his or her difficulties. The final step consists of learning to control the eating disorder mindset, whereby patients learn to identify stimuli that trigger the wish to control one's body and to make a conscious decision to not engage in such control. In a controlled study published in 2009, Fairburn and his colleagues investigated two forms of CBT-E. One form exclusively targets eating disorder psychopathology. The other additionally addresses problems such as mood intolerance, clinical perfectionism, low self-esteem, and interpersonal difficulties. They reported favorable and equivalent treatment effects that were unrelated to specific diagnoses and were sustained at a 60-week follow-up.

BI-CBT for Body Dysmorphic Disorder

In two reviews published in 2008, Buhlmann and colleagues as well as Neziroglu and colleagues summarized the very sparse literature on treatment outcomes for BDD (see Chapter 35). There are few studies, and most are case studies or series, with very little control for treatment modality, length of treatment, and receipt of medication. A recent meta-analysis conducted by Williams and colleagues demonstrated that CBT and behavior therapy alone had equivalent and considerably larger effect sizes than did pharmacotherapy with selective serotonin reuptake inhibitors (SSRIs), although all three interventions were effective. These findings suggest that CBT is an appropriate treatment for BDD. However, as pointed out by Neziroglu and colleagues, the evidence is insufficient to determine which unique components of CBT are effective. Interestingly, the studies conducted by Rosen and colleagues in 1995 and Veale and colleagues in 1996 remain the only randomized controlled trials of BI-CBT for BDD, both of which showed significant gains for treated participants.

Neziroglu and colleagues suggest adjustments to BI-CBT for BDD based on the conceptualization of this disorder as originating from a history of evaluative conditioning, operant conditioning, and biased information processing. They suggest that disputing the accuracy of appearance cognition may be counterproductive. Rather, interventions aimed at modifying attentional biases and effortful thinking, such as rumination, with the goal of distancing the self from irrational cognition and damaging imagery, rather than engaging them, may be more productive. A treatment manual published by Veale and Neziroglu in 2010 details the elements of a CBT program for BDD that integrates this perspective.

Buhlmann and colleagues propose that several characteristics of patients with BDD may be relevant to their treatment such as very high rates of personality disorders, traumatic childhood experiences, delusionality, depression, suicidality, and substance use disorders. Importantly, the latter two often are reported by patients to be connected to their appearance concerns. There is little research investigating the impact of these factors on treatment outcome and how to address them. However, Neziroglu and colleagues have shown that the extent of overvalued ideas about appearance predicts poor treatment outcome.

Components of a BI-CBT Program

The application and evaluation of CBT in the treatment of body image problems began in the 1980s, initiated by Thomas Cash's research group at Old Dominion University and continued by James Rosen's group formerly at the University of Vermont. Treatment protocols evolved over the years, with Cash's most current program being published in 2008 as the revised edition of *The Body Image Workbook*. The program was not developed to be a disorder-specific intervention (i.e., only for persons with eating disorders or BDD). Moreover, unlike previous versions, this contemporary version incorporates mindfulness and acceptance interventions. The structured eight-step protocol is summarized as follows:

• *Step 1*: A thorough multidimensional assessment utilizes scientifically validated tools to pinpoint and provide feedback about the client's body image strengths and vulnerabilities. Assessment includes the body image dimensions of evaluation (satisfaction–dissatisfaction), negative cognitions, contextually cued emotions, self-schematic investment in appearance, coping strategies, and body image quality of life.

• *Step 2*: This element of treatment educates clients about historical determinants of body image development, based on a cognitive social learning framework (see Chapter 5, this volume). Clients engage in a series of expressive writing exercises to elucidate their personal trajectories of body image development.

• *Step 3*: This component moves into the more proximal determinants of day-to-day body image experiences, with a focus on cognitive information processing. Clients engage in diary-recorded self-monitoring and begin to acquire mindfulness and acceptance-based approaches (see Chapter 48) to manage their body image thoughts and emotions. Included in this step are mirror-exposure exercises.

• *Step 4*: This next step addresses common appearance-related schemas or "appearance assumptions" that engender distressing "private body talk." Clients actively engage in dissonance-inducing exercises to begin to alter dysfunctional schemas that reflect and promote overinvestment in appearance as a criterion of self-definition and self-worth.

• *Step 5*: BID entails various errors or distortions in information processing that lead individuals to make faulty inferences and conclusions that instigate dysphoric emotions and maladaptive behaviors. The cognitive change exercises and mindfulness/acceptance strategies are continued and applied to specific cognitive errors or distortions in clients' private body talk.

• *Step 6*: This step targets experiential and behavioral avoidance that perpetuates body image difficulties. Aided by mindfulness and acceptance perspectives and body-and-mind relaxation, clients carry out graduated exposure and response prevention exercises.

• *Step 7*: In this phase, clients identify their "appearance-preoccupied rituals"—appearance checking and appearance fixing. They engage in specific behavioral exercises to gain more control over these rituals.

• *Step 8*: The purpose of this step is the explicit promotion of positive body image experiences, including fitness- and sensory-oriented experiences that are not appearance focused.

Following the eight-step program, clients retake the assessments from Step 1, discern their attained improvements, and identify their needs and plans for continued change, including their prevention of relapse.

Conclusions and Future Directions

The research evidence supports the effectiveness of BI-CBT for BID in nonclinical populations and in individuals with obesity and BDD. Paradoxically, less research has examined the added benefits of BI-CBT for individuals with eating disorders, although the importance of a treatment focus on body image as an etiological and maintaining factor of eating disorders is gaining ground. Research is needed to evaluate a number of questions: Clearly, most outcome research has been conducted with body-dissatisfied women. Does BI-CBT comparably benefit men with body image problems? What is the utility of BI-CBT for persons distressed by their "visible difference," such as congenital or acquired disfigurements (see Chapter 46)? What individual differences predict differences in treatment outcomes? What are the most effective CBT procedures for modifying dysfunctional investment in appearance (i.e., overvaluation or appearance schematicity)? Are contemporary mindfulness and acceptance interventions more effective and lasting than traditional cognitive-behavioral procedures? In this regard, in 2010, Pearson, Heffner, and Follette published a practitioner's guide for acceptance and commitment therapy (ACT) for body image dissatisfaction, despite no published evidence of ACT's efficacy for body image change. Controlled studies with this protocol are welcomed. Finally, at a time of need for cost-effective treatments, self-help BI-CBT is highly relevant. Creativity in the development and delivery of computer-based BI-CBT interventions can be informed by the research literature on such programs for prevention of body image problems (see Chapter 50).

Informative Readings

Buhlmann, U., Reese, H. E., Renaud, S., & Wilhelm, S. (2008). Clinical considerations for the treatment of body dysmorphic disorder with cognitive-behavioral therapy. *Body Image: An International Journal of Research, 5*, 39–49.—A discussion of factors relevant to the assessment and treatment of individuals with BDD, based on empirical evidence and the authors' clinical experiences.

Cash, T. F. (2008). *The body image workbook: An eight-step program for learning to like your looks* (2nd ed.). Oakland, CA: New Harbinger.—A structured manual of CBT suitable for self-help and adaptable for therapist-assisted work.

Fairburn, C. G. (2008). *Cognitive behavior therapy and eating disorders.* New York: Guilford Press.—A description of CBT-E, a treatment based on a clinical formulation of the factors maintaining disordered eating.

Hrabosky, J. I., & Cash, T. F. (2007). Self-help treatment for body-image disturbances. In J. D. Latner & G. T. Wilson (Eds.), *Self-help approaches for obesity and eating disorders* (pp. 118–138). New York: Guilford Press.—A description of Cash's 1997 self-help program for body image and a review of outcome studies of components of this program.

Jarry, J. L., & Berardi, K. (2004). Characteristics and effectiveness of stand-alone body image treatments: A review of the empirical literature. *Body Image: An International Journal of Research, 1*, 319–333.—A descriptive review of empirical studies of stand-alone treatments for body image.

Jarry, J. L., & Ip, K. (2005). The effectiveness of stand-alone cognitive behavioural therapy for body image: A meta-analysis. *Body Image: An International Journal of Research, 2*, 317–332.—A meta-analysis of published and unpublished outcome studies of stand-alone BI-CBT.

Neziroglu, F., Khemlani-Patel, S., & Veale, D. (2008). Social learning theory and cognitive behavioral models of body dysmorphic disorder. *Body Image: An International Journal of Research, 5*, 28–38.—A review of contemporary cognitive-behavioral models of BDD with an emphasis on relational frame theory and information processing.

Ramirez, E. M., & Rosen, J. C. (2001). A comparison of weight control and weight control plus body image therapy for obese men and women. *Journal of Consulting and Clinical Psychology, 69*, 440–446.—A randomized controlled trial comparing BI-CBT combined with a weight loss program to weight loss alone.

Rosen, J. C. (1996). Body image assessment and treatment in controlled studies of eating disorders. *International Journal of Eating Disorders, 20*, 331–343.—A review showing that CBT for bulimia nervosa results in modest improvements in body image.

Rosen, J. C., Orosan, P., & Reiter, J. (1995). Cognitive behavior therapy for negative body image in obese women. *Behavior Therapy, 26,* 25–42.—A randomized controlled trial comparing the effect of BI-CBT to a no-treatment condition in overweight and obese women.

Rosen, J. C., Reiter, J., & Orosan, P. (1995). Cognitive-behavioral body image therapy for body dysmorphic disorder. *Journal of Consulting and Clinical Psychology, 63,* 263–269.—A randomized control trial of BI-CBT for women diagnosed with BDD.

Strachan, M. D., & Cash, T. F. (2002). Self-help for a negative body image: A comparison of components of a cognitive-behavioral program. *Behavior Therapy, 33,* 235–251.—A dismantling study of Cash's (1997) eight-step program comparing psychoeducation and self-monitoring to these two elements combined with cognitive restructuring.

Veale, D., Gournay, K., Dryden, W., Boocock, A., Shah, F., Willson, R., et al. (1996). Body dysmorphic disorder: A cognitive behavioural model and pilot randomised controlled trial. *Behaviour Research and Therapy, 34,* 717–729.—Proposes a cognitive-behavioral model of BDD and formulates hypotheses to test the model.

Veale, D., & Neziroglu, F. (2010). *Body dysmorphic disorder: A treatment manual.* West Sussex, UK: Wiley-Blackwell.—A comprehensive volume on BDD that integrates theory and science and delineates the elements of a CBT treatment.

Williams, J., Hadjistavropoulos, T., & Sharpe, D. (2006). A meta-analysis of psychological and pharmacological treatments for body dysmorphic disorder. *Behaviour Research and Therapy, 44,* 99–111.—A meta-analysis of 15 BDD treatment studies including randomized controlled trials, crossover studies, case series, and series of case studies.

CHAPTER 48

Experiential Approaches to Body Image Change

JUDITH RUSKAY RABINOR
MARION BILICH

Introduction

This chapter describes various forms of experiential therapy aimed at facilitating personal growth or change in body image. The experiential perspective assumes that body image is multidimensional and includes mental representations (thoughts, feelings, and images), as well as sensory (auditory, visual, and kinesthetic) and somatic components. Therefore, if the goal is to change an individual's thoughts, feelings, sensations, and perceptions related to body image, then verbal intervention alone is limited. Direct work with the sensory and somatic bodily experiences must be included in a comprehensive treatment approach. Because the formation of body image begins at a preverbal developmental stage, techniques designed to encourage nonverbal exploration and expression will be effective at creating change at that level. This level of intervention may be particularly important for clients whose body image disturbances stem from early childhood experience.

Experiential techniques can be categorized in relation to their primary orientation to the mind and body. Table 48.1 provides a representative, though not exhaustive, listing of the experiential forms of psychotherapy and personal growth to promote change in body image. Keep in mind that with any attempt at categorization, there will be omissions, oversimplifications, and overlap between the various approaches.

TABLE 48.1. Experiential Approaches and Major Proponents

Techniques	Major proponents	Web resources
Mental representation techniques		
Client-generated imagery	Judith Rabinor Marion Bilich	
Guided body-imagery techniques	Martin Rossman Marcia Hutchinson	*www.academyforguidedimagery.com*
Hypnotherapy	Milton Erickson	*www.erickson-foundation.org*
Journal writing and expressive writing	Kathleen Adams James W. Pennebaker	*www.journaltherapy.com*
Metaphor and poetry therapy	J. J. Leedy	*www.poetrytherapy.org*
Somatic techniques		
Breathing exercises		
Relaxation exercises	Edmund Jacobson Herbert Benson	*www.progressiverelaxation.org www.relaxationresponse.org*
Massage therapy		
Alexander technique	F. M. Alexander	*www.alexandertechnique.com*
Feldenkrais methods	Moshe Feldenkrais	*www.feldenkrais.com*
Sensory techniques		
Music therapy	Helen Bonny	*www.musictherapy.org*
Dance/movement therapy	Rudolf Laban	*www.adta.org*
Art therapy	Mury Rabin Lisa Hinz	*www.arttherapy.org www.art-therapy.us/eating disorders*
Integrated approaches		
EMDR	Francine Shapiro	*www.emdr.com*
Mindfulness approaches	Jon Kabat-Zinn Tiffany Stewart	*www.mindfulnesstapes.com www.thebodyimageproject.com*
Sensorimotor psychotherapy	Pat Ogden	*www.sensorimotorpsychotherapy.org*
Psychodrama	Jacob L. Moreno	*www.asgpp.org*
Bioenergetics	Alexander Lowen	*www.bioenergetic-therapy.com*
Body Talk	John Veltheim Ann Halperin	*www.bodytalksystem.com*
Accelerated experiential dynamic psychotherapy	Diana Fosha	*www.aedpinstitute.com*
Family sculpting	Virginia Satir	
Focusing	Eugene Gendlin	*www.focusing.org*
Gestalt therapy	Fritz Perls	*www.gestalttherapy.net*
Somatic experiencing	Peter Levine	*www.traumahealing.com*
Synergy	Ilana Rubenfeld	*www.rubenfeldsynergy.com*

Basic Assumptions of Experiential Approaches

Experiential approaches to psychotherapy all share an emphasis on the interrelatedness of mind and body; they all assume that the body impacts thoughts and feelings, and vice versa. Experiential approaches share several other assumptions.

• *Assumption 1:* Experiential approaches emphasize present experience. These techniques have as their goal *insight through attention to the here and now.* Hornyak and Baker emphasize that these methods are based on psychological principles and that they usually involve some degree of action on the client's part, either physical or imagined.

• *Assumption 2:* Experiential approaches emphasize working directly with the body. Because experiential techniques are based on the assumption that *the earliest sense of self is rooted in the body,* they target the somatic domain. As early as 1923, Sigmund Freud stated, "The ego is first and foremost a body ego." Before we have the capacity to think in words, the physical body is the vehicle used to explore, understand, experience, and master the world.

• *Assumption 3:* Experiential approaches facilitate nonverbal expression. In her 1998 chapter in *Relational Perspectives on the Body,* Dimen states that body-related conflicts and concerns are so profoundly significant that they often cannot be verbalized. Body image serves as a nonverbal metaphor that provides a psychological "home" for the displacement and projection of intrapsychic and interpersonal conflicts by clients who cannot put emotional conflicts into words.

• *Assumption 4:* Experiential approaches are a "backdoor" to the unconscious. St. John explains that physical sensations provide access to affective states, and that both verbal and nonverbal explorations of these sensations can uncover previously suppressed, repressed, or denied elements of experience. Therefore, when working directly with the body, it is possible to access unconscious as well as preconscious memories and emotions not readily accessible by verbal interaction alone.

Clinical Considerations and Experiential Techniques

The unique characteristics of experiential techniques, which are always integrated into ongoing psychotherapy, require special consideration. First, it is important to be aware that experiential therapies can unleash powerful affective states and memories. Therefore, before any experiential technique is utilized, a climate of safety and trust must be established within the therapy relationship. The therapist, of course, must also consider the client's capacity to tolerate possibly intense levels of affect. Similarly, the therapist must be adequately trained in these techniques and have the temperament as well as the skill to be active and directive in treatment—a role not suited to all therapists. If a referral to an experiential therapist is needed, the primary provider must consider the effects such a referral will have on treatment.

The following sections describe some of the techniques listed in Table 48.1. This is not a comprehensive guide but rather a sampling of techniques that illustrate how and why experiential approaches may be helpful in changing body image. From the wide array of possibilities, one always chooses the techniques that seem most efficient and effective in each clinical situation.

Mental Representation Approaches

These therapies focus on directly changing internal mental representations of the body self. Clinicians working with diverse populations have reported success using *guided imagery*, a particularly powerful approach because body image is an *image* amenable to change. In using this approach, the therapist guides the client to focus on past situations that elicit sensory and affective material and "watch" what unfolds in the mind's eye. Often, deeply repressed material that manifests itself in a negative body image is evoked.

Kearney-Cooke describes the use of theme-centered guided imageries that help clients trace their psychosocial development and identify and rework past experiences of familial and nonfamilial trauma. Specific imageries are used to help clients explore the roots of their feelings about their body at different developmental stages. In this way, the origins of negatively laden body parts are identified. This negativity can also be uncovered during writing exercises in which the client is asked to compose a letter to his or her own body or certain part of his or her body.

In 1982, Hutchinson developed and evaluated a 7-week group program that included guided imagery and journal writing. She found statistically significant improvements in body image and self-image in those who participated in her program. Subsequently, she expanded her protocol to 12-week group meetings lasting 2½ hours each.

Expressive writing, developed by James Pennebaker, has also been applied to modifying dysfunctional body image. In a typical expressive writing exercise, the individual is instructed to write about an emotionally distressing experience for 15–30 minutes on three to five occasions. In his eight-step cognitive-behavioral approach to improving body image (see Chapter 47), Cash assigns writing exercises throughout, but especially to facilitate individuals' discovery of emotion-laden experiences from their developmental body image history.

Somatic Approaches

The somatic experiential approaches change body image by helping the client reconnect to the body in a very concrete manner. These approaches are based on the idea that what we observe in the world depends on our capacity for observation and awareness; expanding our awareness of the body facilitates the capacity to observe and experience life. Techniques such as deep breathing, massage, and yoga, which bring attention back into the body, are especially useful for work with clients whose body image problems include a sense of being disconnected or alienated from body experience. For example, individuals with schizophrenia may benefit from somatic techniques that focus their attention on their body in a nonthreatening way.

Our culture emphasizes the body as a source of beauty and fitness but ignores and discourages awareness of the body as a source of relaxation, comfort, and emotional wisdom. Becoming aware of the "lived experience" of our body, which is central to the somatic approach, is a way of tapping into these positive states. A variety of techniques facilitate self-monitoring of body awareness as a way of perceiving sensations and feelings in this way.

Basic to many experiential and somatic techniques are breathing and relaxation exercises. Breathing exercises focus attention on present bodily experience simply by focusing on one's breathing pattern. Another technique, Jacobson's classic *progressive relaxation method*, involves progressing through the body and tensing and releasing each muscle group before moving on to the adjacent area. The objective is to facilitate awareness of internal sensations, a prerequisite to feeling one's emotions.

Peter Levine's *somatic experiencing*, one of the newer somatic approaches, is particularly useful in healing trauma held in the body. In a series of graded exercises, participants first learn to identify the *felt sense* of the somatic components assumed to be associated with trauma. According to Eugene Gendlin, who coined the term in his book *Focusing*, a felt sense is a "bodily awareness, an internal aura that encompasses all you feel and know about a subject" (p. 35). By learning how to let go of habituated trauma-based bodily responses and replacing them with a more expanded somatic response (e.g., learning to feel sad instead of numb), a healing process is initiated.

Sensory Approaches

Sensory-oriented techniques include dance and movement, art, and music therapy. These various therapies utilize the body's senses—visual, kinesthetic, and auditory—to change body image. Like other experiential techniques, they initially bypass the verbal, thereby reaching a deeper level of consciousness.

Because these approaches reconnect the individual to the body through the use of the senses, the techniques are especially useful for all those in whom the felt sense is distorted, rigid, or traumatized. This population includes people with schizophrenia, eating-disordered individuals, those who have lost a limb or body part to illness or accident, and people who have been sexually or physically abused. Like the somatic techniques described above, these techniques are particularly useful in grounding clients in their body.

Dance therapy focuses on the kinesthetic aspects of body experience through a series of structured and nonstructured movement exercises that increase the client's sensory awareness. Researcher Rosalie Robollo Pratt has suggested that movement may be a primary influence on the development and change in body image especially in women with eating disorders. In the early 1970s, Calloway and Bean found that movement to music was particularly effective in increasing positive body image and awareness of the spatial characteristics of the body. In 2000, Dibbell-Hope published a study of women with breast cancer in which she found that dance therapy promoted a marked improvement in body image and self-esteem.

Improvisational movement and directed movement exercises provide clients with awareness of how long-held emotions are stored in the body and offer new patterns of being in the world. These exercises require one to be open to the unknown, the unexpected, the unfamiliar—and often, the undesired. When one improvises, one accepts as the norm a state of being "lost." When we allow ourselves to experience our spontaneous impulses, we are cut loose from the familiar reference points and become grounded in our body.

Art therapy aimed at body image change can include activities such as clay sculpting or drawings of the body, creation of masks, and collages. These techniques are especially suited to work with children whose body images have been impaired by severe, chronic illness or by trauma, as children naturally choose art as a means of self-expression. They are more comfortable exploring and expressing feelings about their body through this medium. Both Mury Rabin and Lisa Hinz have suggested that through the use of drawing, eating-disordered clients can directly confront body image distortions.

Music therapy is used less frequently in therapies that address body image, but it has been successful with individuals who tend to intellectualize. A music therapy session focused on body image uses rhythm, melody, and harmony to evoke feelings about the body. Receptive activities, such as listening to music, as well as expressive activities, such as music and song writing or playing instruments, may occur. Receptive activities *evoke* memories and associations in the body, while expressive activities facilitate nonverbal *expression* of those memories and associations.

Integrated Approaches

The approaches described above are often integrated into comprehensive treatment programs aimed at changing body image. For example, most use some form of imagery and, even those based in nonverbal expression, such as art and dance therapies, usually have a verbal component, in which clients are encouraged to articulate their newfound awareness.

One of the newer integrative approaches, initially developed to treat posttraumatic stress disorder, is *eye movement desensitization and reprocessing (EMDR)*. It was developed by Francine Shapiro who, while treating trauma survivors, discovered that moving the eyes back and forth decreased the intensity of distressing memories. She hypothesized that in traumatic conditions, the normal patterns of information processing are disrupted and, as a result, the information about the trauma is stored differently from ordinary information. She developed a comprehensive and integrative set of protocols to address and reprocess this dysfunctionally stored information. EMDR has been applauded for its utilization of auditory, visual, kinesthetic, and olfactory descriptors of imagery and sensations. In 1997, Brown, McGoldrick, and Buchanan demonstrated the effectiveness of EMDR in seven clients with body dysmorphic disorder (BDD). In a controlled study in 2008, Bloomgarden and Calogero demonstrated the efficacy of EMDR treatment on some aspects of negative body image in persons with eating disorders.

Mindfulness-based treatment approaches, for example, derived from the work of Jon Kabat-Zinn, emphasize nonjudgmental awareness and experiential acceptance. Tiffany Stewart has delineated a body image treatment program based on mindful awareness and compassion for the self. Delinsky and Wilson have integrated mirror-exposure treatment with mindfulness interventions to reduce body dissatisfaction and shape and weight concerns.

Sensorimotor psychotherapy, founded by Pat Ogden, is based on principles of mindfulness and mind/body/spirit holism and informed by contemporary research in neuroscience, attachment theory, trauma, and related fields. In the late 1970s, Ogden became interested in the correlation between her clients' disconnection from their body, their physical patterns, and their psychological issues. As both a psychotherapist and body therapist, she was inspired to join somatic therapy and psychotherapy into a comprehensive method for healing this disconnection.

Accelerated experiential dynamic psychotherapy, developed by Diana Fosha, is an approach that promotes and accesses disavowed and dissociated affect and visceral experience in the service of metabolizing emotional distress and trauma. Clients are then able to develop a coherent autobiographical narrative and unravel the origins of body image issues.

Psychosomatic integration therapy, developed by Judy Lightstone, integrates body mindfulness with ego state work, EMDR, and feminist relational therapy. Body image issues are seen as resulting from a fundamental split in which the body has become objectified and "forced" to submit to the mind (see Chapter 6). This technique has been used primarily with clients with eating disorders and treatment may include journaling, art, or movement work, and guided fantasies.

In 1989, movement educator Anna Halprin created another integrative approach, *Body Talk*, for women who are HIV positive. This group approach combines movement exercises with psychodynamic exploration to create interventions that operate simultaneously at the verbal and nonverbal levels. Through movement improvisations, these participants grappled with the unknown aspects of their self- and body images, allowing their physical vulnerability and fear of death to coexist with bodily pleasure and engagement with life. Body Talk is particularly useful for individuals confronting severe, chronic, and life-threatening illnesses that bring with them physical changes and shame that adversely affect body image.

Family sculpting and *psychodrama* have value in supporting traditional verbal therapy for family-of-origin work with people with bulimia nervosa. These techniques circumvent the family's well-practiced defenses of minimization, rationalization, and intellectualization, and offer a "corrective experience of living in one's body."

Conclusions and Future Directions

Body image is a multidimensional experience comprised of sensations and feelings that may not have verbal counterparts. Traditional talk therapy does not allow access to the sensory and nonverbal aspects of body image. Experiential approaches initially bypass the verbal arena, allowing for a deeper, richer experience of the body. Each experiential approach is a different manifestation of the principle that therapists can facilitate change in the client's relationship to his or her body and self-image by intervening somatically. A range of experiential techniques are incorporated in contemporary cognitive-behavioral approaches to body image change.

A modest body of clinical literature offers experiential approaches to the improvement of body image. These often focus on clients with eating disorders. However, as other chapters in this book discuss, body image problems occur in a large segment of the population—including people with birth defects, those confronting life-threatening illnesses, accident survivors, and those who suffer with BDD or schizophrenia. Additionally, nonclinical populations—such as adolescents, pregnant women, and aging adults—often experience body dissatisfaction and could benefit from experiential approaches.

Unfortunately, there is a scarcity of well-designed research studies investigating the effectiveness of the experiential approaches to changing body image. Many of the existing studies lack randomized controls and employed too few subjects to draw conclusions. In addition, it can be difficult to evaluate the techniques individually, as they are often used as adjunctive therapies or as components of more comprehensive treatment approaches. However, future research studies will hopefully address which experiential approaches are most effective with which populations.

Informative Readings

Bloomgarden, A., & Calogero, R. M. (2008). A randomized experimental test of the efficacy of EMDR treatment on negative body image in eating disorder inpatients. *Eating Disorders, 16,* 418–427.—A study finding less distress about body image memories and less body dissatisfaction after EMDR treatment.

Cash, T. F. (2008). *The body image workbook: An eight-step program for learning to like your looks* (2nd ed.). Oakland, CA: New Harbinger Publications.—A comprehensive and practical treatment program that contains many experiential exercises—mental imagery, expressive writing, diaphragmatic breathing—to facilitate body image improvement.

Delinsky, S. S., & Wilson, G. T. (2006). Mirror exposure for the treatment of body image disturbance. *International Journal of Eating Disorders, 39,* 108–116.—A controlled study that confirms the efficacy of mindful acceptance with mirror exposure for body image dissatisfaction.

Dimen, M. (1998). Polyglot bodies: Sinking through the relational. In L. Aron & F. Sommer (Eds.), *Relational perspectives on the body* (pp. 65–93). Hillsdale, NJ: Analytic Press.—Articulates a psychoanalytic perspective on body image.

Feldenkrais, M. (1991). *Awareness through movement: Health exercises for personal growth.* San Francisco: Harper.—Though this book does not directly address image change, it provides practical guidelines for implementing the technique.

Gendlin, E. T. (1982). *Focusing.* New York: Bantam Books.—Helpful for teaching clients to unlock "body wisdom," the basis of many experiential approaches to changing body image.

Hinz, L. (2006). *Drawing from within: Using art to treat eating disorders.* London: Jessica Kingsley.—Has an entire chapter devoted to body image, complete with experiential art exercises.

Hornyak, L. M., & Baker, E. K. (Eds.). (1989). *Experiential therapies for eating disorders.* New York: Guilford Press.—A collection of experiential approaches to treating eating disorders, each chapter highlights a different approach.

Hutchinson, M. D. (1988). *Transforming body image: Learning to love the body you have.* Watsonville, CA: Crossing Press.—An experiential program for women's body image change.

Kearney-Cooke, A. (1989). Reclaiming the body: Using guided imagery in the treatment of body image disturbance among bulimic women. In L. M. Hornyak & E. K. Baker (Eds.), *Experiential therapies for eating disorders* (pp. 11–33). New York: Guilford Press.—Gives case material on use of imagery in changing body image among women with eating disorders.

Newman, L. (1992). *Somebody to love: A guide to loving the body you have.* Chicago: Third Side Press.—Guided imagery and writing exercises aimed at exploring women's issues about their body and eating.

Probst, M., Van Coppenolle, H., & Vandereycken, W. (1995). Body experience in anorexia nervosa patients: An overview of therapeutic approaches. *Eating Disorders, 3*, 145–157.—A review of experiential approaches for a difficult-to-treat population.

Pruzinsky, T. (1990). Somatopsychic approaches to psychotherapy and personal growth. In T. F. Cash & T. Pruzinsky (Eds.), *Body images: Development, deviance, and change* (pp. 296–315). New York: Guilford Press.—Summarizes experiential approaches to body image change.

Rabin, M. (2003). *Art therapy and eating disorders: The self as significant.* New York: Columbia University Press.—Describes practical experiential exercises to improve body image.

St. John, M. (1992). Anti-body already: Body oriented interventions in clinical work with HIV positive women. *Women and Therapy, 13*, 5–25.—Describes the "Body Talk" program, an experiential approach to body image problems associated with the stigma of HIV.

CHAPTER 49

School-Based Psychoeducational Approaches to Prevention

JENNIFER A. O'DEA
ZALI YAGER

Introduction

School-based programs to prevent eating disorders and improve body image have evolved since the heavy focus on psychoeducation in the late 1980s. Psychoeducational programs were traditionally based on the adaption of clinical psychological counseling techniques to be implemented in school settings, and they also relied heavily on the didactic presentation of knowledge and information. Most school-based programs now include a range of strategies and preventive approaches combined with traditional psychoeducational strategies, including media literacy, cognitive dissonance, small-group work activities, role play, peer-led teaching, and the use of computer and Internet technology.

Several challenges for school-based prevention impede progress, including disputes over program delivery and content, the personal attitudes and professional training of teachers, and issues of measurement among "normal" populations in natural environments. More evidence is required in order to produce effective programs that can be implemented in a cost-effective manner, throughout the world, among males and females of all ages. This chapter aims to provide an overview of the research in school-based body image programs and to identify the current trends and future directions in this area.

Major Outcomes of Studies through 2004

Examination of the published school-based programs to date reveals several trends over the three most recent decades. A review of school-based health education strategies for the improvement of body image and prevention of eating problems was published in 2005 by O'Dea. This review examines relevant literature dating back 50 years and identified 21 large, randomized, and controlled studies conducted in the United States, Canada, England, Australia, England, Israel, Switzerland, and Italy. The early seminal prevention studies were conceived with a large focus on providing adolescent girls with information about eating disorders, facts about the dangers of dieting, increased nutrition knowledge, analysis of the social construction of cultural body ideals, and construction of the stereotypical ideal body. These early intervention studies resulted in improved knowledge of eating disorders and weight control issues but created little impact upon body image improvement or reduction in eating disorder behaviors.

Despite the lack of substantial behavior change, these early studies were instrumental in paving the way for researchers to design more innovative and successful interventions. The study of Neumark-Sztainer for example, conducted in Israel, provided information about nutrition, dieting, and eating disorders, and also introduced the new topics of behavior modification for weight control, skills in media analysis, and assertiveness. This study resulted in reduced bulimic tendencies and improved eating patterns. Later interventions aimed to educate young people about the media's artificial creation and perpetuation of the "perfect" body via media images and stereotypes of men and women. These studies broadened the preventive approaches to include an investigative critique by students of the many biological, social, and psychological influences on eating behavior and body image.

Later studies were designed to be more student centered, peer led, and educationally interactive with a focus on improving body image via general self-esteem development and rejection of media gender stereotypes. The "Everybody's Different" study implemented by O'Dea and Abraham in 2000 was successful in producing significant and long-lasting impacts among adolescent girls and boys, including those who were "high risk" for eating disorders and those who were overweight. This study deliberately avoided any mention of food, eating, dieting, or body shapes, and instead aimed to improve body esteem by giving the male and female students a "dose" of general self-esteem. The Everybody's Different program simultaneously combined the development of a positive sense of self and stress management with a peer-led analysis and rejection of cultural gender and body image stereotypes and media body image ideals, and encouraged students to develop an acceptance of a diverse range of unique features in themselves and acceptance of diversity among others.

Other school-based interventions also produced moderate levels of success by combining various components including media literacy, self-esteem, sociocultural determinants of body shape and body image, pubertal development, nondieting approaches to weight control, hazards of dieting, genetic diversity, and coping skills; these are summarized in the 2005 review by O'Dea.

Studies from 2005 to 2010

Since 2005 there has been a significant progression toward broader programs that target combined risk factors for obesity and eating disorders and have an additional focus on the reduction of bullying and weight comparison. Another trend is the increased focus on school policy, the school environment and ethos, and the inclusion of parents and the community in line with an ecological approach and the Health Promoting Schools Framework (see Chapter 51). School-based interventions have also been targeted toward intervention at younger age points, and are now more common in primary schools. Finally, programs have investigated the use of new ideas such as the performing arts, yoga, and cooking classes to improve body image, as well as to develop habits for life-long health behaviors.

A recent and effective school-based body image program that has used media literacy is the "Media Smart" program developed in Australia by Wilksch, Wade, and Tiggemann for eighth-grade students. Media literacy refers to a student's ability to identify and critically analyze different types of media and media messages. Students of media literacy also learn how to examine the aims and purposes of media messages and they become skilled at decoding and critiquing media messages. Media Smart participants had lower shape and weight concern, dieting, body dissatisfaction, ineffectiveness, and depression scores than control participants with significant benefits still present at the 2.5-year follow-up. Even single, once-only media literacy lessons from this program were found to be effective in reducing internalization of the media ideals of thinness and muscularity, which is a significant achievement as one-shot programs are not generally known to be effective. In addition, as the recent work by Wilksch and his colleagues suggests, media literacy is believed to be a particularly appropriate way of facilitating body image programs among boys and young men, as it uses a gender-inclusive approach to examining media stereotypes in order to reduce body dissatisfaction.

Many well-designed and effective programs to improve body image have now been conducted in primary schools. Very Important Kids (V.I.K.) and Healthy Schools-Healthy Kids (HS-HK) are two examples of programs that have been conducted over the entire school year with children ages 10–12 years. These programs have a broad focus, and include themes of size acceptance, reduction of weight-based teasing, and healthy living throughout several aspects of the formal and informal curriculum. Shorter school-based programs have also been found to be effective in improving body image with young audiences, including the innovative use of the storybook *Shapesville* and puppetry with children as young as 5 years of age. Ideally, programs to improve body image would be given throughout a child's school career and would target developmentally appropriate risk factors and behaviors.

Studies employing the counterattitudinal advocacy component of the dissonance approach have been successfully developed and implemented by Stice and Shaw among at-risk adolescent girls age 17 years. Results suggest that dissonance-based approaches are suitable in schools with girls 15 years and over, provided that the teachers or facilitators are well trained in the use of this approach. Stice and his colleagues have also confirmed that the dissonance-based eating disorder prevention program is effective when school staff recruit "at-risk" youth. A large efficacy trial found that this intervention produced a 60% reduction in risk for future onset of threshold/subthreshold eating disorders over a 3-year follow-up.

Barriers to Effective School-Based Programs

Iatrogenesis and "First, Do No Harm"

There were some early concerns about the iatrogenic effects of some programs and materials in the area of school-based body image improvement and eating disorder prevention. Researchers and teachers were encouraged to "First, do no harm" when designing and implementing body image programs, as many approaches to teaching about these topics were believed to cause unintended negative effects. Early investigations of the reaction of adolescent girls in Australia to posters that were supposed to improve their body image were found to be alarmingly negative and there is still some controversy over using recovered peers as guest speakers in school-based prevention. Prevention of eating disorders and body image concerns in schools usually employs primary prevention, which aims to avoid the development of the disease, or secondary prevention, which is aimed at early disease detection, thereby increasing opportunities for interventions to prevent progression of the disease and emergence of symptoms.

Although some argue that the recognition of eating disorder symptoms among self and friends is critical to secondary prevention, these approaches have been suggested to be ineffective for primary prevention, as the normalization and glamorization of dieting and eating disorders may lead to adoption of potentially dangerous techniques by previously healthy individuals. It seems that researchers have become more aware of the inadvertent, potentially harmful effects of their programs and are now deliberately evaluating whether programs have in fact done more harm than good. Progress in prevention research needs to ensure that safe, effective, evidence-based, and easy-to-use options are available for schools.

Issues of Program Delivery, Fidelity, and Teacher Training

Even with the best of intentions, many issues with program delivery can reduce program effectiveness. Such issues include teacher deviation from the intended program content, and the training and personal background of those who carry out the program. Most early school-based body image prevention programs were developed and delivered by psychologists and research staff with no education background. Few published programs to date were delivered by classroom teachers or peers, and fewer still provided teacher training about the program. Although meta-analysis of eating disorder prevention programs detect better results from programs that are delivered by researchers, it can be argued that a practical plan for the future of body image prevention programs must involve delivery by the regular classroom teacher in order to achieve widespread dissemination and improvement in body image among all young people.

If teachers are to be asked to deliver body image programs, or any other prevention initiatives, there are several issues that need to be addressed. First, teachers do not have specific skills in delivering prevention programs or encouraging reflective discussion at a personal level. Teachers may not have been exposed to the range of research and information about body image and weight issues that is required to effectively understand the background to and delivery of body image programs. The "Student Body: Promoting Health at Any Size" program designed by McVey, Gusella, and colleagues is the first web-based training tool designed to assist teachers and public health practitioners to deliver programs to improve body satisfaction in schools. This is an important new direction in establishing consistent teacher training for school-based prevention of body image problems.

In addition, teachers (especially those who are young and female) may be experiencing body image issues themselves. Investigations conducted in Australia by Zali Yager have found that university students training to become health and physical education teachers also have a higher prevalence of body image problems and eating and exercise disorders when compared to a control group. These findings mirror those detected among dietitians and fitness trainers. Therefore, it is suggested that teachers undergo suitable training so that they can address both their personal and professional needs. In addition, if preventive programs are to be conducted by regular classroom teachers, some measurement of program fidelity and adherence should be included in the evaluation of the study.

Inclusion of Boys in School-Based Body Image Programs

There are two main reasons for the development of body image programs to include boys. First, they too have body image concerns, and prevalence studies have confirmed that boys and girls are generally equally dissatisfied with their bodies (see Chapters 8 and 10). The second major reason for the inclusion of boys in these school-based programs is that they are an important influence on peer attitudes, and so their attitudes toward sociocultural ideals of thinness must also change to allow improvements in the social environment of girls. Most now agree that boys need to be included in body image programs, but the discussion of whether they should be included in coeducational programs with girls, or have gender-specific programs, still remains.

The most successful mixed-gender program that improved male body satisfaction was Media Smart, which took a media literacy approach and used a male researcher to facilitate the program. Either of these factors may have led to males finding the program relevant and engaged with the activities to a greater level, resulting in improved outcomes. The Everybody's Different program also reported significant improvements in male body dissatisfaction and this program included a media literacy component, as well. It may be that the reaction and discussion between males and females over body image ideals and the resultant realization of more reasonable peer norms may be more powerful than the program content itself.

Conclusions and Future Directions

The development of programs that are aimed at younger children and use age-appropriate educational approaches such as musicals, puppetry, and storybooks are all promising new developments. The latest developments include taking a broader whole-school approach, combining with obesity prevention and healthy living interventions, targeting risk factors for poor body image such as weight teasing, and utilizing the powerful role of parents. Broadly focused ecological programs are providing evidence for school-based prevention of body image problems and these are being appropriately planned and grounded with strong theoretical frameworks of social and emotional learning programs, positive psychology (see Chapter 7), and the Health Promoting Schools Framework (see Chapter 51). Future research should focus on combining several different and complementary longitudinal preventive approaches among a broad age range of students, including males and students of different cultural backgrounds.

Informative Readings

Bruning Brown, J., Winzelburg, A., Absacal, L., & Taylor, C. B. (2004). An evaluation of an internet-delivered eating disorder prevention program for adolescents and their parents. *Journal of Adolescent Health, 35,* 290–296.—An example of a well-designed Internet-based program.

Dohnt, H. K., & Tiggemann, M. (2008). Promoting positive body image in young girls: An evaluation of "Shapesville." *European Eating Disorders Review, 16,* 222–233.—An example of an innovative program that utilizes the application of a storybook approach to prevention among young children.

Haines, J., Neumark-Sztainer, D., Perry, C., Hannan, P. J., & Levine, M. P. (2006). V.I.K. (Very Important Kids): A school-based program designed to reduce teasing and unhealthy weight-control behaviors. *Health Education Research, 21,* 884–895.—Report of an innovative intervention study to reduce teasing and weight-related bullying.

Levine, M. P., & Smolak, L. (2006). *The prevention of eating problems and eating disorders: Theory, research, and practice.* Mahwah, NJ: Erlbaum.—Extensive review of prevention programs including theoretical and methodological issues.

McVey, G. L., Gusella, J., Tweed, S., & Ferrari, M. (2009). A controlled evaluation of web-based training for teachers and public health practitioners on the prevention of eating disorders. *Eating Disorders, 17,* 1–26.—Report of an innovative study that incorporates the involvement of a broad array of educators.

McVey, G. L., Tweed, S., & Blackmore, E. (2007). Healthy Schools-Healthy Kids: A controlled evaluation of a comprehensive universal eating disorder prevention program. *Body Image: An International Journal of Research, 4,* 115–136.—Report of an innovative intervention study conducted among young children.

Neumark-Sztainer, D., Story, M., Hannan, P. J., & Rex, J. (2003). New Moves: A school-based obesity prevention program for adolescent girls. *Preventive Medicine, 37,* 41–51.—Report of an innovative combined approach that addresses both obesity and body image.

O'Dea, J. A. (2000). School-based interventions to prevent eating problems: First do no harm. *Eating Disorders, 8,* 123–130.—A review article describing the potential adverse effects of unplanned eating disorder prevention programs.

O'Dea, J. A. (2005). School-based health education strategies for the improvement of body image and prevention of eating problems: An overview of safe and effective interventions. *Health Education, 105,* 11–33.—A literature review of published strategies and studies up to 2005.

O'Dea, J. A. (2007). *Everybody's different: A positive approach to teaching about health, puberty, body image, nutrition, self-esteem and obesity prevention.* Melbourne: Australian Council for Educational Research.—A review of the evidence base for body image improvement studies. A resource book containing classroom-based teaching activities.

Russell-Mayhew, S., Arthur, N., & Ewashen, C. (2007). Targeting students, teachers and parents in a wellness-based prevention program in schools. *Eating Disorders, 15,* 159–181.—An example of a school-based study in which students, parents, and teachers can become involved.

Stice, E., Marti, C. N., Spoor, S., Presnell, K., & Shaw, H. (2008). Dissonance and healthy weight eating disorder prevention programs: Long-term effects from a randomized efficacy trial. *Journal of Consulting and Clinical Psychology, 76,* 329–340.—A unique report of a longitudinal study of dissonance for eating disorder prevention.

Stice, E., Rohde, P., Gau, J., & Shaw, H. (2009). An effectiveness trial of a dissonance-based eating disorder prevention program for high-risk adolescent girls. *Journal of Consulting and Clinical Psychology, 77,* 825–834.—A unique report of dissonance for eating disorder prevention among early adolescent girls.

Stock, S., Miranda, C., Evans, S., Plessis, S., Ridley, J., Yeh, S., et al. (2007). Healthy Buddies: A novel, peer-led health promotion program for the prevention of obesity and eating disorders in children in elementary school. *Pediatrics, 120,* 1059–1068.—Report of an innovative study that incorporated the involvement of peer educators.

Wilksch, S. M., & Wade, T. D. (2009). Reduction of shape and weight concern in young adolescents: A 30-month controlled evaluation of a media literacy program. *Journal of the American Academy of Child and Adolescent Psychiatry, 48,* 652–661.—Report of a successful and innovative media literacy program.

Yager, Z., & O'Dea, J. (2009). Body image, dieting and disordered eating and exercise practices among teacher trainees: Implications for school-based health education and obesity prevention programs. *Health Education Research, 24,* 472–483.—A descriptive study of the prevalence of body image problems among teachers and how best to deal with such issues via teacher education.

Computer-Based Approaches to Prevention

HANNAH WEISMAN
JAKKI BAILEY
ANDREW WINZELBERG
C. BARR TAYLOR

Introduction

In the past 10 years, a number of programs have been developed to improve body image and reduce weight and shape concerns. This chapter provides an overview of body image enhancement materials available via the computer. We discuss research-evaluated programs for body image enhancement, available evidence on the efficacy of these materials, and outline the advantages and limitations of computer-delivered materials. The chapter includes programs that focus on body image in conjunction with eating disorder *prevention*, but computer-based approaches that focus on clinical *treatment* of eating disorders is not included, although these programs may also contain body image enhancement components. We end this chapter with a discussion on some of the issues still to be addressed about computer-based programs.

Computer-based prevention refers to the broad range of electronic materials, discussion, or interactive feedback available on websites, CD-ROM, smartphones, or downloadable programs or files. The Internet has the most material available on body image, with a surfeit of websites, chat rooms, blogs, discussion groups, social networking pages, videos, audio files, and online programs dedicated to the topic of body image. The majority of information available on the Internet is self-directed rather than part of a specific treatment program. To illustrate the wide range of this material, as of early 2010, Internet users can find tips to improve body image on Something Fishy: Website on Eating Disorders (*something-fishy.org/reach/bodyimage.php*), receive mindfulness-focused tweets from the Body Image Project on Twitter (*twitter.com/bodyimage*), or watch clips from the "Killing Us Softly 4: Advertising's Image of Women" video on YouTube (*youtube.com/user/challengingmedia#p/a/u/0/PTlmho_RovY*).

Although these and other programs developed to improve body image and/or reduce weight and shape concerns are readily available on the Internet, little is known about their impact. In this chapter, the focus is on computer-based, psychoeducational programs for body image enhancement that have been evaluated in research studies. Most research-evaluated programs combine aspects of self-help approaches (where the participant guides and paces him- or herself through material) and clinician-assisted approaches (such as moderated online discussions or chats). The targets of the interventions have generally been weight and shape concerns and preventing eating disorder symptom progression or onset, as well as body image, within this larger objective. Furthermore, the programs have almost exclusively focused on young women, due to the relatively high prevalence of eating disorders in this population.

Are Computer-Based Approaches to Body Image Enhancement Effective?

Given the ubiquitous media attention on body image discontentment, it is surprising how few studies have examined computer-based approaches that focus primarily on body image enhancement. To our knowledge, none of the Internet programs that focus solely on body image enhancement have been evaluated for their clinical impact or with adequate research design; hence, it is difficult to know the scientific impact of these programs. For example, the DOVE Campaign for Real Beauty (*campaignforrealbeauty.com*) aims to improve body image and self-esteem for girls and women worldwide, but the effects of reading material or completing interactive activities on users of their campaign website is unknown.

In terms of clinically evaluated programs, the most extensively researched online body image enhancement and eating disorder prevention program is "Student Bodies," developed at the Stanford University Behavioral Medicine Media Laboratory. Student Bodies is an 8-week psychoeducational program that targets young women with weight and shape concerns, as well as unhealthy eating attitudes and behaviors. Participants assigned to the program have been found to improve their overall body image, reduce their weight and shape concerns, and adopt healthier eating attitudes and behaviors. Variations of the Student Bodies program have been helpful for college and adolescent women across different settings, and have been particularly effective with women at high risk of developing an eating disorder (defined by having high weight and shape concerns). In a sample of college women at high risk of developing an eating disorder, the program significantly lowered weight and shape concerns from pre- to post-tests and the differences were maintained at a 1-year follow-up. Controlled trials of a German version of Student Bodies have found results similar to comparable studies in the United States.

Franko and colleagues developed a 2-hour CD-ROM called "Food, Mood, and Attitude" (FMA) in 2005. The program includes psychoeducational information and accompanying interactive activities, and does not require any facilitation by providers. In a trial of the program, first-year college women at low risk of developing an eating disorder and women at high risk of developing an eating disorder navigated through FMA in two sessions spaced 1–2 weeks apart. Compared to a control group, FMA was effective in reducing body image concerns in the high-risk group at the 10-week follow-up. In a pilot study, the program maintained significant reductions in weight and shape concerns at a 1-year follow-up in a small sample of Latina college women.

In addition, three online body image programs have been developed that utilize synchronous ("real-time") chat functions. In 2004, Zabinski and colleagues used this approach to provide a cognitive-behavioral-based intervention to a group of college-age women with high weight and shape concerns. The women participated in a weekly chat session for 8 weeks, supplemented by psychoeducational readings and homework assignments. Compared to a wait-list control, the program effectively reduced weight and shape concerns at posttreatment and at a 10-week follow-up. Another chat-based program, "My Body, My Life: Body Image Program for Adolescent Girls" was developed in Australia in 2007 by Heinicke, Paxton, McLean, and Wertheim for girls ages 12–18. The program provides a physical manual for each participant and supplements the 6-week program with 90-minute moderated group online chat sessions. Shape concerns decreased significantly at the 2- and 6-month follow-ups for program completers, although the 6-month follow-up data were not significant when the researchers used an intention-to-treat analysis. Finally, Paxton and colleagues in Australia developed a chat-based intervention called "Set Your Body Free." The researchers compared the online program with an analogous in-person treatment group and a control group. Participants were from a community sample of women ages 18–35. Paxton and colleagues found that although both the online and in-person versions were effective compared to a control group at a 6-month follow-up, the improvements were greater for the in-person treatment group.

Taken together, these programs suggest that computer-based prevention approaches have small but consistent effects on reducing weight and shape concerns in adolescent and young adult women, especially women at risk of developing an eating disorder. Both synchronous (real-time chat with a moderator) and asynchronous (self-paced) approaches have demonstrated positive effects on participants' body image. Because of the small number of studies comparing computer-based programs to analogous in-person approaches, it remains unclear whether one of these approaches is more effective. However, as Chapter 47 indicates, it is noteworthy that outcomes of cognitive-behavioral body image treatment programs are better if person assisted than if purely self-help.

Another computer-based approach to improve individuals' body image is developing programs that raise awareness and change behaviors or attitudes within a community. For example, a teacher's weight bias in the classroom may negatively impact students' body image. The program "The Student Body: Promoting Health at Any Size" was created by McVey and colleagues in Canada to raise awareness among teachers and public health educators about how their own behaviors and environment affect students' body image. Compared to a control group, the program significantly improved teachers' knowledge about dieting, peer influences on dieting, and the influence of the media on weight loss; it did not, however, improve their self-efficacy to fight weight bias. Public health practitioners who received the program did not improve on knowledge at postassessment but did increase significantly in self-efficacy to fight weight bias in comparison with the control group. Even though the results from this trial were mixed, the program indicates the potential of combining computer-based and community approaches.

Potentially Harmful Effects of Body Image Websites

Advances in web-authoring programs have simplified the process of creating and posting information on the Internet. It is difficult to determine the accuracy of this information and to censor information that health experts may consider to be wrong, unhealthy, or dangerous. Pro-eating disorder websites have received the most attention in the literature, with "pro-ana," or pro-anorexia sites being the most notorious. It is unclear how frequently these websites are visited, but several recent studies suggest a negative impact from viewing such material.

Many of the pro-ana sites present anorexia nervosa as a lifestyle choice and offer unhealthy "tips and tricks" and "thinspiration" messages (inspirational writings and images to motivate and sustain anorectic behaviors). Researchers have examined the prevalence and effects of visiting pro-ana and other pro-eating disorder sites among eating-disordered patients, as well as among middle school, high school, and college students. The majority of these studies have focused on female populations. Viewing pro-eating disorder websites has been associated with a host of negative body image and behavioral consequences, ranging from restrictive eating to body dissatisfaction and low self-esteem. In general, research in this area suggests that the Internet can be used to share disordered eating behavior and body image attitudes among users, with accordingly harmful effects.

What Are Current Advantages and Disadvantages of These Programs?

Computer-based prevention programs offer a number of advantages to both participants and health care professionals. For participants, they have the potential to be highly interactive and engaging through dynamic presentations of information, tailored messages, feedback, and up-to-date information. In addition, computer-based interventions, particularly those available through portable electronic devices (e.g., smartphones), can offer privacy and convenience. Self-directed interventions are likely to reach audiences that might not think of attending face-to face interventions, as programs can be used anytime and anywhere a computer or the Internet is available. This can be of particular importance for those who are uncomfortable publicly acknowledging body image concerns or those with highly stigmatized or rare conditions such as severe burns or disfiguring surgeries. People with rare body image conditions may have access to a larger group of peers online who face similar specialized body image problems than they would in their local community. In addition, the cost of obtaining programs is minimal, and computer-based programs may be useful to those who cannot afford other forms of treatment such as counseling.

However, computer-based prevention approaches are not a panacea for users. One drawback is that they may disconnect users from person-to-person contact. Also, as Internet and computer technology grow more accessible and it becomes easier to create digital material, it may be difficult for users to distinguish between research-based and non-research-based body image programs or information (such as the pro-ana sites).

Computer-based approaches to body image enhancement have advantages and disadvantages for health care professionals, as well. Information within the programs can be updated quickly to keep up with current research. Computer-based programs can supplement in-person interventions or be provided remotely, with the ability to monitor participants frequently (via program check-ins on smartphones or other portable electronic devices with Internet access). This may help foster greater adherence, engagement, and honesty with respect to sensitive or stigmatized topics. Furthermore, providers can use a stepped-care model by identifying low-risk, high-risk, or clinical populations and tailoring programs to cater to treatment needs.

In theory, programs can be maintained at a low cost after initial startup expenses and are easy to disseminate to a large population. However, in practice we have not always found this to be true. Simple websites that provide information only are inexpensive to maintain, but those that have additional features (e.g., self-monitoring, registration) are more complicated. It can also be costly and time consuming to moderate discussions and provide individualized feedback.

As mentioned, programs that use electronic platforms and mobile technology have the potential to monitor participants frequently throughout a day, such as through smartphone applications. However, collecting frequent data on participants may raise ethical issues for health care professionals. It can be difficult to establish criteria determining when to respond to a significant drop in reported variables (like mood or binge eating) versus when to let things pass as natural fluctuation.

What Important Research Questions Remain Unanswered?

Many important research questions regarding computer-based approaches to body image improvement remain unanswered. The nature and impact of the majority of online body image enhancement materials are unknown. The effects of these materials (e.g., unmoderated Internet-based support groups or the DOVE Campaign for Real Beauty) should be tested, or alternatively, clinical approaches to body image enhancement that do not emphasize eating disorders and eating behaviors could be developed and tested.

The majority of clinically evaluated computer-based body image enhancement programs have been developed for, and used by, teenage or young adult women, with women at high risk of developing an eating disorder showing the most improvement. Our understanding of how to maximize the effectiveness of such programs (e.g., tone, format, or pace of program) is thus based on the experiences of these female populations. Research needs to address how these programs can be tailored to meet the needs of different user demographics (e.g., men, different ages, cultures, literacy levels, or specific body image concerns unrelated to eating disorders). Addressing the concerns of these diverse populations may require significant modification of computer programs for these groups to find them relevant and acceptable. For instance, populations with lower levels of literacy may need more picture-, video-, or audio-based programs.

Little is known about how engaging a community in a program differs in outcome from isolated participation or how these computer-based programs influence broader cultural and group dynamics. The cultural variations of body image ideals within ethnic, racial, and cultural groups (see Chapters 25–28) are not often addressed in programs. The impact of including this cultural-specific information should be tested. Similarly, an area that warrants research is incorporating families into the computer-based prevention process. A program could have a piece for parents to instruct them on how to be less critical of a child's body image, or how to foster a healthy body image environment in the home.

In regard to program components and participant adherence, there are several areas that need to be further explored. Studies that dismantle the computer intervention components are needed to determine which features are most important. Few studies have examined the use of a lay person as a group leader or moderator. It is not known what participant characteristics predict the best outcome of these programs. In particular, little is known about the specific knowledge required of the participant to make attitude or behavior change. We need to discover how self-contained and self-directed approaches can maintain motivation and enhance adherence to the intervention protocol. With the burgeoning industry of mobile technology, it is not clear how best to use text messaging or mobile applications to bolster program adherence and effectiveness. The use of avatars, or digital representations of oneself, may be another avenue to enhance engagement and adherence levels.

Finally, we need to understand how failure while using a computer-based program affects a participant's willingness to seek other assistance. If computer-based interventions are going to be useful in a stepped-care approach, it is important that program failure does not discourage participants from seeking additional assistance.

Conclusions

In summary, the use and impact of the majority of information on body image available on the Internet has not been assessed empirically. Most body image enhancement research has focused on the prevention of eating disorders in young women using psychoeducational and/or chat-based interventions. The evaluations of these programs suggest that they are helpful. Further research is needed to develop programs for demographics beyond young women and to address body image issues within community frameworks. Overall, we are optimistic about the efficacy of computer-based interventions for body image enhancement. As our understanding of the factors that produce improvement and enhance compliance increase, and our ability to integrate self-directed, computer-based approaches into a comprehensive treatment system improve, we are likely to find computer-based approaches to be one of the primary treatments for body image concerns.

Informative Readings

Bardone-Cone, A. M., & Cass, K. M. (2007). What does viewing a pro-anorexia website do? An experimental examination of website exposure and moderating effects. *International Journal of Eating Disorders, 40,* 537–548.—Describes a controlled laboratory study on the harmful effects of viewing pro-anorexia websites.

Custers, K., & Van den Bulck, J. (2009). Viewership of pro-anorexia websites in seventh, ninth, and eleventh graders. *European Eating Disorders Review, 17,* 214–219.—Examines the prevalence of pro-anorexia website use among adolescents and correlations with predictors of anorexia nervosa.

Franko, D. L., Mintz, L. B., Villapiano, M., Green, T. C., Mainelli, D., Folensbee, L., et al. (2005). Food, mood, and attitude: Reducing risk for eating disorders in college women. *Health Psychology, 24,* 567–578.—Evaluates the efficacy of a 2-hour CD-ROM body image enhancement program using first-year college women.

Heinicke, B. E., Paxton, S. J., McLean, S. A., & Wertheim, E. H. (2007). Internet-delivered targeted group intervention for body dissatisfaction and disordered eating in adolescent girls: A randomized controlled trial. *Journal of Abnormal Child Psychology, 35,* 379–391.—Assesses the efficacy of an online chat-based intervention adapted from an in-person version for adolescent girls in Australia.

Lenhart, A., Purcell, K., Smith, A., & Zickuhr, K. (2010). *Social media and young adults: Social media and mobile internet use among teens and young adults.* Retrieved March 11, 2010, from *www.pewinternet.org/Reports/2010/Social-Media-and-Young-Adults.aspx.*—Provides descriptive information on the frequency and character of Internet use by teenagers and young adults.

McVey, G., Gusella, J., Tweed, S., & Ferrari, M. (2009). A controlled evaluation of web-based training for teachers and public health practitioners on the prevention of eating disorders. *Eating Disorders: Journal of Treatment and Prevention, 17,* 1–26.—Assesses an online program that educates teachers and school health practitioners on how to reduce the presence of weight bias in their teaching practices.

Media Education Foundation (Producer), & Jhally, S. (Director). (2010). *Killing us softly 4: Advertising's image of women* [Motion picture]. (Available from Media Education Foundation, *mediaed.org*).—Uses images from advertisements to show how the objectification and idealized thinness of female models can have harmful psychological effects.

Paxton, S. J., McLean, S. A., Gollings, E. K., Faulkner, C., & Wertheim, E. H. (2007). Comparison of face-to-face and internet interventions for body image and eating problems in adult women: An RCT. *International Journal of Eating Disorders, 40,* 692–704.—Uses analogous in-person and online body image programs to compare which is most effective compared to a control group.

Portnoy, D. B., Scott-Sheldon, L. A., Johnson, B. T., & Carey, M. P. (2008). Computer-delivered interventions for health promotion and behavioral risk reduction: Meta-analysis of 75 randomized controlled trials, 1988–2007. *Preventive Medi-*

cine, *47*, 3–16.—Evaluates the effectiveness of computer-based health interventions and examines moderators of behavioral and psychosocial outcomes.

Sinton, M. M., & Taylor, C. B. (2010). Prevention: Current status and underlying theory. In W. E. Agras (Ed.), *Oxford handbook of eating disorders* (pp. 307–330). New York: Oxford.—Provides an in-depth review of eating disorder prevention research, including comprehensive information and references for the work done with the Student Bodies program thus far.

Webb, T. L., Joseph, J., Yardley, L., & Michie, S. (2010). Using the Internet to promote health behavior change: A systematic review and meta-analysis of the impact of theoretical basis, use of behavior change techniques, and mode of delivery on efficacy. *Journal of Medical Internet Research*, *12*, e4.—Examines more recent Internet-based behavior change programs and highlights which theories, methods, and communication techniques yield the largest effects.

CHAPTER 51

Ecological and Activism Approaches to Prevention

NIVA PIRAN
NINA MAFRICI

Introduction

This chapter aims to examine ecological and activism approaches to the prevention of eating disorders by first highlighting the theoretical perspectives that support the shift from individual-focus prevention to systemwide changes. With the goal of delineating paths for further progress, the chapter continues with a brief description of three prevention projects that emphasize ecological perspectives and community activism and discusses shared lessons that can be gleaned from these projects.

Most prevention work to date in the field of eating disorders has occurred at the individual level, centering on changing individuals through enhancing resilience skills and coping strategies. For example, all 66 controlled outcome studies of prevention included in the Stice, Shaw, and Marti meta-analysis of prevention focused on individual-level interventions and changes. This meta-analysis further suggested that universal prevention programs, usually administered to children or youth in early adolescence (up to age 15), yielded low effect sizes (e.g., .06 for changes in body dissatisfaction or dieting). Moreover, the effects of these prevention programs were found to fade over time, likely related to the omnipresent societal pressure to be thin. Indeed, the much larger volume of prevention research with youth in the area of substance abuse clearly suggests the importance of combining systemwide changes with individual-focused interventions in order to achieve a larger effect size, as well as the maintenance of gains. However, the important shift from an almost exclusive focus on individual-level interventions to activism and ecological change has to be grounded in well-examined and developed theoretical perspectives and associated epistemologies.

A key public health concept that can inform both etiological research and ecological interventions in the field of eating disorders is the multilevel nature of causality and the corresponding level of intervention; "macro"-level risk factors, related to social structures and positions such as gender or social class, shape "mezzo"-level risk factors at the community level, and, those, in turn, shape individual-level risk factors. McKinlay and Marceau therefore consider individual-level risk factors as epiphenomena of higher-level risk factors. In the field of eating disorders, for example, Piran has suggested that what may seem as disparate individual-level risk factors, such as dieting, negative body image, internalization of thinness, and negative affectivity, as well as disrupted peer relationships related to social comparisons or "fat talk," can be seen as epiphenomena of social position related to gender and its intersection with social class and ethnicity. McKinlay and Marceau highlight the greater impact of intervening at the higher level instead of pursuing and aiming to prevent multiple lower-level risk factors.

A related key public health construct that supports the importance of ecological and activism approaches to prevention is Rose's distinction between "causes of cases," referring to risk factors that explain the occurrence of a specific disease in a specific individual at a specific time, and "causes of incidence" that include the risk factors that put specific populations at risk. According to Rose, the goal of prevention is to change societal structures and norms so that a whole population is less exposed to risk factors, leading to a large and sustained prevention potential for populations. Regarding eating disorders, gender is the most consistent population risk factor, as girls and women are at a higher risk of negative body image and disordered eating patterns. Research-based models of the way gender, as it intersects with other social variables, shapes body weight and shape preoccupation are being developed, such as the "Adverse Social Experiences Model" (ASEM) to the development of disordered eating patterns or objectification theory (see Chapters 6 and 19). These models can guide the development of ecological and activism interventions aimed at establishing alternative norms at the community and larger societal levels.

To date, relatively few prevention projects have focused on ecological change. In order to support further developments in this domain, it is imperative to examine shared lessons that can be gleaned from these efforts. To this end, the chapter describes three examples of ecological and activism projects in the field of eating disorders and discusses them in relation to key issues in ecological approaches to health promotion.

Community-Based Activism within the Fashion Industry

Interventions aimed at larger social changes in the field of eating disorders can illuminate both possibilities for, and backlash against, change. This section aims to summarize the multiple activism initiatives in one area where consistent efforts have taken place in relation to negative body image and eating disorders: the fashion industry. This industry is considered to have a negative impact on girls' and women's body image through the wide dissemination of idealized images of extremely thin women.

The deaths in 2006 of three South American models from anorexia-related complications, triggered a media frenzy and alerted the public to the grave reality of eating disorders in the fashion industry. The reaction prompted immediate attention from fashion capitals around the world. The response was most decisive in Madrid: Having sponsored a fashion runway show, the regional government in Madrid placed in September 2006 the world's first *mandatory* ban on overly thin models (body mass index [BMI] < 18) in this show. Three months later in Milan, government and fashion industry leaders together developed a voluntary code of conduct stipulating that models should carry a health certificate to participate in fashion shows, be at least 16 years of age, and have a BMI of at least 18.5. In January 2007, the Academy of Eating Disorders (AED) issued guidelines in seven different languages to reform the ideals of the fashion industry and to protect the health and well-being of models. Later that month, a stakeholders group from within the fashion industry, the Council of Fashion Designers' of America (CFDA), formed its first-ever Health Initiative designed to promote awareness and education of the dangers of the fashion industry and to establish *voluntary* guidelines to support a healthier environment for models. Further, in April 2008, the National Assembly in Paris approved a groundbreaking bill prohibiting advertisers, magazines, and websites from promoting extreme thinness. Alongside the bill, French lawmakers and fashion industry executives signed a charter agreeing to discourage eating disorders and promote a healthier body image in the industry.

Calls for change also came through individual activism from within the fashion industry. For example, in June 2009, British *Vogue* editor Alexandra Shulman addressed personal letters of protest to all the major design houses over images of women with no breasts or hips, and protruding bones. Moreover, a number of models, representing yet another stakeholder group of the fashion industry, have since publicly criticized and refused to comply with extreme industry pressures. Indeed, there is a recent increase in the number of covers of magazines such as *Glamour* or *Marie Claire* that depict full-bodied women, or photographs with no digital retouching or photo enhancement, that need to be studied systematically. Although newer designers and designers of more popular fashion have chosen to embrace a healthier and more realistic size of women, to date most elite designers, who play a key role in changing the standards of the industry, have resisted changing their sample sizes arguing that the industry would lose its illustrious appeal and profits. The story of activism in the fashion industry, therefore, is a story of progress propelled by fashion industry stakeholders and governmental and nongovernmental bodies, as well as of backlash by key industry leaders.

Activism within Communities: A School Setting and Sororities on Campus

The use of activism and ecological changes *within* specific settings has been used in the field of eating disorders with promising results that should encourage further study. This section describes two examples: one conducted within a specific school environment, and the other within sororities on a university campus.

The School Community

The school community has been a common site for ecological approaches to health promotion. The Health Promoting School (HPS) Model of the European Network of Health-Promoting Schools is an example of an ecological approach that aims to change all aspects of the school community toward enhanced students' health through the active engagement of all stakeholders of the school community (students, parents, teachers, administrators, and health workers), with a particular emphasis on social justice, equity, and the empowerment of students. This model has been implemented in the prevention of eating disorders among school children. In response to a high prevalence of eating disorders, Piran implemented an ecological prevention program in a competitive residential dance school for students 10–18 years old (the Dance School Participatory Prevention Program [DSPPP]). In addition to the HPS model, this program was informed by the Participatory Action Research (PAR) paradigm, which engages community members in actively researching the targeted health issue and in transforming their environment. Toward this end, in the dance school program, students took part in ongoing gender-cohesive focus groups that examined factors in their school environment that adversely affected their body experiences and engaged in activism projects to make their school environment a more constructive setting. The program also relied on maintaining strong rapport with administration and educational sessions with personnel in order to ensure a receptive response to students' ideas and activism projects.

Adverse body experiences of students were found to be affected by violations of body ownership (e.g., strict external pressures regarding body shape, intrusive "correction" of physical poses during training), restrictive social stereotypes (e.g., girls expected to be "nice" or "demure," whereas boys who expressed feelings were labeled "feminine"), and prejudicial treatment leading to experiences of social disempowerment (e.g., teasing related to weight and gender). Based on their reflections, students initiated and guided changes in their school environment including the establishment of new peer norms (e.g., no evaluative comments by peers regarding body appearance and no teasing related to weight, gender, or other factors), changes to the school curriculum (e.g., having at least one dance class per week in students' choice of clothing and without the objectifying leotard wear), staff changes, and school-implemented policies (e.g., prohibiting sexual harassment in the school), as well as alteration to the physical environment (e.g., making changing rooms safer).

This prevention program was associated with sustained reductions in disordered eating patterns in the school, based on three all-school surveys during a 15-year period (e.g., incidence of Eating Attitudes Test [EAT] > 20 among 16- to 18-year-old dancers was reduced from almost 50 to around 15%), and improvement in different measures of body image (e.g., significant reductions on the Drive for Thinness and Body Dissatisfaction Scales of the Eating Disorders Inventory [EDI]) despite no changes of weight standards in the ballet world during that time frame. The emphasis on dancers' health in this world-class dance school was one propelling factor in implementing health requirements for student competitors in the annual international dance competition in Lausanne, Switzerland. This first extensive and successful ecological program for prevention of eating disorders in a school suggests that establishing a school environment that is more constructive to body and self experiences requires multiple changes in the school community. This approach needs to be studied in a general school setting, employing an experimental design that uses whole schools as randomization units.

University Sororities

At the university level, sororities represent a prime setting for implementing a prevention program related to the scope of its female population, the intense social bonds within sororities, and the opportunity for sorority leaders to encourage broad participation. The development of the Sorority Body Image Program (SBIP), led by Becker, provides a unique example of combining an empirically supported approach initially designed to prevent disordered eating among students preoccupied with body image issues with community activism and broader implementation. Becker et al. initiated the implementation and outcome evaluation of the prevention strategies of cognitive dissonance and media advocacy developed by Stice and colleagues, through ongoing dialogues with sororities on Becker's campus. In this research program, Becker invited sorority members to take an active part in the research process through becoming involved as peer leaders, as advocates for the implementation of the prevention program, and as creative assessors of the program in focus groups.

This extensive collaboration with sorority members has led to the emergence and ongoing revisions of the SBIP that have focused on ecology. As the program was found to be efficacious, responsive to the needs of varied sororities as reflected by its sorority-guided revisions, and respectful of the core values and power of sororities, sororities on campus incorporated this program into their mandatory orientation sessions. In addition to the change in the orientation "curriculum," sororities on campus started to coordinate other projects on campus related to body image, such as a "body image booth" during women's history month. Further, a number of sororities established new policies and peer norms, such as no commenting on appearance. Moreover, peer leaders became activists in their own sororities by embodying what they taught in the program, a stance of resistance to the thin ideal. Throughout, Becker has emphasized the power inherent in sororities. In 2005, Tri Delta, which has 136 chapters in North America, decided to test the SBIP with peer leaders, recognizing the need to tailor the training manuals to different subgroups, such as specific sororities.

This interest in body image issues has led to other initiatives by Tri Delta: "Fat Talk Free Week," as well as "Reflections: Body Image Academy" with training for individuals interested in bringing the revised manual to their campuses. This combined research program and activism in a university community has therefore led to activism in the larger community.

Future Directions

The brief summaries of the three ecological and activism projects in the field of prevention of eating disorders highlight key issues in community-based activism, change, and evaluation that should guide future work in these areas.

• *System theory*: System theory can provide a useful conceptual framework in analyzing varied system factors addressed in all ecological projects, such as organizational power structures, policies and regulations, values and norms, and amenable places of system entry for community change.

• *Community stakeholders and collaboration*: As exemplified in the three projects, favorable changes rely on the combined impact of multiple stakeholders of the community and on the establishment of collaborative partnerships.

- *Community-specific contexts*: In line with the emphasis in system theory on community-specific contexts, processes of change vary in line with specific ecological contexts; for example, in Madrid, the ban on models with BMI < 18.5 can be mandatory due to government subsidy of that event.

- *Knowledge construction*: Ecological perspectives on community change recognize the advantaged epistemological position of community stakeholders most adversely affected by hierarchical systems, and therefore focus on knowledge construction by these community members.

- *Change through empowerment*: Ecological approaches to empower community members to guide changes and project developments in their own community, informed by their "inside" knowledge.

- *The sustainable nature of changes*: As predicted by ecological approaches to health promotion, projects that generate systemic changes (e.g., organizational structures, policies, norms) tend to lead to sustained benefits to community members.

- *Broader and local community links*: Sustained successful local community-based projects extend to projects in the broader community.

- *Epistemological and research challenges in ecological inquiries*: Ecological perspectives to evaluating community change incorporate multiple approaches to research with differing underlying ontological and epistemological assumptions, and include methodologies as diverse as detailed case studies and empirical studies involving random allocation to treatment and control conditions. Further, ecological perspectives highlight different levels of outcome, from more immediate outcomes such as system change (e.g., the creation of the Health Initiative of the CFDA), to intermediate changes (e.g., changed policies and norms), to ultimate outcome (e.g., change in individuals' internalized idealized images). In addition, participatory processes with communities in ecological projects often result not only in shifting time frames but also in local alterations of intervention plans, concurrently enhancing external validity and/or limiting internal validity of planned empirical studies. Another challenging area for ecological paradigms of change in the field of eating disorders is the limited research to date that examines the relationships between risk and protective factors at different levels of causality, and the implications of the multilevel model of causality for the process of eating disorder prevention.

Conclusions

Eating disorder prevention programs that have focused on ecological change, as well as prevention work in domains such as substance abuse, suggest the value of activism and ecological approaches to eating disorder prevention. The shift from individual-focused to community-based interventions requires the consideration of relevant theoretical perspectives, such as the constructs of "multilevel models of causality" and "causes of incidence" advanced by the field of public health, and the application of system theory to health promotion, as articulated within the field of community psychology. Activism and ecological projects in the field of eating disorders conducted to date can serve to delineate the application of these theoretical perspectives to this field. The broadening of theoretical perspectives applies not only to the practice of prevention but also to its evaluation. Activism and ecological approaches to prevention utilize methodologies with differing underlying ontological and epistemological assumptions, ranging from intensive case studies to empirical studies involving random allocation to treatment and control conditions.

Informative Readings

Becker, C. B., Stice, E., Shaw, H., & Woda, S. (2009). Use of empirically supported interventions for psychopathology: Can the participatory approach move us beyond the research-to-practice gap? *Behaviour Research and Therapy, 47,* 265–274.—Collaboration with university sororities facilitates the utilization of the empirically supported cognitive dissonance approach to the prevention of eating disorders in these settings.

Foster-Fishman, P. G., Nowell, B., & Yang, H. (2007). Putting the system back into systems change: A framework for understanding and changing organizational and community systems. *American Journal of Community Psychology, 39,* 197–215.—Discussion of system theory, highlighting normative, resource, regulative, and operational characteristics of systems.

Kraemer Tebes, J., Kaufman, J. S., & Connell, C. M. (2003). The evaluation of prevention and health promotion programs. In T. P. Gullotta & M. Bloom (Eds.), *Encyclopedia of primary prevention and health promotion* (pp. 42–61). New York: Kluwer Academic/Plenum Publishers.—A comprehensive overview of approaches to the evaluation of prevention and health promotion programs, ranging from empirical to descriptive designs.

McKinlay, J. B., & Marceau, L. D. (1999). A tale of 3 tails. *American Journal of Public Health, 89,* 295–298.—Describes implications of the multilevel nature of causality and suggests pitfalls in addressing risk factors at the lower level of causality.

O'Dea, J., & Maloney, D. (2000). Preventing eating and body image problems in children and adolescents using the health promoting schools framework. *Journal of School Health, 70,* 18–21.—Applies the HPS model to the prevention of eating disorders in schools.

Piran, N. (2001). Re-inhabiting the body from the inside out: Girls transform their school environment. In D. L. Tolman & M. Brydon-Miller (Eds.), *From subjects to subjectivities: A handbook of interpretive and participatory methods* (pp. 218–

238). New York: New York University Press.—Case study of a participatory prevention project at a residential dance school that, in addition to positive sustained outcome, also led to the emergence of the ASEM to the development of eating disorders.

Piran, N. (2010). A feminist perspective on risk factor research and the prevention of eating disorders. *Eating Disorders: The Journal of Treatment and Prevention, 18*, 183–198.—Examines risk-factor research and the practice of eating disorder prevention in relation to public health and feminist perspectives.

Piran, N., & Thompson, S. (2008). A study of the Adverse Social Experiences model to the development of eating disorders. *International Journal of Health Promotion and Education, 46*, 65–71.—A structural equation modeling study of the ASEM to the development of eating disorders.

Rose, G. (1985). Sick individuals and sick populations. *International Journal of Epidemiology, 14*, 32–38.—Defines and compares the strengths and weaknesses of prevention activities that aim at "causes of cases" versus "causes of incidence."

Stice, E., Shaw, H., & Marti, C. N. (2007). A meta-analytic review of eating disorder prevention programs: Encouraging findings. *Annual Review of Clinical Psychology, 3*, 207–231.—Suggests higher efficacy for programs that target individuals at risk for the development of eating disorders, who are also older adolescents or young adults.

Trickett, E. J. (2009). Community psychology: Individuals and interventions in community context. *Annual Review of Psychology, 60*, 395–419.—Examines the central importance of context in ecological approaches to prevention and discusses evaluation research methodologies that take context into account.

CHAPTER 52

Public Policy Approaches to Prevention

SUSAN J. PAXTON

Introduction

Public policy is a decision or action of government that addresses a particular problem or issue. Thus, public policy is a course of action or inaction to change what might otherwise occur in relation to a particular issue, taken by any level of government: city, state, or federal. Governments develop public policy in terms of laws, regulations, decisions, allocations of resources, and actions. This chapter addresses public policy approaches around the globe to the prevention of body dissatisfaction, promotion of positive body image, and related concerns. Although public policy initiatives are few, the fact that a chapter on this topic may be written is reason for optimism.

Governments make policy decisions in relation to a mental health problem across the spectrum from prevention and early intervention to treatment. However, they are particularly well placed to engage in prevention policy initiatives for a number of reasons. Philosophically, most governments have an overarching responsibility to ensure the well-being of their populations and prevention interventions are specifically designed for this purpose. As described by the National Research Council and Institute of Medicine, universal prevention interventions (i.e., ones targeted to a whole population regardless of risk status), and selective prevention interventions, (i.e., ones targeted to a population subgroup whose risk of developing the problem is higher than average but has not been identified on the basis of individual risk), are both strategies that address the well-being of the population. Practically, governments are in a position to legislate for, and enforce, environmental changes that may be preventive. In addition, prevention interventions that reach whole populations may not be expensive per capita but nonetheless may be costly.

This chapter first addresses two general issues in relation to public policy approaches to prevention of body dissatisfaction: (1) circumstances under which government action may be achieved, and (2) possible targets for public policy approaches. Next, specific public policy approaches are explored, their strengths and limitations considered, and future extensions are imagined.

Achieving Government Action

In many parts of the world, body image concerns have received little or no public policy attention and reasons for this need to be considered. In some parts of the world there are arguably issues that need to be addressed first, such as poverty. In others, however, mental health issues have been on the government's agenda but body image issues still have not been addressed. There are likely to be a number of reasons for this. Body image problems and eating disorders frequently have been considered the frivolous concerns of adolescent girls. Consequently, the distress associated with body dissatisfaction and the low self-esteem, depression, poor quality of life, and eating disorders that may follow have not been taken seriously. In addition, young people do not typically have a loud voice in the ears of decision makers and are not voters. In this situation, bringing the serious consequences of body image concerns to the attention of policy makers is the top priority.

In countries where public policy approaches have been adopted there has frequently been a long history of advocacy by organizations and individuals who have repeatedly alerted governments to problems associated with poor body image, often in the context of eating disorders. Indeed, the relationship between body dissatisfaction and eating disorders is a key issue in raising awareness of policy makers, as eating disorders, especially anorexia nervosa (AN), may have devastating consequences and treatments can be expensive for governments.

In the presence of a receptive environment, other factors may trigger action. In some countries a tragic event, such as the death of a model from AN, may act as a trigger. In others, a single strong voice within government can play a pivotal role. This was especially evident in Australia when, in 2003, a young, able, female minister in the Victorian government, Jacinta Allan, called for a Parliamentary inquiry into body image among young people. Similarly, strong leadership provided by female politicians in the Quebec and Australian national governments have facilitated public policy action. Committed voices within government are clearly extremely valuable in mobilizing public policy approaches to prevention.

Possible Targets for Public Policy

Importantly, modifiable environmental risk or protective factors need to be identified. Genetic and temperament factors have been implicated as risk factors for body dissatisfaction but these are not readily modified and thus are not appropriate targets for public policy (see Chapter 4). An important risk factor for body dissatisfaction that *is* potentially modifiable is high internalization of the unrealistic media body ideal, that is, a very thin figure for females, and a lean and muscular figure for males (see Chapter 12). Exposure to appearance-focused environments contributes to pressure to conform to the body ideal and increases risk for high internalization of the ideal and consequently risk for body dissatisfaction. These environments may be appearance-focused media/fashion, as well as appearance-focused family and peer environments.

At this early stage in public policy approaches to prevention, the risk factor of internalization of the thin body ideal has been the main focus of intervention. Typically, one of two general approaches has been adopted to do this. First, there have been attempts to reduce the presence of extremely thin female images and to increase diversity in body shapes and sizes presented in media and fashion images as a means of reducing the pressure to conform to an extremely thin body ideal. Second, there have been public policy interventions that aim to assist young people to challenge the unrealistic media ideals with which they are being continually confronted. In addition, there are examples of public policy interventions that aim to address eating disorders that are a consequence of body dissatisfaction and thus have a bearing on body dissatisfaction.

Legislation and Regulation

Legislation and regulation have not been used widely in public policy approaches to prevention of body dissatisfaction. Typically, before legislating, governments must believe they have public support for their law, that the law is entirely justifiable, and that they have the means to enforce the law. Thus, considerable conviction about the importance of body image is required. In this light, it is very interesting that Spain has led the way with legislation specifically designed to try to reduce pressure on children to internalize media ideals.

Responding to extremely high demand for cosmetic surgery in increasingly young girls, in 2010 the Spanish government passed a law to ban broadcasting of television advertisements before 10 P.M. that promote beauty products and treatments that suggest surgical or chemical ways to achieve the perfect body. The government believes that exposure to these advertisements increases internalization of media body ideals and the notion that the perfect body can be achieved. Thus, these advertisements are considered very likely to increase body dissatisfaction and consequently eating disorders. It will be very interesting to see how this is implemented and whether other countries consider a similar approach.

Other legislation considered does not focus specifically on body image but rather has a focus on the prevention of eating disorders. One example is legislation passed by the lower house of the French government in 2008 but yet to pass the upper house (as of April 2010), that would impose heavy fines and a 2-year prison sentence on individuals who or organizations that provoke a person to seek excessive thinness by encouraging prolonged restriction of nourishment to the detriment of his or her health. Effectively, this would be a ban on "pro-ana" websites, but it also means that all media and advertisements could come under scrutiny. This ban might also reduce the normalization of a dangerously thin body and the internalization of this extreme ideal in some situations.

In both France and Spain, at times, regulations have been in place to prevent models with very low body weight from appearing on catwalks (see Chapter 51). This has been an attempt to protect viewers of emaciated models from internalization of extreme thinness as a body ideal but also to protect the health of models. It appears that these interventions have been somewhat inconsistently applied.

The legislation measures described above are pioneering, but are small steps. Legislation that may be considered in the future includes tighter regulation of media presentations of idealized body shapes and sizes. However, in countries where governments oversee the direction of school curricula, regulation that all schools provide evidence-based prevention interventions for children at different developmental phases is likely to be a more powerful intervention.

Working with Industry: Nonbinding Codes for Media and Fashion Industries

Governments may endeavor to change environmental factors that support a thin body ideal through persuasion rather than legislation. In this instance, governments use their leadership role to assert a public policy direction. Government actions of this kind have been mainly through the promulgation of nonbinding codes or charters. Governments that have called on media groups to endorse a code of practice in relation to the portrayal of human images include Italy, France, and the state governments of Quebec, Canada, and Victoria, Australia.

Recognizing the role that media images play in creating unrealistic body ideals and body dissatisfaction, in 2008, the Victorian government in Australia promulgated the Voluntary Media Code of Conduct on Body Image. The Code contained four statements that media and fashion industry representatives were asked to endorse in relation to the responsible presentation of images. Although a number of magazines and fashion houses did endorse the Code, a limitation of the voluntary nature of the Code was such that very many did not. Many argued that advertising and fashion images were not under editorial control and that advertising revenue would be affected if they altered their approach. Others argued that the creation of idealized fashion images was both art and fantasy and that it was inappropriate to interfere with this creative process. Despite these limitations, the Code brought heighted awareness of the role media plays in creating unrealistic body image ideals in the public, in the media, and in fashion. In addition, the Australian government is considering a voluntary code with similar tenets but an emphasis on positive body image content and messaging. A national code with wider reach is likely to be more influential.

In 2009, the Quebec government in Canada promulgated the voluntary Quebec Charter for a Healthy and Diverse Body Image. The Charter includes seven statements related both to body image and healthy eating including a pledge to "Promote a diversity of body images, including different heights, proportions, and ages." A large number of industry leaders and members of the public have pledged their support to the Charter and the fairly general nature of the statements may contribute to this.

By their nature, voluntary codes lack the power to enforce change. However, it is wise to recognize that social change takes time and that an essential first step is to bring about awareness of the problem and recognition of practical actions that can be taken to reduce environmental pressure to conform to a narrow body image ideal. When community and industry attitudes start to shift, communities may be more open to binding legislative initiatives.

Other public policy approaches to working with industry have been proposed by the National Advisory Group on Body Image, Australia. These approaches include providing incentives for promotion of positive body image through industry awards. In addition, governments could encourage public advocacy, providing the public with information about how to make complaints about unhealthy body images. Importantly, governments can also ensure that all their own departments and instrumentalities promote positive body image messages.

Advertising

A strategy frequently used in social marketing campaigns is media advertising that challenges an attitude or behavior and motivates change. Ideally, advertising will be backed-up by community resources that further support individuals to make changes. To date, this approach has not been used for body dissatisfaction. One innovative advertising campaign that was released in 2009 by the Victorian government in Australia was entitled "Real Life Doesn't Need Retouching." This advertisement aimed to reduce internalization of the thin ideal by highlighting the unreality of media advertising images. The advertisement juxtaposed flawless idealized media images of young men and women with natural photographs of young people demonstrating "real friendship," "real laughter," and "real love" with the tag "Real life doesn't need retouching" and "Take a stand against digital manipulation." The advertisement ran for a month on MySpace, a networking site used frequently by young people at the time. Positive aspects of this advertisement were that it had a clear and convincing message and reached the age group for whom it would be most relevant. However, major negative aspects of this campaign were that it didn't last very long and was not shown on a wide variety of media, limiting the number of young people exposed to the message. In addition, it was not backed up by community resources. It is, however, a promising start.

This advertisement followed a media campaign in 2006 entitled "Fad Diets Won't Work" that was designed to raise awareness of the negative effects of crash dieting and prevent the development of eating disorders and obesity. Notably, this advertisement was conducted within a healthy eating and activity initiative. It would be strategic if healthy body image messages could be aligned with this area to capitalize on their frequently large budgets.

School-Based and Community Initiatives

At present, our most successful strategy for preventing or reducing body dissatisfaction is through school-based curricula (see Chapter 49). Governments could mandate and fund the dissemination of evidence-based body dissatisfaction prevention programs. As a step in this direction, the Victorian government in Australia has provided modest funding for training of teachers and other professionals in a brief self-esteem and media literacy curriculum. If extended, this approach has the capacity to reach a very large number of the young people. However, it is essential that governments support programs that have been shown to be most effective.

Public policy to promote positive body image may also be demonstrated through government financial support for community activities. Illustrating this approach, the Victorian government offers 50 highly sought-after small grants annually to fund creative community-based activities that promote positive body image and self-esteem in their Positive Body Image Community Grants program.

If the number of young people exposed to these approaches is extended, they have the potential to reduce body image problems. However, even greater impact is likely to be achieved by a concerted school–community approach supported by government funding and resources. With this in mind, in 2009, the National Advisory Council on Body Image in Australia recommended that the government provide support and resources for whole-school prevention approaches in which school policy is attuned to body image issues, teachers are given training related to body image concerns, prevention interventions are provided at each school level, and parents are provided with information to help them build positive body image in their children.

Governments could also support body image prevention by facilitating sharing of prevention resources so that existing resources can be used more efficiently. It would be especially valuable if parents of young children could be given information to assist them in providing a positive body image environment for their children.

Support for Research

Although some universal and selective prevention strategies have been identified that are effective in reducing risk factors for body image concerns, there is enormous need to extend these options. An essential public policy approach to prevention is to provide significant funding for prevention research and evaluation of existing approaches.

Conclusions

Public policy approaches to prevention of body image concerns are in their infancy. Before governments will take thorough and consistent action on prevention they need to be convinced of the seriousness of body image concerns and their consequences. Unfortunately, in many countries this first step has yet to be achieved. However, in others, a number of creative initiatives have been implemented. To be most effective in preventing body image concerns it is likely that ongoing interventions of all kinds will be required. Advocates and researchers in our field need to work closely with governments to provide them with the motivation and the means to implement public health initiatives.

Informative Readings

Department of Health, Victorian Government. (2006). *Fad diets won't work*. Retrieved November 16, 2010, from *www.goforyourlife.vic.gov.au/hav/articles.nsf/pages/*

Fad_diets?OpenDocument.—An advertisement illustrating an evidence-based advertising campaign to reduce disordered eating and obesity.

Department of Planning and Community Development, Victorian Government. (2008). *Voluntary media code of conduct on body image.* Retrieved November 16, 2010, from *dpcd.vic.gov.au/youth/positive-body-image.*—An illustration of a voluntary media code of conduct designed to alter the way in which images are portrayed.

Department of Planning and Community Development, Victorian Government. (2009). *Real life doesn't need retouching.* Retrieved November 16, 2010, from *www.youthcentral.vic.gov.au/News+&+Features/Body+Image/Body+Image+Ad.*— An advertisement illustrating ways in which governments can use social marketing to prevent body dissatisfaction.

Family and Community Development Committee. (2005). *Inquiry into issues relating to the development of body image among young people and associated effects on their health and wellbeing.* Melbourne, Australia: State Government of Victoria. Retrieved November 16, 2010, from *www.parliament.vic.gov.au/images/stories/ committees/fcdc/inquiries/55th/bi/report/FCDCBI-Report.pdf*—Summarizes the findings of the Parliamentary inquiry that preceded policy developments to prevent body dissatisfaction.

National Advisory Group on Body Image. (2009). *A proposed national strategy on body image.* Canberra: Commonwealth of Australia. Retrieved November 16, 2010, from *www.youth.gov.au/Documents/Proposed-National-Strategy-on-Body-Image.pdf.*—A summary of proposed public policy initiatives to prevent body dissatisfaction in Australia.

National Research Council and Institute of Medicine. (2009). *Preventing mental, emotional, and behavioral disorders among young people: Progress and Possibilities.* Washington, DC: National Academics Press.—Provides a background to the rationale for prevention of mental health problems in general.

Neumark-Sztainer, D., Paxton, S. J., Hannan, P. J., Haines, J., & Story, M. (2006). Does body satisfaction matter? Five-year longitudinal associations between body satisfaction and health behaviors in adolescent females and males. *Journal of Adolescent Health, 39,* 244–251.—Demonstrates reasons why prevention of body dissatisfaction is important.

Paxton, S. J., Neumark-Sztainer, D., Hannan, P. J., & Eisenberg, M. E. (2006). Body dissatisfaction prospectively predicts depressive mood and low self-esteem in adolescent girls and boys. *Journal of Clinical Child and Adolescent Psychology, 35,* 539–549.—Demonstrates reasons why prevention of body dissatisfaction is important.

Quebec Charter for a Healthy and Diverse Body Image. (2009). Retrieved November 16, 2010, from *www.ijoinonline.com/en/charter.php.*—Illustrates initiatives of the Quebec government to prevent body dissatisfaction.

Ricciardelli, L., McCabe, M., Mussap, A., & Holt, K. (2009). Body image in preadolescent boys. In L. Smolak & J. K. Thompson (Eds.), *Body image, eating disorders, and obesity in youth: Assessment, prevention, and treatment* (2nd ed., pp. 77–96). Washington, DC: American Psychological Association. Describes risk factors for body dissatisfaction among young boys.

Richardson, S. M., & Paxton, S. J. (2010). An evaluation of a body image intervention based on risk factors for body dissatisfaction: A controlled study with adolescent girls. *International Journal of Eating Disorders, 43,* 112–122.—Illustrates potentially valuable prevention strategies that could be implemented in schools.

Smolak, L. (2009). Risk factors in the development of body image, eating problems, and obesity. In L. Smolak & J. K. Thompson (Eds.), *Body image, eating disorders, and obesity in youth: Assessment, treatment, and prevention* (2nd ed., pp. 135–156). Washington, DC: American Psychological Association.—A consideration of biological and sociocultural risk factors.

Wertheim, E. H., Paxton, S. J., & Blaney, S. (2009). Body image in girls. In L. Smolak & J. K. Thompson (Eds.), *Body image, eating disorders, and obesity in youth* (2nd ed., pp. 47–76). Washington, DC: American Psychological Association.—Chapter describing risk factors for body dissatisfaction in girls.

Wilksch, S. M., & Wade, T. D. (2009). Reduction of shape and weight concern in young adolescents: A 30-month controlled evaluation media literacy program. *Journal of American Academy of Child and Adolescent Psychiatry, 48,* 652–661.—Describes potentially valuable prevention strategies that could be implemented in schools.

PART IX

CONCLUSIONS AND DIRECTIONS

CHAPTER 53

Future Challenges
for Body Image Science,
Practice, and Prevention

LINDA SMOLAK
THOMAS F. CASH

Introduction

There has been substantial and exciting progress in the understanding of body image since the 2002 edition of this handbook. In this chapter, we seek to highlight several major gaps in the research. Our goal is to emphasize broad themes rather than to be specific about each of the preceding 52 chapters. We do, however, hope to identify issues for research, theory, clinical practice, and prevention efforts.

As in the concluding chapter of the previous edition, we organize this discussion around the seven major sections of the book: (1) conceptual foundations, (2) developmental perspectives and influences, (3) body image assessment, (4) individual and cultural differences, (5) body image dysfunctions and disorders, (6) body image issues in medical contexts, and (7) changing body images. As is always true, these divisions are somewhat artificial. We encourage people to look for the relationships among these topics, a perspective we have tried to emphasize both throughout the book and in the present chapter.

Conceptual Foundations

• A century of body image theory and research has been largely pathology focused, seeking to understand an impaired or dysfunctional body image. A growth in conceptual perspectives and research on positive, adaptive, or healthy body image is essential to the future of the field.

• It is evident that researchers and theorists have expanded their view of body image in certain ways. Most notably, biologically based explanations, particularly in the forms of genetic and evolutionary perspectives, have gained in importance. However, as was true in the previous edition, theoretical explanations continue to be heavily focused on weight and shape concerns.

• Relatedly, interest in eating disorders continues to fuel much of the body image theorizing. Eating disorders are, of course, an important mental and physical health concern. Furthermore, body image is an important component of the eating disorders, particularly anorexia nervosa and bulimia nervosa. However, body image is a richer, more varied construct than simply weight and shape concerns in eating-disordered women. This bias has resulted in a disproportionate amount of data on adolescent and emerging adult women.

• Theorizing has focused on appearance. However, as a broader construct, body image also includes function. Competencies related to strength or athletic abilities, as part of the masculine gender role, might be commonly related to body image satisfaction among boys and men. Nonappearance athletic competency might also help girls and women feel more satisfied with their body, though if it conflicts with a sexuality version of femininity, the relationship is more complicated than in men. Similarly, changes in physical competencies, including perhaps health, may be associated with developmental shifts in body image.

• Although many sociocultural variables such as media or peer conversations have been integrated into theories, theorists have been less thorough in discussing the effects of macro-level influences such as ethnicity, gender, and social class. Indeed, considering such macro-level factors may require the inclusion of new variables, such as acculturation, individual identity (e.g., gender and ethnic identities), and physical functioning.

• Most theories address body image as a trait. More work on the meaning of, influences on, and consequences of state body image is needed. Indeed, some of the most widely investigated risk factors in the body image literature, such as media, probably influence both trait and state body image. Without appropriate theory, it will be difficult to develop strong assessment tools or to fully understand body image influences and consequences.

Developmental Perspectives and Influences

• Like the theories, much of the developmental research has focused on weight and shape concerns among girls. This is slowly changing but much of the research on young children, including boys, continues to apply theories, assessments, and variable identification from the literature examining body image and disordered eating among adolescent and young adult women.

• In a similar vein, we need more qualitative work that permits us to hear the voices of young children (under about age 8), boys, working-class and poorer children, and children from ethnic minority groups in order to understand what their body image strengths and concerns are.

• More attention needs to be paid to developmental patterns or trajectories. When do various components of body image emerge? When do traitlike components become stable? How do influences and outcomes change over time?

• Over the past decade, research on media influences on body image has greatly expanded. Much of this research focuses on momentary media effects. Future studies must examine cumulative and lasting effects, and the variables that predict self-exposure to these influences.

• More research is also sorely needed investigating body image in people who are middle-aged or older. Do important body image components, such as satisfaction and investment, change? Are the causes of body dissatisfaction similar across the lifespan? How do functional changes influence body image? Both qualitative and quantitative investigations are needed. Such research needs to be designed to effectively separate cohort and age effects.

• Research examining the complex relationships among biological, sociocultural, and individual psychological variables' influence on body image across the lifespan is needed. Understanding the changes in these relationships is crucial for designing interventions, including prevention programs.

• These and other developmental questions require longitudinal, prospective data to ascertain not only patterns of development but also possible causal relationships. We are in particular need of longer-term prospective data (i.e., 5 or more years) as well as longitudinal data from groups other than White adolescent girls.

Body Image Assessment

• Although it is widely held that body image is a multi-dimensional construct, too many researchers use only a single measure (and sometimes a single-item measure) to assess body image. Most commonly, this is a measure of body dissatisfaction, a choice rooted in the frequent interest in disordered eating. As we expand our definition of body image, researchers need to consider including assessments of multiple aspects of body image in their studies. Drawing upon the wisdom of Cronbach and Meehl articulated over 50 years ago, body image requires a more sophisticated "nomological network," one that incorporates biophysical, cognitive, behavioral, and affective dimensions. For example, the inclusion of cognitive and behavioral body image investment variables alongside body image evaluation variables holds promise.

• There are numerous psychometrically sound measures of various aspects of body image that can be used with young adult women. There are also many assessment tools available for use with adolescent girls. Many fewer are designed for use with children, especially very young children. Many of the extant measures have also not been directly validated with older adult samples. Developmentally appropriate body image measures are needed.

• Many of the available measures were designed for use with girls or women. It is not clear how directly applicable these are to boys and men. On the other hand, several new measures have been developed for boys and men. It is not clear how directly applicable these are to girls and women. It is always important to select gender-appropriate measures. Right now, that is particularly challenging if the researcher is interested in comparing males and females. Measures that are appropriate for each gender but also for both genders need to be developed.

• It is increasingly clear that there are ethnic and cultural differences in body image. More work needs to be done to ascertain which existing measures can be appropriately used with various ethnic and cultural groups. Thus, research to evaluate "measurement invariance" of these assessments across such groups is imperative. At the same time, measures that reflect the body image functioning of specific ethnic and cultural groups are also crucial.

• We need more context-specific body image assessments as well as standardized, general dispositional assessments that bridge the needs of researchers and clinicians (including prevention program designers). Moreover, an important research direction utilizes technology for the ecological momentary assessment of body image experiences "where people live." Capturing the elements of these experiences within the contextualized flow of daily life can be an edifying research endeavor.

Individual and Cultural Differences

• It is obvious that body image is gendered in terms of its scope, form, risk factors, and implications. It is time to understand what about gender roles and lived experiences contribute to these differences. Such information is absolutely essential if we are to design effective prevention and intervention programs for girls as well as boys.

• Sociocultural models have long dominated the body image literature. Cross-cultural and cross-ethnic research studies are an effective way
to test such models. Continued growth in such research is valuable.

• Cross-cultural, ethnic, sexual orientation, and gender research can
be a good way to identify potential protective factors. Research has long
focused on risk factors. Understanding why some groups have better
body image than others helps us to better promote positive development
among at-risk youth and adults.

• It is almost incredible that programs aimed at helping obese individuals target either weight loss or body image. This dichotomy reflects
the debate within the field as to whether weight loss programs might
trigger eating disorders, whereas enhancing body image might facilitate
increased obesity. Both fears have likely been misplaced. Researchers need
to better understand the developmental course and implications of body
image (both positive and negative) among overweight and obese individuals. It is critical that these studies represent the range of cultural, ethnic,
age, social class, and gender groups affected by obesity.

Body Image Dysfunctions and Disorders

• Despite the extensive research on eating disorders, the role of
body image in these disorders is still not well explicated. More research is
needed on the role of body image in the development of eating disorders,
recognizing that this role may vary across cultural groups. In addition,
interventions that recognize and address the role of body image in the
eating disorders, including binge-eating disorder, need to be developed
and evaluated.

• Compared to the eating disorders, other disorders and problems
in living that might involve body image, such as gender identity disorder,
body dysmorphic disorder, use of appearance- and performance-enhancing
drugs, or somatic delusional disorder, have received little attention in the
body image literature. Much more research is needed concerning the role
of body image in the development and successful treatment of these and
other disorders.

• The prospective contribution of body image to other disorders,
such as sexual dysfunction, depression, or social phobia, needs to be
investigated. This research requires a broad, inclusive definition of body
image rather than a simple focus on weight and shape concerns or body
dissatisfaction. This inclusive definition must then be translated to specific
dimensional measures.

Body Image Issues in Medical Contexts

• All too often, medical conditions are treated only as physical symptoms and consequences. Psychological and behavioral components are sorely neglected, often to the chagrin and detriment of patients. Therefore, the most fundamental change must be to provide the descriptive research that leads to a reconceptualization of these problems as biopsychosocial rather than solely medical. This reconceptualization should include a greater recognition of the role of body image in coping with serious medical conditions and injuries.

• Such descriptive research needs to be nuanced enough to identify which patients suffering from cancer, arthritis, dermatological conditions, and other medical disorders are particularly likely to develop problems with body image. Theoretical models need to be developed to facilitate this research.

• Multisite studies with large samples need to be conducted with an eye toward assessing prospective risk and protective factors in body image problems within particular disorders.

• Measures need to be developed that assess the body image disorders specific to different medical conditions. These measures should include not only appearance but function and investment in body image.

• There are interventions designed to assist victims of burns as well as other medical conditions. However, most of these have not been rigorously evaluated. This research is essential.

Changing the Body: Medical, Surgical, and Other Approaches

• As body-changing options for body image change continue to expand, we must investigate whether and how the promotion of these "solutions" undermine body acceptance among certain populations.

• The prospective roles of body image in decisions for body art, exercise, and cosmetic surgery need to be elucidated. Such decisions are clearly multifactorial in their motivations. The foci of body image (e.g., appearance, functional, evaluative, affective) that might influence such decisions need to be specified.

• The unintended influence of body changes, such as weight loss or body art, on body image has received some empirical attention. However, more research is needed to help people fully understand and prepare for these changes. In the same vein, we need research that identifies psychological and sociocultural factors that affect body image after these bodily changes.

• Some of these interventions, including the treatment of disfigurement and surgical and nonsurgical cosmetic procedures, are often assumed to automatically and permanently improve body image. These assumptions need to be tested more rigorously in longer-term prospective designs. Furthermore, variables that affect the likelihood of a positive or adverse impact on body image need to be ascertained. The set of variables should include features of the intervention as well as psychological, social, and cultural factors.

Changing Body Images: Psychosocial Interventions for Treatment and Prevention

• In general, both treatment and prevention interventions need to be designed to be effective with groups other than White adolescent and young adult girls and women. Most studies have focused on these groups but do not provide efficacy information for any other group. These other groups include different ethnicities and cultures but also different ages. Boys' and men's needs also must be addressed.

• Prevention programs continue to dodge the question of how to include boys. Boys clearly contribute to body image problems among girls. But it is equally evident that boys can have serious body image issues of their own. Imaginative approaches to resolving these seemingly conflicting issues need to be developed and evaluated.

• We need to stop debating whether one intervention is *the* best and understand under what conditions different interventions might be effective. The preferred method of treatment or prevention may vary with age, gender, ethnicity, social class, or body image history.

• While cognitive-behavioral body image therapy has considerable empirical support, its support does not have follow-up evidence beyond a few months. Moreover, clinical trials with this therapeutic approach and other approaches seem to have stagnated in the past decade. A renewal of body image treatment outcome research is greatly needed.

• We need to develop treatment and prevention programs that are effective and can be delivered at a relatively low cost. We must then demonstrate that these programs retain their effectiveness when delivered inexpensively.

• Intervention programs should address the context within which body image problems develop rather than focusing exclusively on the "pathology" of the individual. If, as many theories suggest, body image is rooted in sociocultural factors, body image problems can only be fully addressed when those factors are changed.

• Given the advances in communication technologies and the power and popularity of the Internet and social media, there is great potential for innovation in the delivery and evaluation of body image interventions. Such interventions can be interactive and can be tailored to the assessed characteristics of the individual.

Conclusions

There have been substantial improvements in our knowledge about body image since the 2002 publication of the first edition of this handbook. There are better assessment tools, a growing recognition of body image issues among boys, more attention to ethnic and cultural group differences, and more efficacious treatment and prevention programs. During this period, a peer-reviewed publication, *Body Image: An International Journal of Research*, has emerged. Though we happily acknowledge these advances, there also continue to be important gaps in the literature. These gaps represent at least three broad themes: (1) there has been continued failure to recognize the multidimensional nature of body image; (2) more attention needs to be given to diverse ethnic, age, cultural, gender, sexuality, and social class groups, as well as to those who suffer from various physical and mental health issues; and (3) assessment tools need to be more sensitive to the goals of intervention, as well as to developmental, gender, and ethnic/cultural differences. This chapter has aimed to identify some specific questions that should be the focus of future research. Our hope is that another decade of solid science and its innovative application will bring continued advancement of the field.

Index

An *f* following a page number indicates figures; a *t* indicates tables.